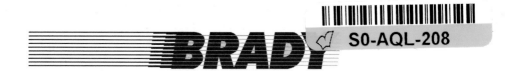

ALS Case Studies in Emergency Care

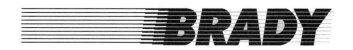

ALS Case Studies in Emergency Care

Edward T. Dickinson, MD, NREMT-P, FACEP
Assistant Professor of Emergency Medicine
Director of EMS Field Operations
Department of Emergency Medicine
Hospital of the University of Pennsylvania
Philadelphia, Pennsylvania

Andrew W. Stern, NREMT-P, MPA, MA
Senior Medic/Flight Medic
CME Coordinator
Town of Colonie Emergency Medical Services
Colonie, New York

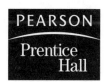

Upper Saddle River, New Jersey 07458

Library of Congress Cataloging-in-Publication Data
Dickinson, Edward T.
    ALS case studies in emergency care / Edward T. Dickinson, Andrew W. Stern.—1st ed.
    p. ; cm.
    ISBN 0-13-094317-7
    1. Emergency medicine—Case studies. 2. Emergency medical services—Case studies.
    [DNLM: 1. Emergency Treatment—Case Report. 2. Emergency Medical Services—Case Report.
WB 105 D553a 2004] I. Title: Case studies in emergency care. II. Stern, Andrew W. III. Title.
    RC86.7.D549 2004
    616.02'5—dc22

                                                            2003021753

Publisher: Julie Levin Alexander
Publisher's Assistant: Regina Bruno
Executive Editor: Marlene McHugh Pratt
Assistant Editor: Monica Moosang
Senior Managing Editor for Development: Lois Berlowitz
Senior Marketing Manager: Katrin Beacom
Channel Marketing Manager: Rachele Strober
Marketing Coordinator: Janet Ryerson
Director of Production and Manufacturing: Bruce Johnson
Managing Editor for Production: Patrick Walsh
Production Liaison: Jeanne Molenaar
Production Editor: Cindy Miller/Carlisle Publishers Services
Manufacturing Manager: Ilene Sanford
Manufacturing Buyer: Pat Brown
Creative Director: Cheryl Asherman
Senior Design Coordinator: Christopher Weigand
Cover Designer: Christopher Weigand
Composition: Carlisle Communications, Ltd.
Printing and Binding: R. R. Donnelley & Sons
Cover Printer: Coral Graphics

Pearson Education LTD.
Pearson Education Australia PTY, Limited
Pearson Education Singapore, Pte. Ltd
Pearson Education North Asia Ltd
Pearson Education Canada, Ltd.
Pearson Educación de Mexico, S.A. de C.V.
Pearson Education—Japan
Pearson Education Malaysia, Pte. Ltd

Studentaid.ed.gov, the U.S. Department of Education's website on college planning assistance, is a valuable tool for anyone thinking of pursuing higher education. The website presents information on applying to and attending college as well as on funding your education and repaying loans.

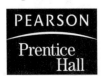

10 9 8 7 6 5 4 3 2 1
ISBN 0-13-094317-7

CONTENTS

PREFACE

ALS Case Studies in Emergency Care is intended to be a paramedic-level, multi-purpose learning tool. There is a uniqueness to prehospital emergency care that requires providers to perform difficult tasks in uncontrolled environments, often with limited personnel, and often under specific time constraints.

The intent of this book is to challenge those who use case studies as a learning technique to expand their ability to be more thorough in assessments, flexible when interpreting clinical findings, and ultimately be prepared to provide the best clinical care possible. To optimize learning for both new and current providers, each case is presented in the same easy-to-follow format. The *Case Presentation* describes the history, physical findings, and basic interventions that may be applied in a real-life situation. This is followed by *Questions* regarding intervention and pathophysiology/mechanisms of action. The *Discussion* includes a presentation of pathology, key prehospital interventions to optimize care, and controversial issues regarding management. The *Return to the Case* returns to the scenario to describe the use of the intervention and patient's response.

Case studies provide a methodology for looking at an entire EMS call from initial dispatch until transition of care to the emergency department. Integrating this information is important to both the provider and the patient. The process of planning and preparing to give care starts with dispatch information. As a call progresses, additional data is provided from first responders, family members, and the patient. All this information needs to be processed in order to develop a full clinical picture of the patient's presenting problems and to determine what treatment options should be considered. Case studies make students and active field providers sort information and frequently reevaluate decisions.

Please note that the case studies contained in this book reflect generally acceptable clinical treatment approaches and modalities. There is usually more than one clinically acceptable way to treat patients. There are variances that field providers must always take into account such as local or regional protocol as well as different approaches to care based on training and local resources. EMS is evolving. As more and more research is being conducted, some current practices may change. Finally, be open to change and realize that the evolution of new standards and interventions is an essential part of the dynamics of prehospital care.

Edward T. Dickinson
Andrew W. Stern

ACKNOWLEDGMENTS

CONTRIBUTORS

We wish to acknowledge the following people who contributed to *ALS Case Studies in Emergency Care*. Individually, they offered instruction and insight that will prove to be of great value in the classroom. Together, they form a team of talented professionals who have upheld a high standard of EMS instruction.

Jill M. Baren, M.D., FACEP, FAAP Assistant Professor of Emergency Medicine and Pediatrics, University of Pennsylvania School of Medicine; Attending Physician, Department of Emergency Medicine, Hospital of the University of Pennsylvania; Division of Emergency Medicine, The Children's Hospital of Philadelphia, Philadelphia, Pennsylvania

Jonathan L. Burstein, M.D., FACEP Assistant Professor of Medicine, Harvard Medical School; Assistant Professor of Population and International Health, Harvard School of Public Health, Boston, Massachusetts

Jonnathan Busko, M.D., MPH, EMT-P Carolinas Medical Center, Department of Emergency Medicine, Center for Prehospital Medicine, Charlotte, North Carolina

Steven J. Busuttil, M.D., FACS Assistant Professor, Division of Vascular Surgery, University of Maryland Medical Center; Chief Section of Vascular Surgery, VA Maryland Health Care System, Baltimore, Maryland

Ken Campbell, R.N. Flight Nurse—PennStar Flight, Hospital of the University of Pennsylvania, Philadephia, Pennsylvania

Richard A. Cherry, M.S., EMT-P Clinical Assistant Professor of Emergency Medicine, Assistant Residency Director for Education, Department of Emergency Medicine, SUNY Upstate Medical University, Syracuse, New York

Arthur Cooper, M.D., FACS, FAAP, FCCM Associate Professor of Clinical Surgery, Columbia University College of Physicians and Surgeons; Director of Trauma and Pediatric Surgical Services, Harlem Hospital Center, New York, New York

Kevin M. Curtis, M.D. Assistant Professor, Director of Research, Department of Emergency Medicine, Dartmouth–Hitchcock Medical Center, Lebanon, New Hampshire

Michael W. Dailey, M.D. Assistant Professor of Emergency Medicine, Albany Medical College, Albany, New York

Elizabeth M. Datner, M.D., FACEP Assistant Professor, Department of Emergency Medicine, Hospital of the University of Pennsylvania, Philadelphia, Pennsylvania

Francis DeRoos, M.D., FACEP, FACMT Residency Director, Department of Emergency Medicine, Hospital of the University of Pennsylvania; Assistant Professor, University of Pennsylvania School of Medicine, Philadelphia, Pennsylvania

Daniel S. Gabbay, M.D. Attending Physician, Saint Vincent's Medical Center, New York, New York

Claudia E. Goettler, M.D. Assistant Professor, East Carolina University, Department of Surgery, Division of Trauma and Surgical Critical Care, Brady School of Medicine, Greenville, North Carolina

Vicente H. Gracias, M.D., FACS Assistant Professor, Division of Trauma and Critical Care, Department of Surgery, Hospital of the University of Pennsylvania, Philadelphia, Pennsylvania

Howard A. Greller, M.D. Senior Fellow–Medical Toxicology, New York City Poison Control Center, New York, New York

Shamai A. Grossman, M.D., M.S. Associate Chief, Department of Emergency Medicine, Beth Israel Deaconess Hospital (Needham Campus); Director, The Cardiac Emergency Center, Clinical Decision Unit, Department of Emergency Medicine, Beth Israel Deaconess Medical Center; Instructor of Medicine, Harvard Medical School, Boston, Massachusetts

Rajan Gupta, M.D., FACS Assistant Professor, Division of Trauma and Critical Care, Department of Surgery, Hospital of the University of Pennsylvania, Philadelphia, Pennsylvania

Jonathan S. Halpert, MD, NREMT-P Attending Physician, Department of Emergency Medicine, St. Peter's Hospital, Albany, New York

Joseph J. Heck, D.O., FACOEP, FACEP President/Medical Director, Specialized Medical Operations, Inc., Henderson, Nevada

Patrick Hinfey, M.D. Assistant Residency Director, Department of Emergency Medicine, Newark Beth Israel Medical Center, Newark, New Jersey

Judd Hollander, M.D. Professor of Emergency Medicine, Department of Emergency Medicine, Hospital of the University of Pennsylvania, Philadelphia, Pennsylvania

Vivian Hwang, M.D. Instructor in Emergency Medicine, Department of Emergency Medicine, Hospital of the University of Pennsylvania; Fellow in Pediatric Emergency Medicine, Department of Pediatrics, Division of Emergency Medicine, The Children's Hospital of Philadelphia, Philadelphia, Pennsylvania

Alexander P. Isakov, M.D., MPH Co-Director, Section of Prehospital And Disaster Medicine, Department of Emergency Medicine, Emory University School of Medicine, Atlanta, Georgia

Troy R. Johnson, M.D., MAJ, MC, USA Assistant Professor, Department of Military and Emergency Medicine, Uniformed Services University of Health Sciences, Bethesda, Maryland

Owen M. Lander, M.D. Harvard Affiliated Emergency Medicine, Residency Program, Beth Israel Deaconess Medical Center, Boston, Massachusetts

Steve Larson, M.D. Associate Professor of Emergency Medicine, Department of Emergency Medicine, Hospital of the University of Pennsylvania, Philadelphia, Pennsylvania

Craig T. Lauder, D.O. Clinical Instructor, Penn State University, Milton S. Hershey Medical Center, Hershey, Pennsylvania

Richard Levitan, M.D. Assistant Professor of Emergency Medicine, Department of Emergency Medicine, Hospital of the University of Pennsylvania, Philadelphia, Pennsylvania

Daniel Limmer, AS, EMT-P Instructor/Clinical Coordinator, Southern Maine Community College, South Portland, Maine Paramedic, Kennebunk Fire Rescue, Kennebunk, Maine

Dan Mayer, M.D. Professor of Emergency Medicine, Theme Leader, Evidence Based Health Care, Albany Medical College, Albany, New York

James P. McCans, B.S., NREMT-P, FP-C PennSTAR Flight, Hospital of the University of Pennsylvania, Philadelphia, Pennsylvania

C. Crawford Mecham, M.D., FACEP Associate Professor, Department of Emergency Medicine, Hospital of the University of Pennsylvania; Medical Director, Philadelphia Fire Department, Philadelphia, Pennsylvania

Zack Meisel, M.D. Chief Resident, Department of Emergency Medicine, Hospital of the University of Pennsylvania, Philadelphia, Pennsylvania

Dan S. Mosely, M.D., MAJ, MC, FS, USA EMS Director and Attending Faculty, Walter Reed Army Center, Washington, D.C.

Lawrence Mottley, M.D., MHSA, FACEP Assistant Professor, Harvard Medical School; Vice Chair for Quality, Emergency Department, Beth Israel Deaconess Medical Center, Boston, Massachusetts

Robert E. O'Connor, M.D., MPH Professor of Emergency Medicine, Director of Education and Research, Department of Emergency Medicine, Christiana Care Health System affiliate of Thomas Jefferson University, Newark, Delaware

Susan A. O'Malley, M.D. Assistant EMS Coordinator, Department of Emergency Medicine, Brookhaven Memorial Hospital Medical Center, Patchogue, New York

Eric W. Ossmann, M.D. Assistant Professor, Department of Emergency Medicine, Emory University; Medical Director, Grady Emergency Medical Service; Associate Medical Director, EmoryFlight, Atlanta, Georgia

Jeanmarie Perrone, M.D., FACEP, FACMT Assistant Professor, Department of Emergency Medicine, Director, Division of Toxicology, Hospital of the University of Pennsylvania, Philadelphia, Pennsylvania

Jon Politis, BA, NREMT-P Chief, Colonie EMS Department, Colonie, New York

Charles N. Pozner, M.D., FACEP Medical Director, Metropolitan Boston EMS Council; Director of EMS, Brigham and Women's Hospital/Harvard Medical School, Boston, Massachusetts

Thomas J. Rahilly, Ph.D., EMT-CC Administrative Manager, Department of Emergency Medicine, North Shore University Hospital, Manhasset, New York; Center for Emergency Training and Development, Garden City, New York

Iris M. Reyes, M.D., FACEP Associate Medical Director, Assistant Professor of Emergency Medicine, Department of Emergency Medicine, Hospital of the University of Pennsylvania, Philadelphia, Pennsylvania

Carlo L. Rosen, M.D. Program Director, Harvard Affiliated Emergency Medicine Residency Program, Beth Israel Deaconess Medical Center, Boston, Massachusetts

Raquel M. Schears, M.D., MPH, FACEP Clinical Faculty, Department of Emergency Medicine, Assistant Professor of Emergency Medicine, Mayo School of Medicine, Rochester, Minnesota

Thomas A. Sweeney, M.D., FACEP EMS Medical Director, New Castle County, Delaware; Associate Chairman, Emergency Medicine, Christiana Care Health System, Newark, Delaware

Derek J. tenHoopen, M.D., FACOG Clinical Instructor, Department of Obstetrics and Gynecology, University of Rochester School of Medicine and Dentistry; Attending and Clinical Faculty, Department of Obstetrics and Gynecology, Rochester General Hospital, Rochester, New York

Owen T. Traynor, M.D., FAAEM Director of Prehospital Care, St. Clair Hospital; EMS Physician, UPMC Health System; Medical Director of Paramedic Education, Center for Emergency Medicine of Western Pennyslvania, Pittsburgh, Pennsylvania

Paul A. Werfel, NREMT-P Director, Paramedic Program, Assistant Professor of Clinical Emergency Medicine, Health Science Center, State University of New York at Stony Brook, Stony Brook, New York

Roger D. White, M.D., FACC Mayo Clinic, Departments of Anesthesiology and Internal Medicine, Division of Cardiovascular Diseases, Rochester, Minnesota

Douglas M. Wolfberg, J.D. Attorney-at-Law, Page, Wolfberg & Wirth, LLC, Mechanicsburg, Pennsylvania

REVIEWERS

The reviewers of *ALS Case Studies in Emergency Care* provided many excellent suggestions and ideas for improving the text. Their reviews have been a major aid in the revision of the manuscript, and their assistance is greatly appreciated.

Glen Mayhew, MSEd, NREMT-P Director, Assistant Professor, Emergency Health and Fire Science Department, College of Health Sciences, Roanoke, VA

Becky Tyler, NREMT-P EMT-I Instructor, Marietta, GA

Dawn Bidwell, EMT-P EMS Educator, North Memorial EMS Education, Robbinsdale, MN

Louis Robinson West Virginia State College, Institute, WV

NOTICES

NOTICE ON CARE PROCEDURES

It is the intent of the authors and publisher that this textbook be used as part of a formal education program taught by qualified instructors and supervised by a licensed physician. The procedures described in this textbook are based upon consultation with EMT and medical authorities. The authors and publisher have taken care to make certain that these procedures reflect currently accepted clinical practice; however, they cannot be considered absolute recommendations.

The material in this textbook contains the most current information available at the time of publication. However, federal, state, and local guidelines concerning clinical practices, including, without limitation, those governing infection control and universal precautions, change rapidly. The reader should note, therefore, that the new regulations may require changes in some procedures.

It is the responsibility of the reader to familiarize himself or herself with the policies and procedures set by federal, state, and local agencies as well as the institution or agency where the reader is employed. The authors and the publisher of this textbook and the supplements written to accompany it disclaim any liability, loss, or risk resulting directly or indirectly from the suggested procedures and theory, from any undetected errors, or from the reader's misunderstanding of the text. It is the reader's responsibility to stay informed of any new changes or recommendations made by any federal, state, or local agency as well as by his or her employing institution or agency.

NOTICE ON GENDER USAGE

The authors have made great effort to treat the two genders equally, recognizing that a significant percentage of EMTs are female. However, in some instances, male pronouns may be used to describe both males and females solely for the purpose of brevity. This is not intended to offend any readers of the female gender.

NOTICE RE "CASE STUDIES"

The names used and situations depicted in the case studies throughout this text are fictitious.

ABOUT THE EDITORS

Edward T. Dickinson, MD, NREMT-P, FACEP, is currently Assistant Professor and Director of EMS Field Operations in the Department of Emergency Medicine of the University of Pennsylvania School of Medicine in Philadelphia. He is Medical Director of the Malvern Fire Company, the Berwyn Fire Company, and the Township of Haverford paramedics in Pennsylvania. He is a residency-trained, board-certified emergency medicine physician who is a Fellow of the American College of Emergency Physicians.

Dr. Dickinson began his career in emergency services in 1979 as a firefighter-EMT in upstate New York. He has remained active in fire service and EMS for the past 25 years. He frequently rides with EMS units and has maintained his certification as a National Registry EMT-Paramedic. He has served as medical editor for numerous Brady EMT-B and First Responder texts and is the author of *Fire Service Emergency Care* and coauthor of *Emergency Care—Fire Service Edition* and *Emergency Incident Rehabilitation*.

Andrew W. Stern, NREMT-P, MPA, MA has been working in EMS for over 25 years as a provider, educator, and administrator. He has authored over 25 articles, book chapters, and instructor manuals. He holds intrustor certifications in BCLS, ACLS, PALS (AHA), as well as for PHTLS and PEPP. Currently affiliated with the Town of Colonie Emergency Medical Services in New York State as a Senior Paramedic/Flightmedic, also serving as their CME coordinator. Mr. Stern's involvement in emergency services extends to membership in DMAT-2 (NY) and New York Rapid Response Team-1 (USAR). He is an associate of the Prehospital Care Research Forum and is a member of the National Association of EMS Educators.

MEDICAL
EMERGENCIES

Craig T. Lauder, DO

1

ACUTE CHEST PAIN

CASE PRESENTATION

You and your partner are dispatched to the house of a 58-year-old male complaining of substernal chest pain for the past 45 minutes. You are met at the door by his wife who states he looks like he did when he had a heart attack 3 years ago. As you maneuver your way to the back bedroom you learn from the wife that he has a history of hypertension, congestive heart failure, high cholesterol, and tobacco abuse. She hands you a list of his medications, which include Norvasc, Lasix, and Zocor.

As you enter the back bedroom, you note a pale, diaphoretic, obese male lying propped up in bed. He states that the chest pain woke him from sleep and has not gone away since it started. You note that his respirations are labored and he is clutching his chest. You proceed to get a first set of vital signs as your paramedic partner listens to his heart and lungs. Vital signs are heart rate 98, respiratory rate 28, blood pressure 122/64, and room air pulse oximetry 96%. Your partner tells you that the patient's lungs are clear and his heart rate is regular with no murmur. The patient is placed on 4 liters (L) oxygen by nasal cannula, and ECG monitor, and an 18-gauge IV is established in the right antecubital fossa (AC). Your paramedic partner obtains a 12-lead ECG (Figure 1-1) as you give the patient two baby aspirin and proceed to give him sublingual nitroglycerin (0.4 milligrams [mg]) for his substernal chest pain which the patient rates at 10 out of 10 (10/10). A few minutes later you note that the patient's blood pressure is 80/40.

QUESTIONS

1. What is your clinical impression of the above patient?
2. What is the interpretation of the 12-lead ECG?
3. Why did the patient's blood pressure drop after the administration of the nitroglycerin and what is the treatment for the patient?

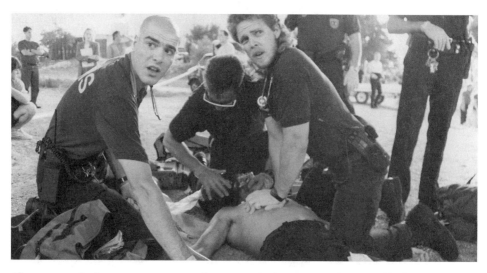

Chest pain may be the presenting symptom of various medical emergencies that can suddenly result in cardiac arrest.

DISCUSSION

Acute coronary syndrome (ACS) refers to the continuum of ischemic cardiac disease that includes stable angina, unstable angina, and acute myocardial infarction (AMI). In the prehospital environment, ACS should also include patients with chest pain who have the presence of ischemia or infarction (T-wave inversions, ST-segment depressions, ST-segment elevations) on 12-lead ECG or symptomatic patients with known cardiac disease.

AMI is the development of myocardial necrosis due to an imbalance between oxygen supply and myocardial demand. The diagnosis of AMI requires two of three criteria: clinical history, ischemic ECG changes, or positive cardiac enzyme markers. Until recently, prehospital diagnosis of AMI was largely presumptive. The paramedic providers' diagnosis relied heavily on the patient's history and physical findings. New technologies including portable 12-lead ECGs and rapid cardiac enzyme diagnostic tests have evolved to help make a reliable diagnosis of AMI in the prehospital setting.

Electrocardiograms (ECGs) are the most frequently utilized screening tool in the emergency department in evaluating patients with chest pain. Over the past few years, they have become increasingly used in the prehospital setting and today have become the standard of care in some progressive Emergency Medical Service (EMS) systems. Studies have shown that prehospital ECGs are easily obtainable, accurately interpreted by trained personnel, easily transmitted via VHF radio link to the receiving facility, and lead to a more rapid commencement of reperfusion therapy without delaying the out-of-hospital time.

The ECG in Figure 1-1 indicates the patient is indeed having an AMI localized to the inferior wall based on the distribution of ECG abnormalities. Inferior AMIs are characterized by ST-segment elevation in at least two of the inferior leads (II, III, aVF). The ECG shows ST-segment elevation in all three of the inferior leads. In 90% of patients, the right coronary artery (RCA) supplies both the atrioventricular (AV) node and infe-

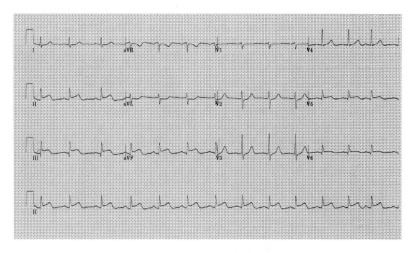

Figure 1-1 Tracing from a patient with an acute inferior wall infarct.

rior wall of the left ventricle. Thus, if an atheromatous plaque ruptures and thrombus formation occurs in the RCA, this will result in a reduction of blood supply to a portion of the inferior wall of the left ventricle and cause an AMI.

Prehospital treatment of patients with AMI includes oxygen, aspirin, nitroglycerin, and morphine. Nitroglycerin causes relaxation of the vascular smooth muscle of the coronary arteries, peripheral arterial bed, and venous capacitance vessels. Simply, it causes a decrease in blood pressure. Potential complications of nitroglycerin include systemic hypotension as well as extreme bradycardia (heart rate less than 50) or tachycardia. Nitroglycerin can be administered sublingually, topically, or intravenously. It is indicated for the symptoms and ischemia with AMI in patients with systolic blood pressure (SBP) over 90 mm Hg. However, nitroglycerin should be used with caution in patients with inferior wall AMI. The reason is that right ventricular infarcts may occur in up to half of patients with inferior wall AMI. Patients with right ventricular infarcts have increased right ventricular filling pressures which results in decreased left ventricular end diastolic pressure and thus reduced cardiac output. Consequently, agents that reduce preload (nitroglycerin) should be avoided because it can cause severe hypotension.

Detection and diagnosis of right ventricular infarcts is achieved by obtaining an ECG of the right precordial lead (V_4R). If ST-segment elevation of 1 millimeter (mm) or more is noted in the V_4R lead, then right ventricular infarct can be diagnosed. Clinical findings of right ventricular infarct include jugular-venous distention (JVD), Kussmaul's sign, and hypotension. However, these findings are seen in only 15% of patients. Another clinical scenario is a patient with an inferior wall infarction, hypotension, and clear lung sounds. These findings strongly suggest right ventricular wall involvement, as with the patient in our case. Treatment of a patient with an inferior wall infarction and hypotension includes the cessation of nitroglycerin and the administration of a 500 centimeter (cc) bolus of normal saline. Up to 2 L can be administered, but serial lung examinations must be performed in order to note pulmonary congestion or edema.

RETURN TO THE CASE

En route to the hospital, you transmit the 12-lead ECG to the receiving facility while your paramedic partner secures a second IV. You administer a 500 cc bolus of normal saline. After the bolus, you note the SBP to be 88/46. Lung exam remains clear to auscultation. You notify the receiving hospital about the patient and that you are 10 minutes away. Medical control informs you that the cardiac catheterization team is being notified and the physician orders a second IV bolus. You administer a second 500 cc bolus of normal saline and the SBP rises to 106. Lung exam, again, remains clear. You and your partner enter the emergency department and wheel the patient to the resuscitation bay where you are met by the emergency medicine physician, two nurses, and the cardiology nurse. The patient is swiftly brought up to the "cath lab" where he undergoes a cardiac catheterization. The cardiologist notes a 100% occlusion of the RCA. Angioplasty and stenting of the lesion is performed. Blood flow through the artery returns to normal and the patient is transferred to the intensive care unit. Vital signs remain stable and the patient is discharged to home on day 4. The patient continues to do well with no further interventions.

REFERENCES

American Heart Association and International Liaison Committee on Resuscitation. "Guidelines 2000 for Cardiopulmonary Resuscitation and Emergency Cardiovascular Care." *Circulation* 102 (August 2000 Suppl.): I-1–384.

Bledsoe, Bryan E., Robert S. Porter, and Richard A. Cherry. *Medical Emergencies.* Vol. 3 of *Paramedic Care: Principles & Practice.* Chapter 2, "Cardiology." Upper Saddle River, NJ: Brady/Prentice Hall Health, Pearson Education, 2001.

O'Connor, R., D. Persse, B. Zachariah, J. P. Ornato, R. A. Swor, J. Falk, C. M. Slovis, A. B. Storrow, and J. K. Griswell. "Acute Coronary Syndrome: Pharmacotherapy." *Prehospital Emergency Care* 5, no. 1 (January–March 2001): 58–64.

Perina, P. and S. Braithwaite. "Diagnosis and Treatment of Acute Myocardial Infarction: Acute Myocardial Infarction in the Prehospital Setting. *Emergency Medicine Clinics of North America* 2, no. 2 (May 2001).

Paul A. Werfel, NREMT-P

2

ACUTE MYOCARDIAL INFARCTION

CASE PRESENTATION

It is a beautiful spring day and you are working with your regular partner. The fishing season is in full swing and your thoughts are turning to hooking the big ones when the dispatcher calls your unit to the nursing home for a male with chest pain.

As your vehicle moves through the traffic you recall that this nursing home has quite the infamous reputation among your coworkers. You arrive and, after some delay, are directed to the patient's bedside.

A gentleman of about 80 is complaining of chest pain. He says that the pain began about 2 hours ago and you note that it does not change with position or breathing. In fact, nothing makes it better or worse. The pain is squeezing in quality and is in the middle of his chest. There is radiation to the arm and jaw. He denies any shortness of breath or nausea. The patient also denies a heart history (which the staff corroborates) or any recent trauma that could have caused this. He does, however, admit to an ulcer history and was hospitalized several years ago for a bleeding perforated ulcer. The staff tells you that his only medication is Pepcid and that he has no known allergies. His skin is warm and dry, and he is alert and oriented times three. Your initial impression is that this patient may have a potential acute myocardial infarction (AMI). The patient's vital signs are blood pressure 98/72, pulse is 54 and regular, the ventilations are regular at 20, and the lung sounds are clear. Your partner places the 12-lead ECG on the patient and sinus rhythm at 54 is demonstrated. You also note deep Q waves and ST-segment elevation evident in leads II, III, and aVF. The patient is administered high-flow oxygen via a nonrebreather mask and an IV is started in the antecubital fossa with normal saline at a keep vein open (KVO) rate. You and your partner are now deciding on what therapy may be indicated for this patient.

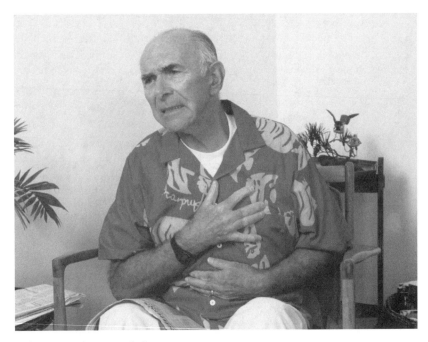

Male patient in his 80s with chest pain.

QUESTIONS

1. What information would lead you to believe that this man is in the midst of an acute myocardial infarction (AMI)?
2. What therapy is available for this patient?
3. What is the significance of the ECG changes?

DISCUSSION

Although not everybody who complains of chest discomfort is aggressively treated as a myocardial infarct, there are very clear cases that sing out for prehospital intervention. This is one of those. What is it about this patient's complaint that worries us? The patient's story is a good one. He is complaining of chest heaviness that does not change with movement or positioning. In fact, there is radiation of the pain to the arm and jaw. This presentation is very suspicious and highly suggestive of myocardial infarction (MI). Other things that could be suspected would include pulmonary embolism, thoracic aneurysm, or ulcer pain.

Pulmonary embolus (PE) should always be considered when a patient has chest discomfort. Symptoms that strongly suggest PE would be chest pain that was more pleuritic in nature. In addition, you would probably expect to see tachypnea, tachycardia, and possibly hypotension and cyanosis in the PE patient.

Could this be a thoracic or abdominal aneurysm? Again, probably not. With an aneurysm, the patient is typically a male. Aortic aneurysm is actually 10 times more prevalent in males in their 50s or 60s. Although cases do occur in older folks, the patient usually complains of a "ripping, tearing, or boring" pain that goes to the back. In addition, the vast majority of patients with aneurysms have long-standing hypertensive as well as smoking histories.

Could this be an ulcer? Probably not, as ulcer pain is usually of a "gnawing nature" and tends to change with position and meals. There are many other causes of chest discomfort, but it is always best to think of horses and not zebras when you hear hoof beats.

Because patient apprehension and fear drive the myocardial oxygen demand upward, and can actually increase the size of the infarct, pain relief is of prime importance in MI patients. Always remember the advanced cardiac life support (ACLS) dogma that "MONA greets all patients." The new ACLS recommendations are that MONA— morphine, oxygen, nitroglycerin, and aspirin—are appropriate therapies for *all* patients with ischemic chest pain. This includes patients with ST-segment elevation, patients with ST depression, as well as those with nonspecific ECG changes.

Morphine sulfate is a very potent narcotic analgesic that has many dosage recommendations. For patients with chest pain from cardiac ischemia, most clinicians start with an initial dose in the range of 2–4 mg and repeat small doses of 2 mg every few minutes until the pain is relieved or side effects occur (namely, respiratory depression or hypotension). Although its analgesic and sedative effects are well known, morphine also has hemodynamic properties that are beneficial for the patient. Morphine "unloads" the heart by being a vasodilator. One result of this increased venous capacity is decreased venous return and lowered blood pressure. The up-side of this is that the patient's myocardium has less work to do and thereby needs less oxygen. This is of great importance in a patient who, by the presence of ischemic chest pain, is demonstrating that he does not have the myocardial oxygen supply to meet the demand.

Because there are no contraindications for the use of oxygen, its use is indicated in all situations where hypoxemia may be encountered. In giving patients oxygen, you increase alveolar oxygenation resulting in increased hemoglobin saturation. This makes more oxygen available for the tissues. In these cases, oxygen should be given at high flow rates. To avoid mucosal drying, humidification is recommended when oxygen is given at flow rates of 6 liters per minute (L/min) or more. Patients should be monitored for improvement as well as the respiratory depression that is occasionally seen in chronic obstructive pulmonary disease (COPD) patients.

Nitroglycerin is a drug that has long been a staple in the treatment of chest pain. Its potent vasodilatory effects reduce blood pressure and myocardial workload. In addition, this vasodilation (to a lesser degree) affects the coronary arteries resulting in improved myocardial blood flow. The main concern with this drug is that many patients develop a tolerance to it. Obviously, it should not be given to patients who are hypotensive or have elevated intracranial pressure. Side effects include hypotension, tachycardia, dizziness, and headache. Once exposed to air, nitroglycerin has a very short shelf life and should be protected from light, as it is light sensitive. Dosing is one 0.4 mg sublingually via tablet or spray. The dose can be repeated in 3 to 5 minutes as required and as long as the patient maintains stable vital signs. The dose of nitroglycerin paste is usually 0.5 to 1.0 inch of ointment.

Aspirin, the common everyday nonsteroidal anti-inflammatory drug, is quite a wonder when it comes to MI patients. Aspirin blocks platelet aggregation and localized vasoconstriction by blocking a substance that causes the platelets to congregate (thromboxane A_2). The early administration of aspirin has been demonstrated to significantly reduce mortality in MI. Its only contraindication is known hypersensitivity. It can be used in cases like this where the patient has ulcer disease if the benefits outweigh the risks. The recommended dosage of aspirin is 160–325 mg. Patients need to chew the drug for maximal effect and for this reason, baby aspirin is used.

To answer the final question—What is the significance of the ECG changes?—deep Q waves and ST-segment elevation in leads II, III, and aVF are consistent with an inferior wall infarction. The posterior left coronary artery is most often involved but, less commonly, the left circumflex or left coronary artery can be the culprit. This is important to know because patients with this particular event are very susceptible to heart blocks, bradycardia, hypotension, and cardiogenic shock. Knowing this fact may help you to maintain vigilance of the patient's vital signs during treatment and transport. Of clinical importance is that patients with inferior wall AMIs who are hypotensive are more likely to respond well to judicious IV fluid boluses than patients with anterior wall AMIs. This is because inferior wall MIs often affect the right ventricle which responds well to preload volume to increase cardiac output and thus increase blood pressure.

With all prehospital MIs, it has been demonstrated that prehospital 12-lead ECG may significantly reduce time to thrombolytic therapy and limit or reverse ischemic damage.

RETURN TO THE CASE

You now administer 0.4 mg of sublingual nitroglycerin to the patient under standing orders. The patient tells you that he gets a burning sensation under the tongue. (This assures you of the drug's potency.) In addition, as your partner retakes vitals, the patient tells you that he is getting a headache. This is to be expected from the drug, as is the patient's heart rate increasing to 78. The blood pressure is unchanged.

After again confirming that the patient is not allergic to it, 160 mg of baby aspirin are given, also under standing orders. Although you are aware that the patient's ulcer history is a caution for aspirin, you realize that the major problem here is the myocardial ischemia and possible infarction and aspirin could reduce his chances of mortality up to 25%.

Another set of vitals is obtained and does not demonstrate any change. Medical control is contacted and you request a repeat of the sublingual nitroglycerin, 0.5 inch of nitropaste, and 2 mg of morphine sulfate with repeats every 5 minutes, monitoring the respiratory rate closely, until the chest pain is relieved or as long as the vital signs remain stable. The physician agrees and the medications are given. The patient's vital signs remain stable as transportation is started. When you inquire, he tells you the pain is diminished substantially and no more medication is administered to him. Upon arrival at the hospital, a history and physical are done and the ECG still indicates an inferior wall infarct. The patient is hustled up to the interventional cardiology lab for emergency angioplasty with the placement of a stent. The patient has an uneventful recovery and is discharged several days later.

REFERENCES

Bledsoe, Bryan E., Dwayne E. Clayden, and Frank J. Papa. *Prehospital Emergency Pharmacology*. 5th ed. Upper Saddle River, NJ: Prentice Hall, 2001.

Bledsoe, Bryan E., Robert S. Porter, and Richard A. Cherry. *Medical Emergencies*. Vol. 3 of *Paramedic Care: Principles & Practice*. Chapter 2, "Cardiology." Upper Saddle River, NJ: Brady/Prentice Hall Health, Pearson Education, 2001.

Hennekens, C. H., M. A. Jonas, and J. E. Buring. "The Benefits of Aspirin in Acute Myocardial Infarction: Still a Well-Kept Secret in the US." *Archives of Internal Medicine* 154 (1994): 37–39.

Krumholz, H. M., M. J. Radford, E. F. Ellerbeck, J. Hennen, T. P. Meehan, M. Petrillo, Y. Wang, T. F. Kresowik, and S. F. Jencks. "Aspirin in the Treatment of Acute Myocardial Infarction in Elderly Medicare Beneficiaries: Patterns of Use and Outcomes." *Circulation* 92 (1995): 2841–2847.

Second International Study of Infarct Survival (ISIS-2) Collaborative Group. "Randomised Trial of Intravenous Streptokinase, Oral Aspirin, Both, or Neither among 17,187 Cases of Suspected Acute Myocardial Infarction: ISIS-2." *Lancet* 2 (1988): 349–360.

Troy R. Johnson, MD

3

Acute Myocardial Infarction with Bradycardia

CASE PRESENTATION

You and your partner are working during the evening and are called to the scene of a 56-year-old male having chest pains. You arrive within 5 minutes at a house in a middle-class neighborhood. There are family members both out in front and inside the house and the scene appears to be safe. Family members usher you into the house where you find a middle-aged man lying supine on the floor breathing heavily.

Your initial impression is of a middle-aged conscious man in moderate distress. As your partner places your equipment around the patient, you introduce yourself to the patient and ask him what is wrong. The patient tells you that he is experiencing 6/10 dull substernal chest pain associated with shortness of breath and nausea. Family members tell you that shortly after the start of his pain he felt lightheaded and they placed him on the floor.

Your initial survey reveals his airway to be patent and without abnormality. He has a Glasgow Coma Scale (GCS) of 15. His breathing is labored at a rate of 25 with an oxygen saturation of 90% on room air and he has bibasilar rales. You instruct your partner to place the patient on 100% oxygen with a nonrebreather (NRB) mask that raises the oxygen saturation to 100%. Your cardiovascular examination reveals a blood pressure of 110/70 with a pulse rate of 40. You note normal heart sounds without murmurs or gallops. Jugular-venous distention or lower extremity edema is absent. You place him on your monitor with 12-lead capability and note a heart rate of 40 with a third-degree atrioventricular block (AVB). There are 2 millimeter (mm) ST elevations in leads II, III, and aVF.

You quickly place a peripheral IV and package the patient for transport. You notify medical control that you suspect this patient has an acute myocardial infarction with hemodynamically stable third-degree heart block and they instruct you to proceed to the nearest hospital. While you get the patient in the ambulance you ask the family for additional information. You find out that he has a past medical history for only hypertension

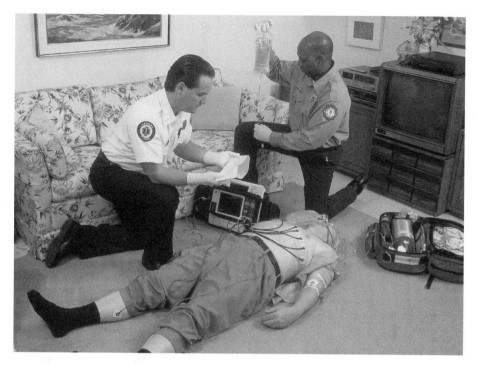

Paramedics obtain a 12-lead ECG on a patient with chest pain and bradycardia.

and elevated cholesterol. He does not take any medications and has no allergies. He has never had heart problems in the past.

Once the patient is loaded in the ambulance you give him an aspirin and repeat your vital signs. His heart rate is now 35, blood pressure 90/40, respiratory rate 20, and oxygen saturation is 100% on 100% NRB mask. He is less responsive but still maintaining his airway control. The ECG is unchanged except the heart rate.

QUESTIONS

1. What are the various options available to the paramedic for the treatment of myocardial infarction?
2. What is the role of atropine in the treatment of symptomatic bradycardia in the face of a myocardial infarction?
3. What other options are available in the field setting for symptomatic bradycardia?

DISCUSSION

Every year, approximately 1,250,000 persons in the United States experience an acute myocardial infarction (AMI). Of these, more than 50% die before reaching a medical facility with the majority of these deaths occurring within 1 hour of the onset of acute symptoms.

Studies indicate that 50% to 60% of these patients will use the EMS system; thus it is imperative that EMS personnel are prepared and knowledgeable about this topic and complications associated with this disease. Rapid interventions and transport can greatly lessen the devastating impact of AMI.

Although some interventions for AMI available to the paramedic may seem basic, they can have a far-reaching impact overall. Aspirin, for example, has been shown to be the most beneficial intervention for patients experiencing a myocardial infarction. Aspirin has also been shown to be very safe in this setting and does not contribute to major bleeding. In addition, oxygen and IV access are important interventions that can ensure maximal oxygenation and provide a reliable route for medications.

Nitroglycerin has been shown to reduce chest pain in patients, but with a significant downside of potential rapid drops in blood pressure. In this patient with hypotension, this intervention is not indicated and can be potentially harmful. Rapid transport for suspected AMI patients to facilities that can perform thrombolytic therapy or cardiac catheterization has also been shown to greatly improve outcome. Paramedic personnel must be very sensitive to the impact of on-scene time in this setting.

Ninety percent of patients with acute myocardial infarction will have some cardiac rhythm abnormality during the course of their infarction. Almost any rhythm disturbance can be associated with acute myocardial infarction, including bradyarrhythmias, supraventricular tachyarrhythmias, ventricular arrhythmias, and atrioventricular block. Of these arrhythmias, bradycardia encompasses approximately 25% to 30%. Table 3-1 outlines the types of bradycardia and symptomatic bradycardia seen in AMI. In this case, the patient presents with hemodynamically stable third-degree AV block, meaning that the patient is still able to perfuse his tissues even though his heart rate is slow. However, once transport was initi-

TABLE 3-1

BRADYCARDIA IN AMI

TYPE OF BRADYCARDIA	PERCENTAGE
Sinus bradycardia	40%
Junctional rhythm	20%
First-degree AV block	15%
Second-degree AV block	12%
Third-degree or complete heart block	8%
Idioventricular rhythm	5%
SYMPTOMATIC BRADYCARDIA	PERCENTAGE
Complete heart block	40%
Sinus bradycardia	25%
Junctional rhythm	20%
Other	15%

Source: From W. J. Brady and R. A. Harrigan, "Diagnosis and Management of Bradycardia and Atrioventricular Block Associated with Acute Coronary Ischemia." *Emergency Medicine Clinics of North America* 19, no. 2 (May 2001): 371–384.

ated he decompensated. The interventions available to the paramedic are atropine, isoproterenol, dopamine, and epinephrine, and, in most systems, transcutaneous pacing.

Atropine is a drug that blocks the parasympathetic (slowing) innervation of the sinoatrial and atrioventricular node and enhances the conduction through the electrical system of the heart. Early use of this drug is recommended by the American Heart Association's *Guidelines 2000 for Cardiopulmonary Resuscitation and Emergency Cardiovascular Care* and is a mainstay in the treatment of symptomatic bradycardia in the ACLS protocol. An initial dose of 0.5–1.0 mg IV repeated every 5 minutes is recommended. Some authors recommend a minimum dosage of 0.6 mg for adults due to the potential for paradoxical bradycardia that can occur with low doses of this medication. The maximal effective dose is 0.04 milligram per kilogram (mg/kg) or approximately 3.0 mg for the average adult. Many studies have shown atropine to be beneficial in greater than half of patients who receive it in the prehospital setting. This response was increased with additional doses of atropine; however, the vast majority of patients who responded to atropine did so on the initial dose.

Even though the side effect profile of atropine in this setting is very low, there are some concerns with its use in the setting of an acute myocardial infarction. As a parasympathetic blocker it increases the heart rate. This in turn will increase the oxygen requirements on the heart, which could potentially worsen the cardiac ischemia. The other concern with the use of atropine is the potential unmasking of tachycardia. Its mechanism is thought to be due to the unopposed effect of catecholamines (e.g., epinephrine) once the inhibitory mechanism is blocked with atropine. This effect can be seen in 2% to 4% of patients treated with atropine.

Other medications such as isoproterenol, epinephrine, and dopamine all exert their effect by beta-receptor stimulation. Whereas effective at increasing heart rate, this greatly increases myocardial oxygen demand and these drugs should be used only in situations where atropine is ineffective, transcutaneous pacing is unavailable, and transport times are prolonged. Refer to ACLS protocol for dosing measurements.

Transcutaneous pacing is gaining greater usage and is becoming the treatment of choice for symptomatic bradycardia unresponsive to atropine. Transcutaneous pacing is a temporizing procedure to increase heart rate and stabilize the patient until more definitive treatments can be administered (e.g., transvenous pacing). It is important to remember that this procedure is painful to the patient and pain control measures or sedation should be given as soon as possible.

RETURN TO THE CASE

After confirming the change in the vital signs, you administer 1 mg of atropine IV. You notice the patient becomes more arousable, and repeat vital signs are pulse rate 55, blood pressure 120/60, respiratory rate 20, and O_2 oxygen saturation 100% on 100% NRB. You rapidly transport the patient while transmitting a copy of the 12-lead ECG and give an initial report to the receiving facility.

On arrival at the emergency department you give a verbal report to the emergency physician. The patient is quickly moved to a monitored bed, transcutaneous pacer pads are placed on the patient, and a right internal jugular central catheter is placed with a transvenous pacer. The cardiology team arrives quickly, evaluates the patient, and the patient is taken to emergency cardiac catheterization where a proximal right coronary artery thrombus is identified and stented. Five days later the patient is discharged in good condition and will undergo outpatient cardiac rehabilitation.

REFERENCES

American Heart Association and International Liaison Committee on Resuscitation. "Guidelines 2000 for Cardiopulmonary Resuscitation and Emergency Cardiovascular Care." *Circulation* 102 (August 2000 Suppl.): I-1–384.

American Heart Association. *Heart Facts*. Dallas, TX: American Heart Association, 1992.

Antiplatelet Trialists' Collaboration. "Collaborative Overview of Randomized Trials of Antiplatelet Therapy I: Prevention of Death, Myocardial Infarction, and Stroke by Prolonged Antiplatelet Therapy in Various Categories of People." *British Medical Journal* 308 (1994): 81–106.

Aufderheide, T. P. "Arrhythmias Associated with Acute Myocardial Infarction and Thrombolysis." *Emergency Medicine Clinics of North America* 16, no. 3 (August 1998): viii, 583–609.

Bledsoe, Bryan E., Robert S. Porter, and Richard A. Cherry. *Medical Emergencies*. Vol. 3 of *Paramedic Care: Principles & Practice*. Chapter 2, "Cardiology." Upper Saddle River, NJ: Brady/Prentice Hall Health, Pearson Education, 2001.

Brady W. J., and R. A. Harrigan. "Diagnosis and Management of Bradycardia and Atrioventricular Block Associated with Acute Coronary Ischemia." *Emergency Medicine Clinics of North America* 19, no. 2 (May 2001): 371–384.

Brady, W. J., G. Swart, D. J. DeBehnke, O. J. Ma, and T. P. Aufderheide. "The Efficacy of Atropine in the Treatment of Hemodynamically Unstable Bradycardia and Atrioventricular Block: Prehospital and Emergency Department Considerations." *Resuscitation* 41, no. 1 (June 1999): 47–55.

Fibrinolytic Therapy Trilists' (FTT) Collaborative Group. "Indications for Fibrinolytic Therapy in Suspected Acute Myocardial Infarction: Collaborative Overview of Early Mortality and Major Mobidity Results of All Randomized Trials of More than 1,000 Patients." *Lancet* 343 (1994): 311–322.

National Heart, Lung, and Blood Institute. *Morbidity and Mortality: Chart Book on Cardiovascular, Lung, and Blood Diseases*. Bethesda, MD: U.S. Department of Health and Human Services, Public Health Service, 1992.

"Randomised Trial of Intravenous Streptokinase, Oral Aspirin, Both, or Neither among 17,187 Cases of Suspected Acute Myocardial Infarction: ISIS-2." *Lancet* 2 (1988): 349–360.

Second International Study of Infarct Survival (ISIS-2) Collaborative Group. "Randomised Trial of Intravenous Streptokinase, Oral Aspirin, Both, or Neither among 17,187 Cases of Suspected Acute Myocardial Infarction: ISIS-2." *Lancet* 2 (1988): 349–360.

Swart, G. L., W. J. Brady Jr., D. J. DeBehnke, O. J. Ma, and T. P. Aufderheide. "Acute Myocardial Infarction Complicated by Hemodynamically Unstable Bradyarrhythmia: Prehospital and ED Treatment with Atropine." *American Journal of Emergency Medicine* 17 (November 1999): 647–652.

Weaver, W. D., R. J. Simes, A. Betriu, C. L. Grines, R. Zijlstra, E. Garcia, L. Grinfeld, R. J. Gibbons, E. E. Ribeiro, M. A. DeWood, and F. Ribichini. "Comparison of Primary Coronary Angioplasty and Intravenous Thrombolytic Therapy for Acute Myocardial Infarction: A Quantitative Review." *Journal of the American Medical Association* 278 (1997): 2093–2098.

Jill M. Baren, MD

4

ACUTE SEVERE ASTHMA EXACERBATION

CASE PRESENTATION

A 22-year-old female with a history of asthma attends a holiday party in a crowded apartment with a wood-burning stove. She suddenly feels short of breath and realizes she has forgotten her inhaler. She leaves the party to return to her own apartment to administer an albuterol treatment from her home nebulizer. Fifteen minutes later her husband finds her severely short of breath and lethargic and he dials 911. You arrive on scene within 5 minutes. The patient is pale, sweaty, and unable to utter more than a single word at a time. She has paradoxical chest wall movement, nasal flaring, and decreased breath sounds in both lung fields with occasional faint wheezes. Pulse is 135 with respirations at 36. Your estimated time of arrival (ETA) to the nearest hospital is 10 minutes. The patient's husband informs you that the last time this happened the patient almost died, required intubation, and was admitted to the ICU for 2 weeks.

QUESTIONS

1. What physical exam findings indicate the severity of an acute asthma exacerbation?
2. Which medications are immediately indicated in the setting of asthma with moderate to severe respiratory distress?
3. What are the options for asthma patients in severe distress who do not respond to initial therapy?

DISCUSSION

EPIDEMIOLOGY/PATHOPHYSIOLOGY

Asthma is a common chronic disease in the United States. Approximately 2 million individuals with asthma seek emergency care annually. Emergency department visits for acute asthma expend considerable resources. Surveillance of mortality data has revealed that asthma deaths increased from 1980 to 1990. These disturbing statistics remain despite advances in our knowledge of the pathophysiology and treatment of asthma.

Asthma is a chronic inflammatory disease characterized by exacerbations and remissions. During exacerbations, bronchial inflammation, hyperactive smooth muscle activity, and airflow obstruction occur and are partially reversible with medications. Most individuals experiencing an asthma exacerbation will complain of acute shortness of breath, coughing, wheezing, or chest tightness. Exposures to smoke, air pollutants, other allergens, and respiratory viruses are important precipitating factors for acute asthma.

Paramedics who encounter asthmatics who report a past medical history of prolonged hospitalizations for asthma—especially those who required intubation—should be especially diligent in their assessment and aggressive management of these patients, since previous intubation is a "red flag" that the patient is at high risk for respiratory failure again.

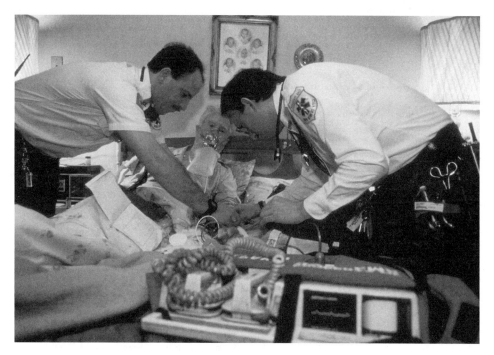

Managing a patient with acute shortness of breath.

Typical physical exam findings during an asthma exacerbation are tachypnea, tachycardia, accessory muscle use (intercostal, subcostal, and supraclavicular retractions), wheezing or other abnormal breath sounds, and decreased aeration. The younger the patient, particularly children, the easier it is to appreciate accessory muscle use because of the increased compliance of the chest wall. Absence of wheezing at any age, along with other signs of respiratory distress, may indicate very poor air entry and a severe exacerbation.

The overall assessment of respiratory distress should reflect both ventilation and oxygenation. Tachypnea and accessory muscle use are indications of impaired ventilation. Adequate oxygenation can be assessed by nasal flaring, color change, and changes in mental status (irritability, confusion) in addition to direct measure by pulse oximetry. Markedly altered mental status, like lethargy or unresponsiveness, may indicate elevated carbon dioxide levels and hypoxia and is a sign that respiratory failure may soon occur with immediate need for intubation.

KEY PREHOSPITAL INTERVENTIONS

Oxygen

Most patients who present with mild to moderate asthma exacerbations will not require supplemental oxygen. According to nationally published guidelines, those who present with initial pulse oximetry of less than 90% should be given oxygen by whichever route is best tolerated. All pregnant patients, children, and patients with comorbid conditions like heart disease may also need supplemental oxygen.

Inhaled Beta-agonists

Inhaled beta-agonists are the standard first-line therapy for the management of acute asthma. They are the most effective way to relieve airflow obstruction, with a rapid onset of action of 5 minutes. Albuterol is the most frequently used beta-agonist in the United States. It causes bronchodilation by relaxing airway smooth muscle.

Recommended prehospital dose of albuterol is 2.5 mg. Albuterol is often available with saline in premixed vials. It can be given intermittently and the most common dosing interval is every 15–20 minutes; however, it can be given more frequently, and even continuously if needed. It is also acceptable to administer albuterol through a metered dose inhaler (MDI). Dose recommendations range between two and eight puffs every 5 minutes. An MDI delivers the drug efficiently, but it may be difficult for some patients to coordinate their breathing with this apparatus when in distress.

Other Medications

Systemic steroids (prednisone, Solu-Medrol) are indicated for most patients with an asthma exacerbation, but their administration is often held until the patient arrives in the ED. Corticosteroids speed the resolution of airflow obstruction, potentiate the effects of beta-agonist therapy, and have the potential to decrease hospitalization for sicker patients. Ipratropium bromide (Atrovent) is an anticholinergic medication delivered by the inhaled route. It also causes bronchodilation and is often administered to more severe asthmatics. An increasing number of EMS systems have elected to carry this medication. The recommended dose is either 250 or 500 micrograms (mcg).

Recent studies have indicated that intravenous magnesium sulfate is a useful adjunct in the management of moderate and severe asthma attacks. Although carried by many EMS units as an antiarrhythmic drug, its prehospital use for acute asthma is limited since it is not considered a first-line drug and its 2 to 3 gram dosage is normally infused over 20 to 30 minutes.

MANAGEMENT OF SEVERE ASTHMA

Many patients will respond to ß-agonists, anticholinergics, and steroids in the initial stages of therapy. For the small percentage of patients who do not, there are additional therapeutic agents that can be added. Systemic ß-agonists should be considered in patients with severe asthma exacerbations who have failed to respond to maximal inhaled therapy. Options for subcutaneous administration include terbutaline or epinephrine. Subcutaneous epinephrine is dosed at 0.3 cc for an adult patient. Aggressive airway and ventilatory management is warranted for severe asthma due to the high morbidity associated with respiratory failure, but intubation should be viewed as a last resort. There are numerous complications associated with intubation of asthmatics such as pneumothorax and cardiac arrest.

If intubation is required the patient should initially be preoxygenated with 100% oxygen. Some authors have advocated ketamine as a preferred sedative agent as it is also a bronchodilator; however, this is rarely carried by EMS systems. Midazolam and diazepam are acceptable alternatives. Next, a paralytic agent should be administered using a rapid sequence intubation protocol. After intubation, careful attention should be given to the ventilatory rate to allow adequate time for expiration (typically 8–12 breaths per minute). Buildup of pressure in the thorax can lead to airway leak as well as cardiac arrest due to impaired venous return. ß-agonist therapy should continue for the intubated patient via the endotracheal tube.

RETURN TO THE CASE

You allow the patient to remain sitting upright in a position of comfort and immediately supply 100% oxygen by face mask. Next, you administer a nebulized albuterol treatment (2.5 mg). Intravenous access is also obtained and you are able to give Solu-Medrol 125 mg IV. Despite these therapies, the patient becomes increasingly agitated and is unable to coordinate her rapid breathing with the nebulized treatment. You decide to administer 0.3 mg epinephrine subcutaneously. Several minutes later the patient is more responsive and cooperative. You can now hear loud, coarse bilateral inspiratory and expiratory wheezes. You continue with nebulization therapy, oxygen, and monitoring. You begin rapid transport to the nearest hospital.

In the ED, the patient is placed on continuous albuterol. Pulse oximetry is 88% on room air but responds well to oxygen. A chest radiograph shows hyperinflation but no evidence of pneumonia. She is admitted to a telemetry unit for close observation. She is discharged from the hospital 5 days later on a steroid taper and multiple inhalers and is instructed to attend an asthma education class to learn about symptom recognition, avoidance of asthma triggers, and proper use of rescue medications.

REFERENCES

Bledsoe, Bryan E., Robert S. Porter, and Richard A. Cherry. *Medical Emergencies*. Vol. 3 of *Paramedic Care: Principles & Practice*. Chapter 1, "Pulmonology." Upper Saddle River, NJ: Brady/Prentice Hall Health, Pearson Education, 2001.

Brenner, B. E., ed. *Emergency Asthma*. New York: Marcel Dekker, 1999.

Emond, S. D., C. A. Camargo Jr., and R. M. Nowak. "1997 National Asthma Education and Prevention Program Guidelines: A Practical Summary for Emergency Physicians." *Annals of Emergency Medicine* 31, no. 5 (May 1998): 579–589.

Richard Cherry, MSI, EMT-P

5

ACUTE STROKE

CASE PRESENTATION

You and your partner are working your normal shift for a low-volume, rural EMS agency when a call for an ill person at an assisted-living complex interrupts your dinner. As you arrive, first responders are taking vital signs on an elderly gentleman who is sitting on the floor, leaning to one side and staring into space. The staff states that he was walking down the corridor and slowly slumped to the ground. You direct your partner to obtain more history from the staff as you begin to evaluate your patient.

The man is in his 80s and appears alert but unable to speak. His airway is clear and he is moving good air. He has regular bounding peripheral pulses, rate of 100, and his skin is warm and pink. Per the first responder, his blood pressure is 200/112. You immediately direct the first responders to administer oxygen with a nonrebreather mask at 15 L/min and place him on the cardiac monitor. You also ask them to set up equipment for an IV (normal saline) while you continue your examination.

Your patient is an otherwise healthy-looking man in no apparent distress. He has no signs of difficulty breathing. His lungs are clear bilaterally, and he has no signs of peripheral edema. You perform the Cincinnati Prehospital Stroke Scale exam. He has an obvious left arm drift, left-sided facial paralysis from the eyebrows down, and is aphasic. His fingerstick reads 120 milligrams per deciliter (mg/dl), his arterial blood oxygen saturation (SpO_2) is 98% on room air, and his ECG shows normal sinus rhythm. When your partner returns you learn that the patient has a long history of coronary artery disease and diabetes. He takes Lotensin (beta-blocker), Lipitor (anticholesterol), isosorbide (antianginal), warfarin (anticoagulant), and insulin. He is a lifetime smoker (75 pack/years) and has a positive family history for hypertension. At this point your field diagnosis is an acute stroke.

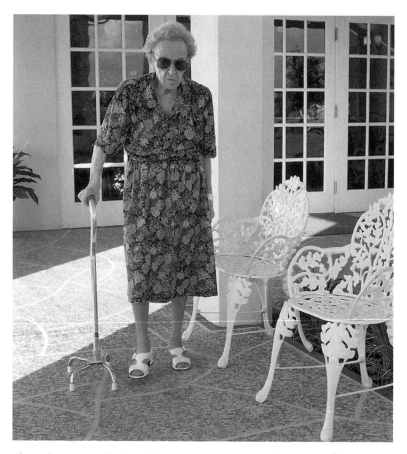

The stroke patient will often suffer paralysis affecting the extremities on one side of the body.

QUESTIONS

1. What crucial information is missing from the history?
2. Will you attempt to reduce the patient's blood pressure? Why or why not?
3. What is the appropriate facility for this patient?

DISCUSSION

Stroke is the third leading cause of death and a frequent cause of disability in elderly and middle-aged patients. Until just recently, prehospital stroke management consisted of supportive care and managing the resulting cardiac or respiratory complications. There was no emphasis on rapid transport or invasive interventions. Even in the hospital, no therapy was available to alter the course or severity of the stroke.

In recent years, however, we have seen dramatic changes in the management of the acute stroke patient. The federal Food and Drug Administration approved the use of clot-busting drugs (fibrinolytics) on certain types of strokes. Fibrinolytic therapy now provides the opportunity to limit the severity of neurological damage and improve the outcome up to 30% in certain stroke patients. For this reason, a new prehospital emphasis on stroke identification and rapid transport to a stroke center has evolved. This chapter discusses the major role of prehospital providers in the management of the acute stroke patient.

The American Heart Association has developed the Stroke Chain of Survival and Recovery consisting of seven key links. The first three links occur in the prehospital phase. These are detection, dispatch, and delivery. First, the patient and family or bystanders must be educated to recognize the signs and symptoms of an acute stroke. Second, someone must summon EMS immediately and emergency medical dispatchers must dispatch the appropriate response. Finally, responders must support the ABCs (airway, breathing, and circulation), make an accurate field diagnosis of an acute stroke, rapidly transport the patient to the appropriate facility, and notify the receiving facility of the time of onset of symptoms.

The brain is a greedy organ. It demands a constant supply of oxygen and nutrients and the efficient elimination of waste products. It consumes 17% of cardiac output and 20% of all available oxygen. When deprived of these essentials, even for a few minutes, severe neurological symptoms occur and, if left uncorrected, brain cell death is imminent. Circulation to and perfusion of the brain occurs via four main feeds—the two internal carotid arteries and the two vertebral arteries, which become the basilar artery. These arteries meet at the Circle of Willis at the base of the brain, an arterial manifold that ensures a redundant delivery of blood if one of the main arteries becomes obstructed. From the Circle of Willis, branch arteries reach all lobes of the brain, bringing nourishment and removing waste products. Branch arteries off the vertebrobasilar system perfuse the cerebellum.

A stroke occurs when blood supply to an area of the brain is interrupted. The severity of the stroke depends on the size of the artery involved and the presenting signs and symptoms depend on the area deprived of oxygen. Strokes are caused either by ischemia (85%) or hemorrhage (15%).

Ischemic strokes occur when a blood clot or foreign matter blocks a cerebral artery, resulting in tissue ischemia and, if not corrected, infarction. Ischemic strokes are caused by either a thrombus (stationary blood clot) or an embolus (moving blood clot). Atherosclerotic plaque deposits on the arterial wall form a thrombus, much like coronary artery disease process. An embolus arises usually from the carotid arteries or from abnormally functioning valves in the heart. Often atrial fibrillation, a precursor to the formation of blood clots, is a contributing factor. In certain cases, the effects of an ischemic stroke can be reversed with fibrinolytic therapy.

Hemorrhagic strokes are classified as intracranial (within the brain) or subarachnoid (between the dura and the brain). Both appear to arise from chronic hypertension or congenital abnormalities, such as an aneurysm or arteriovenous malformation (AVM). These are often preceded by a severe headache and sometimes result in increasing intracranial pressure. Hemorrhagic strokes require surgical repair, if possible.

Assessment of the stroke patient begins, as always, with the ABCs—recognizing and correcting any life-threatening conditions. Common chief complaints of a stroke include unilateral weakness or paralysis, unilateral numbness, speech and language disturbances, painless vision loss in one eye, vertigo, and ataxia. The key feature of the history of present illness is the time of onset of symptoms. This is critical because the administration of fibrinolytics must occur within 3 hours of the onset of symptoms. The focused history is aimed at identifying those components associated with stroke risk factors. These include hypertension, coronary artery disease, diabetes, and prior strokes or transient ischemic attacks. Other contributing factors include smoking, family history, a high-stress lifestyle, carotid bruits, and atrial fibrillation. Your patient's medications may include antihypertensives, insulin, anticholesterol drugs, antianginals, anticoagulants, and antidysrhythmics. The more risk factors present, the higher your suspicion for an acute stroke.

The Cincinnati Prehospital Stroke Scale was designed to identify any of the three classic physical signs suggesting a stroke: abnormal speech, facial droop, and arm drift. Simply ask your patient to repeat a simple phrase while you assess for speech problems. Then ask him to show his teeth in a wide smile while you look for symmetrical facial movement. Finally, ask him to shut his eyes and hold both arms straight out as if he were sleepwalking while you watch for arm drift. If any one of these positive signs is new, suspect a stroke.

On-scene management of an acute stroke is supportive and includes placing the patient in the recovery (laterally recumbent) position to facilitate the drainage of secretions; ensuring the ABCs and providing the appropriate airway, ventilatory, and circulatory support; protecting paralyzed extremities; monitoring for signs of increasing intracranial pressure; and providing continual reassurance to the patient who may hear and understand but cannot respond. Rapidly transport all patients still within the 3-hour window to a facility that can begin fibrinolytic therapy within 1 hour. Notify the receiving facility of the time of onset of symptoms and your estimated time of arrival. This notification is crucial so that the receiving facility can notify the stroke team, saving valuable time.

En route to the hospital, reassess and support the ABCs. Evaluate your patient's blood glucose and administer 50% dextrose if your patient is hypoglycemic. Otherwise, avoid glucose-containing IV solutions. Monitor your patient's neurological status and look for changes in mental status, motor and sensory function, and vital signs. If time allows, you may conduct a thorough neurological exam including cranial nerves and fine motor coordination (e.g., rapid alternating movements, point-to-point, heel-to-shin).

Avoid the impulse to reduce your patient's high blood pressure in the field. Remember that although hypertension may be the cause of your patient's stroke, it also may be a stress reaction to the event, or a physiological response to decreased brain perfusion. Hypertension may reflect the brain's attempt to perfuse itself in the presence of occluded areas. For this reason, lowering the blood pressure may, in fact, worsen your patient's condition. Lowering the patient's blood pressure should occur in the hospital under more controlled conditions.

RETURN TO THE CASE

Your patient is brought to the emergency department of a tertiary care hospital where the remaining four steps in the stroke chain occur. First, he is triaged at the door and the triage nurse confirms signs and symptoms of an acute stroke. Second, the patient is wheeled immediately to an examination room where a quick assessment is completed by the emergency physician. During the examination, blood samples for a complete blood count (CBC), electrolytes, and coagulation studies are drawn and sent to the lab. With the neurological exam completed, the emergency physician immediately pages the stroke team to respond to the emergency department. The patient is then wheeled away for a noncontrast computerized tomography (CT) scan of his brain. The CT is normal with no signs of hemorrhage or previous infarct. The stroke team, comprised of a neurologist and a nurse, arrives while the patient is still on the CT scan table and immediately evaluates the patient for any contraindications or exclusions to initiating fibrinolytic therapy. Because the patient's hypertension exceeds their thrombolytic protocol guidelines, the team administers labetalol (a beta-blocker) to lower the patient's systolic blood pressure. With the patient's blood pressure controlled, tissue plasminogen activator (TPA) is then administered to the patient exactly 2 hours and 11 minutes after the onset of his cerebrovascular accident (CVA) symptoms. The patient is admitted to the neurologic intensive care unit and recovers with no permanent neurological deficits.

Eighty-five percent of strokes occur at home, yet currently only one-half of stroke patients use the EMS system. The public must be educated to recognize the signs and symptoms of an acute stroke and call 911. Emergency medical dispatchers should be trained to ask the appropriate questions to ascertain the possibility of an acute stroke and to dispatch the appropriate advanced life support response. Last, paramedics must immediately identify the signs and symptoms of a stroke, confirm the time of onset of symptoms, and immediately transport the patient to a facility that can rapidly and comprehensively evaluate the patient. In cases where all the components of the Stroke Chain of Survival are combined with a patient who meets all the strict criteria for fibrinolytic therapy, the administration of fibrinolytics can rapidly reverse the devastating effects of an acute stroke.

REFERENCES

American Heart Association and International Liaison Committee on Resuscitation. "Guidelines 2000 for Cardiopulmonary Resuscitation and Emergency Cardiovascular Care." *Circulation* 102 (August 2000 Suppl.): I 1–384.

Bledsoe, Bryan E., Robert S. Porter, and Richard A. Cherry. *Medical Emergencies*. Vol. 3 of *Paramedic Care: Principles & Practice*. Chapter 3, "Neurology." Upper Saddle River, NJ: Brady/Prentice Hall Health, Pearson Education, 2001.

National Institute of Neurological Disorders and Stroke. *Rapid Identification and Treatment of Acute Stroke*. Bethesda, MD: National Institutes of Health, 1997.

Charles Pozner, MD

6

ANAPHYLAXIS

CASE PRESENTATION

You are dispatched for an unresponsive female at the home of a young couple who have been working out in the garden. Both have been in good health, neither taking any medications. You are met at the front of the house by a frantic neighbor who is eager to bring you to the patient. As you gather your proceed-out equipment and move quickly to the rear of the residence, you try to ask the neighbor some questions. All she can tell you is that her friend is lying on the grass, and won't wake up. A broad differential begins to run through your mind, including cardiac dysrhythmias, pulmonary embolism, syncope, an intracerebral event, seizure, trauma, and toxic exposure.

As you approach the patient, you see a female in her 20s, lying supine on the grass. A male in his 20s is attempting to provide mouth-to-mouth breathing. You immediately ask him to move, and you assess the airway. It appears that the patient is making efforts to breathe, though her depth of respirations is shallow. Her carotid pulse is weak, but present, at a rate of approximately 120. You immediately place a nonrebreathing mask on the patient, and attempt to assess her ability to respond; there is no response. You are able to place an oropharyngeal airway. While your partner is setting up his equipment to intubate this patient, you place her on the ECG monitor, examine the patient, and gather data from the husband.

The husband tells you that his wife was having a normal day in the garden. They were thirsty and he went inside to get something for both of them to drink. After approximately 10 minutes he came out to find his wife unresponsive. This had never happened before. Her breathing had become progressively labored and all he could think to do, after summoning his neighbor, was to give her mouth-to-mouth.

The patient's blood pressure is palpable at 60 at the brachial artery, and the oxygen saturation monitor provides neither a reading nor an adequate waveform. At this point you attempt to assist ventilations with a bag-valve-mask (BVM), and find extreme resistance when squeezing the bag. While your partner is attempting to intubate, you cut off the patient's shirt and you see a generalized erythema with some welts on the patient's chest.

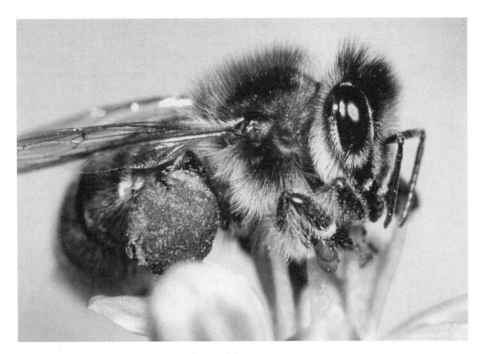

Bee envenomation is a common trigger for anaphylaxis.

Your partner proclaims that the airway is red and distorted, and he cannot visualize the cords. He quickly begins to prepare for a surgical cricothyrotomy.

You immediately draw up 0.3 mg of epinephrine 1:1000 and inject it into the sublingual venous plexus. You obtain an 18-gauge antecubital line, opening normal saline (NS) to wide open, and draw up 0.2 mg of epinephrine 1:10,000, diluting it with 8 cc of NS. You are about to inject this when the patient begins to have stridor, with better air movement, her blood pressure is now systolic of 90 by palpation, and she spits out the oral pharyngeal airway (OPA).

QUESTIONS

1. What pathophysiologic mechanisms take place to create the clinical picture seen in this case? Does anaphylaxis always present the same way?

2. What is the approach and management of patients presenting with anaphylaxis?

DISCUSSION

A severe multisystem allergic reaction, anaphylaxis is the result of exposure to an allergen leading to the release of mediators that may cause increased secretions from mucous membranes, increased bronchial smooth muscle tone, decreased vascular smooth muscle tone, or increased capillary permeability. Although the clinical manifestations may present with varying severity, the full-blown clinical manifestations result in oropharyngeal, laryngeal, and lower airway edema, bronchospasm, hypotension, edema (including edema of the GI tract), and skin manifestations (commonly urticaria).

Classically, mediators of anaphylaxis are released in response to an antigen (allergen) that binds to antigen-specific immunoglobulin E (IgE) receptors that are affixed to the cell membranes of previously sensitized immune cells (basophils and mast cells). Within seconds to minutes, binding results in the release of mediators of anaphylaxis including histamine, leukotrienes, prostaglandins, platelet activating factor, and proteases. It is at the end organs (e.g., skin, mucous membranes, lungs, blood vessels, and GI tract) that these mediators "wreak their havoc." In anaphylactoid reactions, mediator release occurs directly upon exposure to the allergen, without necessitating binding of antigen-specific IgE.

The most common inciting agents in the prehospital setting are bee stings and food allergies. Other agents (e.g., oral antibiotics and nonsteroidal anti-inflammatory agents) may also initiate this reaction. Some cases are idiopathic. Although many at risk have a known prior exposure to the inciting agent, a minority will have no known risk. The frequency in the United States is unknown, largely due to the lack of a precise case definition; however, less than 100 fatal reactions to bee stings are reported in the United States each year, the majority being less severe. Food allergy, though most commonly mild, may cause severe anaphylaxis. The foods most commonly associated with anaphylaxis are peanuts and shellfish. Risk of mortality is highest in elderly people due to the many comorbid conditions that complicate their presentation and management.

The severity of clinical manifestations varies depending on the degree of host sensitivity as well as the dose, route, and rate of exposure to the allergen. Manifestations may include

1. **Dermal:** 90% of reactions result in skin manifestations including a combination of urticaria (red or raised lesions with irregular borders of varying size), erythema, and pruritis.

2. **Eyes:** Itching and tearing may occur.

3. **Upper Respiratory Tract:** Common manifestations include nasal congestion, rhinorrhea, and sneezing. More severe upper airway symptoms relating to edema of the tongue, oropharynx, or larynx may result in coughing, hoarseness, and stridor (patient has trouble getting air in), portending significant airway obstruction.

4. **Lower Respiratory Tract:** Bronchospasm and increased lower airway secretions may result in dyspnea and wheezing (trouble getting air out).

5. **Cardiovascular:** Tachycardia with or without hypotension may occur. Lightheadedness from hypotension occurs due to vascular smooth muscle relaxation and capillary leak resulting in a distributive shocklike state. Tachycardia may be due to a compensatory response to hypotension or from intrinsic catecholamine release without hypotension. Dysrhythmias and myocardial infarction may occur due to increased catechols or systemic hypotension. In rare cases there can be normal vital signs, and bradycardia has been reported in very severe cases.

6. **Neurological:** Anxiety is the chief neurological presentation. Syncope may result from sudden loss of vascular tone resulting in cerebral hypoperfusion. Alteration in mental status may also occur due to the hypoxemia related to airway obstruction.

7. **GI Tract:** Cramping abdominal pain, thought to be related to bowel edema, may occur. Nausea and vomiting are less common.

As in most life-threatening patient presentations, diagnosis and management are best performed in parallel, by multiple rescuers. The rescuers must quickly assess and manage the airway, breathing, and circulation. If the patient is breathing, which is the most common circumstance, it is important to place the patient on high-flow oxygen. Care should be taken not to exacerbate any anxiety that could adversely affect the airway. If breathing is inadequate, attempts at ventilation with BVM may be the prudent airway maneuver while medications are administered and given a chance to alleviate any obstruction. If one is unable to adequately ventilate the patient with the BVM, the rescuer may attempt intubation. If unsuccessful, an airway must be obtained percutaneously.

In the prehospital setting there are six pharmacological therapies to be considered in the management of anaphylaxis:

1. **Epinephrine:** Due its combined effects of mitigating mediator release from basophils and mast cells as well as its sympathomimetic effects on end organs, epinephrine remains the primary therapy for moderate to severe cases of anaphylaxis. Epinephrine's alpha-receptor properties cause peripheral vasoconstriction, resulting in shrinkage of edematous tissues and improvement in blood pressure. Its beta effects cause increased chronotropy, inotropy, and bronchial smooth muscle relaxation. Common side effects include tachycardia, hypertension, palpitations, headache, and agitation.*

Adult Dosing:	0.3–0.5 ml (1:1000) SC q15min
	1ml (1:10,000; diluted in 10 cc NS) IV; slowly; repeat prn
	1.0 ml (1:1000) ET in approximately 10 cc NS
	IV infusion: 0.1–1.0 mcg/kg/minute
Pediatric Dosing:	0.01 ml/kg (1:1000) SC q15min (minimum 0.1 ml)
	0.01 ml/kg (1:10,000) IV prn (minimum 0.1 ml)
	0.01 ml/kg (1:1000) ET in 1–3 cc NS (minimum 0.1 ml)
	IV infusion: 0.1–1.0 mcg/kg/minute

When administering epinephrine, it is critical that the 1:1000 mixture is never given intravenously, as this may result in severe hypertension and tachycardia leading to cerebral, cardiac, and retinal complications.

2. **Antihistamines:** A mediator released from basophils and mast cells, histamine primarily results in cutaneous manifestations in anaphylaxis. Although its primary effects are on the cutaneous manifestations, some feel that

antihistamines may help antagonize other effects and should be used routinely in all cases of anaphylaxis. Diphenhydramine is the drug of choice:

Adult Dosing: 25–50 mg IV/IM

Pediatric Dosing: 1–2 mg/kg IV/IM q4–6h

3. **Inhaled beta-agonists:** By acting to relax bronchial smooth muscle, inhaled beta-agonists are thought to benefit the lower airway manifestations of anaphylaxis. Albuterol is most commonly employed:

Adult Dosing: 0.5 ml 0.5% sol in 2.5 cc NS nebulized q15minutes

Pediatric Dosing: 0.03–0.05 ml/kg 0.5% sol in 2.5 cc NS nebulized q15minutes

4. **Glucagon:** Patients taking beta-blocking agents may be resistant to the effects of epinephrine or other adrenergic agents used to treat the cardiovascular effects of anaphylaxis. Glucagon may be effective in these patients but should be used in addition to, not substituting for, epinephrine.

Adult Dosing: 1–10 mg IV/IM/SC; typically 1–2 mg q5minutes to effect

Pediatric Dosing: Not established

5. **Crystalloid:** Because there may be considerable vascular leak and loss of systemic vascular resistance, anaphylaxis may manifest as a distributive-like shock with refractory hypotension. IV crystalloid is a primary treatment in this setting.

Several other issues must be considered in the pharmacological management of anaphylaxis. The route of administration of medications may vary depending on the hemodynamic status of the patient. Intramuscular or subcutaneous injections will have unpredictable absorption in the setting of peripheral hypoperfusion, and should be avoided in the hypotensive patient. Many patients with a known history of anaphylaxis will carry autoinjectors containing epinephrine, and may inject this prior to your arrival. This dose, however, may not reach the central circulation until the hemodynamic status of the patient improves; therefore, patients should be closely monitored after administration of all medications, especially in this setting. This should never preclude you from administering epinephrine in patients with life-threatening anaphylaxis.

Although steroids are an integral part of the management of anaphylaxis, their onset of action (measured in hours) commonly precludes their effects being appreciated in the prehospital setting. If IV steroids are available to the paramedic, they can be administered in the setting of anaphylaxis after other pharmacologic interventions such as epinephrine and antihistamines have been administered.

In patients that have hemodynamic compromise (hypotension) refractory to epinephrine and IV fluids, one may consider other IV sympathomimetics. In this situation, dopamine should be considered the prehospital agent of choice.

RETURN TO THE CASE

The patient's respiratory rate increases as does both stridor and wheezing. You place the patient back on 100% oxygen by nonrebreathing mask and extricate her to the ambulance. Your partner sets up an albuterol nebulizer, while you administer 50 mg of diphenhydramine IV. Recheck of her blood pressure reveals a systolic pressure of 100. The monitor shows a sinus tachycardia at 110 and her oxygen saturation is 98%. You make an entry notification to the receiving facility, with an ETA of approximately 20 minutes. You continue to closely monitor the patient and she continues to improve. She tells you that while putting on her glove she felt a sting, and reveals to you an edematous, warm welt on the medial side of her right hand.

As you and your partner discuss the case, you reflect on the differential diagnosis of her initial presentation of syncope. Your quick assessment and management skills allowed you to make this difficult diagnosis and save this patient's life. You vow to at least consider anaphylaxis in all patients with a syncopal presentation.

As you leave the hospital the patient's husband pulls you aside and thanks you profusely for the expert life-saving care that you administered to his wife. She is given steroids and is admitted for observation. The next day she is discharged with both an Epi-pen and an appointment with an allergist.

REFERENCES

Bledsoe, Bryan E., Robert S. Porter, and Richard A. Cherry. *Medical Emergencies*. Vol. 3 of *Paramedic Care: Principles & Practice*. Chapter 5, "Allergies and Anaphylaxis." Upper Saddle River, NJ: Brady/Prentice Hall Health, Pearson Education, 2001.

Krause, R. S. *Anaphylaxis*, 2001. Available on the emedicine Web site at http://www.emedicine.com.

Thomas A. Sweeney, MD

7

CARDIAC ARREST

CASE PRESENTATION

You are dispatched to a private residence for a 46-year-old male collapsed. The emergency medical dispatcher began telephone cardiopulmonary resuscitation (CPR) instructions to the patient's wife who witnessed the patient collapse without warning. This CPR was difficult because the patient was profusely bleeding from a mouth laceration sustained as he fell. On arrival 6 minutes later you find that you have been preceded by a local volunteer fire company ambulance lieutenant who was in his car not far from the address when the call was dispatched. He quickly reached the house and had already defibrillated the patient once with his automatic external defibrillator (AED).

As you approach the patient in the living room, you note an unresponsive male of average build with blood around the nose and mouth. He appears mottled through the neck and upper chest. The EMS lieutenant is performing chest compressions. Your paramedic partner begins bag-valve-mask ventilation with oxygen and suctions the airway for blood and secretions with the help of additional fire department personnel who arrive just behind your unit. You connect the monitor-defibrillator and upon stopping CPR note pulseless electrical activity (Figure 7-1). You instruct the fire lieutenant to resume CPR.

In the meantime, your partner finishes basic airway maneuvers and oxygenation and intubates the patient with an 8.5 endotracheal tube. After visualizing passage through the cords she applies an esophageal detector device which promptly refills. She replaces it with the end-tidal carbon dioxide Easy Cap detector and as a firefighter-EMT begins bag-valve-mask ventilations she auscultates first over the epigastrium and then over the left and finally the right chest. You note symmetrical rise and fall of the chest and misting of the tube as your partner calls out "no epigastric, but equal breath sounds; Easy Cap is still dark." Given the patient's hypoperfused state, neither of you expects enough carbon dioxide from the patient to change the Easy Cap colorimetric monitor, but the other indicators of correct tube placement are reassuring.

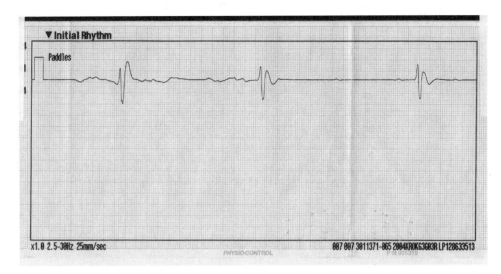

Figure 7-1 Initial paramedic ECG after first responder AED use: Pulseless Electrical Activity (PEA).
Courtesy of Thomas A. Sweeney, MD.

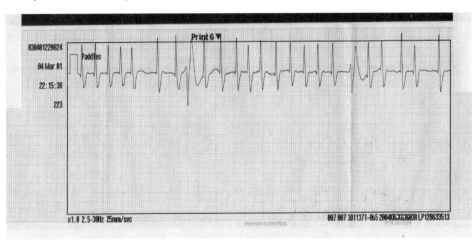

Figure 7-2 Supraventricular tachycardia (SVT) after intubation.
Courtesy of Thomas A. Sweeney, MD.

Once the tube position is ensured you hand your partner 2 mg of epinephrine to place down the endotracheal tube (ETT). While your partner is hyperventilating the patient, you start a 16-gauge IV in the left forearm and begin to run in a 500 cc bolus of normal saline.

Suddenly you note that the patient is in a narrow complex rhythm at a rate of 190 beats per minute (bpm), which appears to be supraventricular tachycardia (SVT) (Figure 7-2). You feel for a carotid pulse which is still absent. You hit the synchronization button on the monitor-defibrillator and provide synchronized cardioversion at 100 joules (J). The patient briefly goes into normal sinus rhythm at a rate of 80 with a pulse. Then SVT is noted once again at 220 bpm which you synchronize cardiovert again but this time at 200 J. The patient remains in a normal sinus rhythm with a rate of between 90 and 140 bpm. The colormetric carbon dioxide detector is now gold and there are palpable carotid and radial pulses.

QUESTIONS

1. What are the main objectives of prehospital care in a newly resuscitated cardiac arrest patient?
2. What information do paramedics need to collect to allow a newly resuscitated cardiac arrest patient to receive life-saving definitive care?

DISCUSSION

Rapid defibrillation of cardiac arrest victims is key to survival and, as shown in this case, first responders can play a vital role in reversing sudden cardiac death. Meticulous paramedic care is beneficial for further stabilization and evaluation of the rapidly defibrillated cardiac arrest victim.

The main objectives of prehospital care in a newly resuscitated cardiac arrest patient include maintenance of the airway and circulatory status.

Information that paramedics need to collect to allow a newly resuscitated cardiac arrest patient to expeditiously receive potentially life-saving care includes historical factors as to whether the arrest might be of cardiac origin and 12-lead ECG acquisition to determine whether an acute myocardial infarction exists based on ECG criteria.

AIRWAY MAINTENANCE

Airway maintenance and protection are paramount. Basic airway maneuvers and competent bag-valve-mask ventilation with oral or nasopharyngeal airways are as important as intubation skills. Once an endotracheal tube has been placed, its actual location must be verified with multiple techniques, as no one technique is completely accurate under all circumstances.

Rarely, an ETT may be misplaced even when the operator reports "direct visualization." Esophageal intubations can easily occur through ETT displacement. Neck flexion can cause 3–5 centimeter (cm) of ETT movement that can easily result in tube dislodgement from the trachea. Thus, great care must be taken to verify tube placement, maintain tube position, and monitor tube placement.

The esophageal detector device should be used immediately after intubation but before ventilation. This self-inflating bulb or 60 cc syringe takes advantage of the anatomical differences between the trachea and the esophagus, namely that under suction the trachea will not collapse and air can be easily and continuously aspirated, whereas the esophageal wall easily collapses onto the ETT, obstructing the aspiration of air. Although sometimes inaccurate, it serves as a valuable adjunct in the cardiac arrest patient where end tidal carbon dioxide may not be readily detected.

End-tidal carbon dioxide detection is valuable in patients with adequate perfusion. In cases of cardiac arrest such as the beginning of this case, colorimetric devices may not function even with good ventilation and CPR because the amount of carbon dioxide (CO_2) exhaled is minimal. Waveform CO_2 detectors, even though much more costly, detect much lower levels of CO_2 and are useful in cases of recent cardiac arrest with good CPR.

Verification of proper ETT placement should consist of multiple observations including visualization of ETT passage through the cords, esophageal detector device aspiration initially, end-tidal CO_2 reading, absence of epigastric sounds, bilateral breath sounds with chest rise and fall, and tube misting on inhalation. Any one of these indicators has the potential to be misleading, but taken in combination, they assure proper endotracheal tube placement (ETT).

It is important to secure the ETT firmly in place. This can be accomplished by skilled use of tape or any number of commercially available devices. It may be beneficial to take active steps such as utilizing a cervical collar and hard spine board to limit neck flexion and extension. The placement of the ETT should be reevaluated after every movement of the patient.

CIRCULATORY STATUS

The patient was defibrillated to pulseless electrical activity. The key function of defibrillation is to stop ventricular fibrillation, which consumes significant amounts of oxygen and nutrients from the heart. Whether the patient then regains a perfusing rhythm depends on factors such as the prearrest status of the myocardium and the duration of hypoxia and circulatory standstill. Prehospital providers can greatly increase the chances of successful resuscitation from cardiac arrest with intact neurologic survival if the EMS system can provide rapid defibrillation. Great attention to airway maintenance and oxygenation will also be of benefit.

This patient was fortunate in that he had never suffered any previous heart damage and his time to defibrillation was within 4 minutes of collapse. The development of pulseless supraventricular tachycardia requiring synchronized cardioversion was unusual but fortunately responded to direct cardioversion. More commonly seen are recurrent ventricular fibrillation or ventricular tachycardia.

Epinephrine, now considered of indeterminate value by the American Heart Association's *Guidelines 2000 for Cardiopulmonary Resuscitation and Emergency Cardiovascular Care*, actually appeared to play a role in this resuscitation. There is, however, little convincing scientific evidence that epinephrine is helpful to the cardiac arrest patient and high doses of epinephrine are now suspected to cause harm in adults.

Antiarrhythmics also have proarrhythmic properties and thus should be used with care. They should not be combined, but rather only one antiarrhythmic should be selected for each patient if used at all. Lidocaine is considered of indeterminate value in a postarrest situation if no ventricular ectopy is present. Other options available include amiodarone if the patient exhibits persistent ventricular fibrillation or tachycardia; however, this drug has been shown only to increase return of spontaneous circulation, not intact neurologic survival at discharge from the hospital. Magnesium sulfate should be considered for torsade de pointes or persistent ventricular fibrillation/ventricular tachycardia associated with suspected hypomagnesemia.

TWELVE-LEAD ECG AND OPTIONS FOR REPERFUSION

Acute myocardial infarction can precipitate cardiac arrest as in this case. If the ongoing infarction is not reversed, significant myocardial damage and recurrent cardiac arrest are likely. A prehospital 12-lead ECG allows early identification of those cardiac arrest patients who are also demonstrating an acute infarct.

There are two strategies to achieve myocardial reperfusion: thrombolytic therapy and percutaneous coronary angioplasty (PTCA) with stenting. PTCA requires not only the immediate availability of a properly trained cardiologist but also the ability to mobilize the entire cath lab team. For these reasons, early PTCA intervention is not available at most hospitals. After significant CPR, thrombolytic therapy is contraindicated due to the risk of internal bleeding from chest wall and pericardial trauma.

In the patient presented here, a prehospital 12-lead ECG diagnostic for AMI could allow the medical control physician to summon a qualified cardiologist and the catheterization team even before the patient had arrived at the emergency department. If a patient is located closer to a community hospital that is not capable of such specialized cardiac care, he could be diverted directly to the regional cardiac center. This type of diversion can extend the prehospital time, but could avoid the need for the time-consuming transfer of the patient from the community emergency department to the regional PTCA center.

RETURN TO THE CASE

You contact medical control. The online physician listens to the report and your desire to now rapidly transport the patient to the hospital. The physician advises you to check a blood pressure and a 12-lead electrocardiogram and recontact her before initiating transport.

Your partner turns over bag-valve-mask ventilation to a firefighter-EMT with instructions that he securely hold the newly taped endotracheal tube at the 23 cm mark. She measures the blood pressure as 180/100. You hook up the leads and perform a 12-lead electrocardiogram (Figure 7-3). You and your partner examine the 12-lead and note 3 mm of

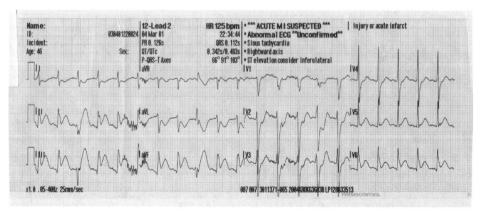

Figure 7-3 Post-resuscitation 12-lead ECG showing acute inferior wall myocardial infarction. Courtesy of Thomas A. Sweeney, MD.

ST-segment elevation in the inferior leads (II, III, and AVF) with 3–5 mm of ST-segment depression in the anterior leads (V_1–V_3) and 2–3 mm ST depression in the lateral leads (I and aVL). These depressions are also known as reciprocal changes and confirm that the ST elevation actually does represent an acute myocardial infarction.

You recontact medical control who agrees that this is consistent with an inferior wall myocardial infarction. She states that she will activate a "heart alert" immediately to summon the catheterization team and a cardiologist trained in angioplasty (using a balloon catheter to dilate clots out of the coronary artery). Regarding your query as to whether you should administer an antiarrhythmic (you carry lidocaine, amiodarone, and magnesium sulfate), she advises to defer as the patient is currently in a sinus tachycardia without ectopy.

The fire department crew assists you with moving the patient onto a Reeves Sleeve® flexible litter for removal down a tight hallway with a sharp turn. Upon exiting the house you reconfirm the airway by noting the Easy Cap showing gold—carbon dioxide, no epigastric sounds, equal lung sounds present and the tube at 23 cm, and oxygen is still attached to the Ambu-bag. The cardiac rhythm is still a narrow complex sinus tachycardia at 120 bpm. A radial pulse is present. With the ABCs intact you move from the house to the ambulance and, after loading, you recheck the ABCs. While proceeding to the hospital you check the patient's blood sugar, which is 220. You complete your secondary exam that is unremarkable except for some persistent oozing from an upper lip laceration and a blood pressure of 170/85.

On arrival at the emergency department you instruct the firefighter-EMT to disconnect the Ambu-bag while the patient is removed from the ambulance to the ground. Ventilation is then resumed and you proceed into the resuscitation bay. As the patient is lifted over to the hospital gurney on the flexible Reeves litter, the patient's head extends as the litter bends. When the physician begins his assessment he suddenly calls out, "Why is the carbon dioxide detector purple?" He rapidly listens for epigastric sounds and orders that ventilations through the endotracheal tube be stopped.

The patient's head had flexed and extended during transfer to the hospital gurney with displacement of the ETT into the esophagus. The emergency physician confirms the lack of end-tidal CO_2 using the colorimetric detector and auscultation. The ET tube is immediately withdrawn and BVM ventilation with 100% oxygen is begun. Once the pulse oximeter shows a 100% reading the paralytic succinylcholine and the sedative midazolam are administered to relax the patient's jaw and he is reintubated. The intubation is somewhat difficult due to pooled blood in the hypopharynx from the patient's upper lip laceration that requires suctioning.

The patient is taken emergently to the cardiac catheterization laboratory where a completely occluded right coronary artery is identified. This is reopened with balloon angioplasty and a metal stent is deployed to hold the vessel open. Acute ECG changes are resolved with this procedure.

Over the next several days the patient gradually awakens and is extubated and released from the intensive care unit. Some initial confusion felt secondary to mild hypoxic encephalopathy resolves by day 4 of his hospitalization. He is also treated with antibiotics for mild aspiration pneumonia. The cardiologist starts him on a beta-blocker (atenolol), a nitrate agent (isosorbide mononitrate), and two platelet agents (aspirin and clopidogrel). Seven days after admission he is discharged to home in excellent condition

with the diagnosis of acute inferior wall myocardial infarction complicated by ventricular fibrillation.

REFERENCES

Bledsoe, Bryan E., Robert S. Porter, and Richard A. Cherry. *Medical Emergencies*. Vol. 3
of *Paramedic Care: Principles & Practice*. Chapter 2, "Cardiology." Upper Saddle
River, NJ: Brady/Prentice Hall Health, Pearson Education, 2001.

Cummins, R. O., W. Thies, J. Paraskos, et al. "Encouraging Early Defibrillation: The
American Heart Association and Automated External Defibrillators." *Annals of
Emergency Medicine* 19 (1990): 1245–1248.

Kudenchuk, P. J., L. A. Cobb, and M. K. Copass. "Amiodarone for Resuscitation after
Out-of-Hospital Cardiac Arrest Due to Ventricular Fibrillation." *New England
Journal of Medicine* 341 (1999): 871–878.

O'Connor, R. E., and R. A. Swor. "Verification of Endotracheal Tube Placement Following Intubation." *Prehospital Emergency Care* 3 (1999): 248–250.

Robert O'Connor, MD, MPH

CATHETERS/PICC LINES

CASE PRESENTATION

You are called to a private residence to treat a 36-year-old female with right arm pain and swelling. Emergency medical dispatch verifies that the patient has no respiratory distress and is awake, alert, and conversant.

As you approach the residence, the patient answers the door. The patient states that she has noted progressive swelling of her right arm over the past 12 hours. She has a history of leukemia and is currently receiving chemotherapy through a peripherally inserted central catheter (PICC) line that was inserted in her right arm 2 weeks ago. She denies fever, chills, nausea, or vomiting. She has no chest pain.

You ask her to have a seat on a chair just inside the door so that you can perform an assessment and take vital signs. On exam, you note marked swelling of the patient's right arm. Pitting edema is present. The skin color appears normal, with no evidence of infection. Capillary refill of the fingers is less than 2 seconds. Radial pulse is intact and her vital signs are stable. The patient is concerned about the swelling, but states that she would prefer not to go to the hospital unless it is necessary.

QUESTIONS

1. What are your primary concerns with this patient? Why is her arm swollen?
2. Does she need to go to the hospital? If so, what should she expect to have done at the hospital?

DISCUSSION

PICC LINES

The PICC is a thin, flexible catheter about 60 cm long, which is inserted via the superficial veins of the upper arm until its tip lies in the superior vena cava just above the heart. Insertion, which involves just one cannulation, can be carried out in the home as well as in the hospital. Risks of the procedure are minimal, but include bleeding from the needle puncture site and temporary tendon or nerve injury. After insertion, the line can remain in place for up to a year.

PICC lines are becoming commonplace in outpatient intravenous therapy because they permit prolonged venous access, offer a means to administer medications that would otherwise be irritating to peripheral vessels, and can be used to provide parenteral nutrition. Perhaps the most common use of PICC lines is for prolonged courses of intravenous antibiotics. These central lines provide life-saving therapy, are easily inserted, cost effective, and convenient. Although there are many benefits to using these catheters, patients must remain acutely aware of the risks involved with placement of PICC lines so that complications can be minimized. Prevention of insertion site infection and sepsis is always a priority, and several measures can be implemented to reduce this risk, including scrupulous aseptic technique, knowledgeable selection of the insertion site, and consistent daily care. Other complications such as a venous clot (thrombosis), extravascular collection of fluid due to catheter migration or blockage, vessel perforation, and line leakage may occur. Careful catheter tip placement and conscientious ongoing monitoring can assist in reducing morbidity as well as mortality related to PICC lines.

Venous thrombosis is a particularly common complication in patients with PICC lines in place. Clinically, venous thrombosis results in diffuse swelling and often some associated pain in the affected extremity due to the blockage of venous drainage and engorgement of the distal venules. Reported symptomatic venous thrombosis rates associated with PICC lines are based solely on clinical signs, and symptoms range from 1% to 4%. It is not uncommon that patients who are receiving IV medications through a PICC line will require removal and replacement of the original line during the course of therapy. In one study, problems with device breakage, thrombophlebitis, and line occlusion necessitated replacement in the majority of cases, with patients receiving an average of three PICC insertions during the course of the study.

CENTRAL CATHETERS: HICKMAN, BROVIAC, GROSHONG, AND OTHERS

Central catheters are ideal for infusing medications that may be irritating, or ones that require prolonged infusion. These devices are widely used in patients who are receiving chemotherapy treatments for cancer. The Hickman catheter is a modification of an earlier catheter developed by Broviac in 1973 for the purpose of infusing total parenteral nutrition over prolonged periods. The Hickman has a wider tube and thicker tube wall than the Broviac catheter, and is more widely used today. Hickman catheters are used for patients who require ongoing intravenous therapy, whether it is for parenteral nutrition, chemotherapy, or antibiotic administration. The Hickman consists of a long internal tube that extends from a vein above the heart through a subcutaneous tunnel in the chest wall through the exit site.

Central catheters may have one or more separate lumens branching from the catheter, each of which is 4 or 5 inches long and ends in an access port. When the catheter is used, a needle is inserted into the port. The lumens are looped and taped to the chest when not in use.

The Groshong catheter is a newer version of the Hickman, in which the internal catheter tip is closed, using a one-way valve instead. The valve remains closed when not in use; however, during infusion, pressure opens the valve, which then closes when the infusion is stopped. When suction is applied (usually by a syringe), this negative pressure causes the valve to open inward, letting blood flow through the catheter into the syringe. A Groshong catheter does not need heparin flushes, slightly simplifying routine maintenance procedures. The Groshong's tube caliber is not as wide as the Hickman's, and, as a result, more time is needed for procedures such as transfusions.

The PORT-A-CATH® is another type of central intravenous access device. The PORT-A-CATH differs from the Groshong and Hickman devices in that the port's access is implanted subcutaneously, and clinically appears as a round lump under the skin in the upper chest, in contrast to the other devices that have traditional-appearing IV tubing and ports exposed, with only the distal catheter burrowed under the skin into the central vein. PORT-A-CATHs have to be accessed with specialized right-angle needles called Huber point needles.

The most common complication of central catheters is infection, usually termed "line sepsis." In line sepsis, bacteria are inadvertently introduced into the blood resulting in a potentially life-threatening infection that clinically may present as fever and may be associated with pain at the site where the catheter is inserted under the skin. Full-blown line sepsis can result in overwhelming infection, shock, and death.

Central catheters (including the Hickman, PORT-A-CATH, and Groshong) are also prone to the development of thrombus that may not only occlude the lumen of the device but also cause obstruction of venous return from the upper extremity because of deep vein thrombosis (DVT).

In immediate life-threatening situations such as cardiac arrest or profound shock, where peripheral access cannot be obtained, it is appropriate to aseptically access catheters such as the Groshong or Hickman for drug or fluid administration. Such access should either be authorized as part of established EMS protocols or done under direct contact with the base station physician.

RETURN TO THE CASE

The patient possibly has catheter-induced thrombosis of the right subclavian vein. She needs to go to the hospital for definitive diagnosis by ultrasound or venography. You tell her that if thrombosis is confirmed, fibrinolytic therapy might be administered to restore subclavian patency. She agrees to go to the hospital.

On hospital arrival, she undergoes ultrasound, which confirms thrombosis of the subclavian vein. Interventional radiology infuses TPA through the PICC line and confirms dissolution of the thrombus. Blood cultures are drawn that are negative. The patient's CBC and platelet count are normal. She is started on anticoagulation and is discharged home after a 1-day hospital stay, with the original PICC line still in place.

REFERENCES

Allen, A. W., J. L. Megargell, D. B. Brown, F. C. Lynch, H. Singh, Y. Singh, and P. N. Waybill. "Venous Thrombosis Associated with the Placement of Peripherally Inserted Central Catheters:" *Journal of Vascular and Interventional Radiology* 11, no. 10 (November–December 2000): 1309–1314.

Bledsoe, Bryan E., Robert S. Porter, and Richard A. Cherry. *Medical Emergencies*, Vol. 3 of *Paramedic Care: Principles & Practice*. Chapter 2, "Cardiology." Upper Saddle River, NJ: Brady/Prentice Hall Health, Pearson Education, 2001.

Camara, D. "Minimizing Risks Associated with Peripherally Inserted Central Catheters in the NICU." *MCN, American Journal of Maternal Child Nursing* 26 (January–February 2001): 17–21.

Haire, W. D., R. P. Lieberman, J. Edney, W. P. Vaughan, A. Kessinger, J. O. Armitage, and J. C. Goldsmith. "Hickman Catheter-Induced Thoracic Vein Thrombosis. Frequency and Long-Term Sequelae in Patients Receiving High-Dose Chemotherapy and Marrow Transplantation." *Cancer* 66, no. 5 (September 1, 1966): 900–908.

O'Neill, V. J., T. R. Jeffrey Evans, J. Preston, J. Moss, and S. B. Kaye. "A Retrospective Analysis of Hickman Line-Associated Complications in Patients with Solid Tumors Undergoing Infusional Chemotherapy." *Acta Oncologica* 38, no. 8 (1999): 1103–1107.

Sariego, J., B. Bootorabi, T. Matsumoto, and M. Kerstein, "Major Long-Term Complications in 1,422 Permanent Venous Access Devices." *American Journal of Surgery* 165, no. 2 (February 1993): 249–251.

Judd E. Hollander, MD

9

COCAINE-RELATED CHEST PAIN

CASE PRESENTATION

Your unit is dispatched to attend to an agitated 32-year-old male who is pacing the street outside a crack house. Police have secured the scene prior to your arrival. On arrival you find that the patient is quite anxious, grasping his chest and complaining of chest pain that has worsened over the past 4 hours and was not relieved by self-medication with alcohol and crack cocaine. The pain began several hours after his last use of crack cocaine. The primary survey reveals an agitated male, holding his midsternum, breathing easily and yelling for pain medications. The patient agrees to treatment and sits down on the curb as you begin your assessment and treatment. Initial vital signs include a blood pressure of 200/110 mmHg; pulse 132 bpm; and a respiratory rate of 24. The patient does not have any jugular-venous distention, his lungs are clear, and his heart is tachycardic but regular. His abdomen is soft and nontender and he does not appear to have focal neurological deficits. You place the patient on the monitor while your partner begins an intravenous line with normal saline, and then you load the patient into the back of the ambulance.

QUESTIONS

1. What is the differential diagnosis for chest pain in a cocaine user?
2. What are the cardiovascular effects of cocaine?
3. What is the most important treatment that can be administered to the patient with cocaine-related chest pain prior to hospital arrival?

DISCUSSION

The differential diagnosis of patients with cocaine-associated chest pain includes all the conditions that you must consider for patients with chest pain that is unrelated to cocaine. The main caveat is that cocaine-using patients with chest pain are much more likely to have serious conditions than noncocaine users of the same age. The differential diagnosis includes acute coronary syndromes or ACSs (AMI and unstable angina), pulmonary infarction, pneumothorax, pneumomediastinum, and aortic dissection, in addition to less serious causes such as muscular chest wall ischemia, rhabdomyolysis (breakdown of skeletal muscle), pneumonia, peptic ulcers, and so on. In general, the approach to patients with cocaine-associated chest pain should be to presume the most serious etiologies are the cause of the chest pain until proven otherwise and to treat accordingly with aggressive prehospital care.

The cardiovascular effects of cocaine include acute coronary syndrome (myocardial infarction or ischemia), cardiomyopathies leading to congestive heart failure, endocarditis, and dysrrhythmias (both tachy and brady). A "normal" 12-lead ECG does not exclude ACS. ECG monitoring is, however, essential to detect the presence of dysrhythmias.

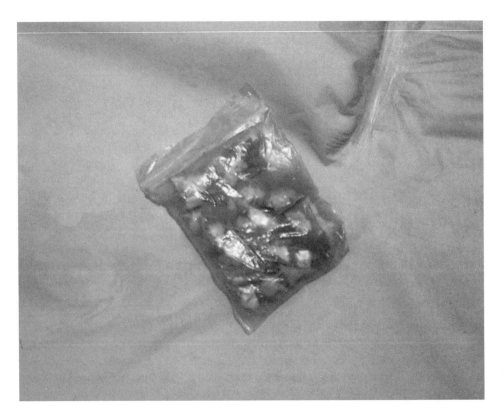

Crack cocaine.
Courtesy of Edward T. Dickinson, MD.

Myocardial ischemia and infarction (ACS) occur secondary to cocaine use. They are unrelated to the route or amount of cocaine used, patient age, or presence of a hyperdynamic (increased heart rate and blood pressure) state. Patients with cocaine-associated myocardial infarctions frequently have atypical chest pain or chest pain delayed for hours to days after their most proximate use of cocaine. Myocardial ischemia is most common shortly after cocaine use. The risk of MI increases twenty-fourfold in the hour after cocaine use. The exact duration of time that cocaine increases risk for ACS is not clear. One study, using ambulatory ECG (Holter) monitoring in patients admitted to an inpatient detoxification center, demonstrated that spontaneous episodes of ST-segment elevation occurred for up to 6 weeks after withdrawal of cocaine. Thus, the effects of cocaine might be very long lasting.

Patients with cocaine-associated acute coronary syndromes may or may not have initial ECG abnormalities, so there does not appear to be tremendous value to single-lead monitoring, other than identification of dysrrhythmias.

Cocaine causes myocardial ischemia through a complex pathophysiology resulting from its acute and chronic effects. Acutely, cocaine results in coronary artery vasoconstriction, tachycardia, hypertension, increased myocardial oxygen demand, platelet aggregation, and thrombus formation. Chronic cocaine users develop accelerated atherosclerosis and left ventricular hypertrophy, which can further exacerbate the oxygen supply-demand mismatch. Myocardial ischemia and infarction have occurred in patients using cocaine without any underlying atherosclerotic disease or other evidence of preexisting heart disease.

Low-dose cocaine may result in bradycardias, whereas higher doses have been associated with virtually all types of tachydysrrhythmias. Sinus tachycardia, atrial fibrillation/flutter, other supraventricular tachycardias, premature ventricular contractions, ventricular tachycardia, and ventricular fibrillation may be the direct result of cocaine use. In addition to the direct effects of cocaine that may result in dysrhythmias, dysrhythmias may also occur secondary to cocaine-induced acute coronary syndromes.

Chronic cocaine use can also lead to the development of a dilated cardiomyopathy either from recurrent or diffuse ischemia with subsequent "stunned" myocardium or from a direct effect of the cocaine on the heart muscle.

Finally, cocaine use can lead to aortic dissection and rupture. It is presumed that dissection and rupture result from the increase in shear forces that result from cocaine-induced hypertension and tachycardia.

It is important to realize that the treatment of hyperdynamic patients with cocaine-associated acute coronary syndromes is different from the treatment of patients with ACS unrelated to cocaine. The largest prehospital differences are that patients with recent cocaine use should receive treatment with benzodiazepines (e.g., diazepam) and should *not* get treatment with beta-adrenergic blockers (e.g., propanolol or metoprolol).

There is a direct relationship between cocaine's neuropsychiatric and cardiovascular complications. Proper management of the neuropsychiatric manifestations almost always improves cardiovascular abnormalities, at least from an emergent or initial care perspective. Sedation with a benzodiazepine is most efficacious and improves symptoms of agitation and anxiety as well as cardiovascular abnormalities. Other agents often used in agitated patients, such as neuroleptics (e.g., haloperidol) should not be given to agitated patients who are cocaine intoxicated. Neuroleptic agents impair heat dissipation and may, in some cases, lower the seizure threshold. Diazepam or another benzodiazepine, such as lorazepam, should be used intravenously for initial management of severe agitation. Even patients with cocaine-associated chest pain, in the absence of agitation, should receive benzodiazepines. They have been shown to relieve chest pain as rapidly as nitroglycerin in this group of patients.

The hemodynamic effects of cocaine often do not require specific treatment. Treatments aimed at the resolution of anxiety, agitation, and ischemia will often lead to resolution of the abnormal hemodynamic parameters. When necessary, treatment with benzodiazepines aimed at the central effects of cocaine will usually lead to reduction in blood pressure and heart rate. When hypertension fails to respond to sedation, it is usually best managed in the ED setting, where it can be treated with sodium nitroprusside or phentolamine, if needed.

Treatment of the vascular manifestations of cocaine intoxication should focus on the reversible causes of oxygen supply-demand mismatch: specifically, coronary artery vasoconstriction, platelet aggregation, thrombus formation, hypertension, and tachycardia.

Studies in the cardiac catheterization laboratory have helped determine the mechanisms of coronary artery vasoconstriction and have evaluated several treatment options. In these studies, adults without prior cocaine use who were undergoing coronary catheterization for evaluation of underlying coronary artery disease were given 2 mg/kg of intranasal cocaine. Patients were demonstrated to have an increase in heart rate, blood pressure, and coronary vascular resistance. Coronary arterial diameter was diffusely narrowed by approximately 13%. Following infusion of phentolamine (0.4 milligrams per minute [mg/min]), an alpha-adrenergic agent, these parameters returned to baseline. This suggests that cocaine-induced vasoconstriction is caused through an alpha-adrenergic mechanism and that phentolamine may be useful for treatment of cocaine-induced myocardial ischemia. Nitroglycerin has also been shown to reverse cocaine-induced vasoconstriction and relieve chest pain in patients with cocaine-induced chest pain.

Coronary artery vasoconstriction is exacerbated by propranolol, a beta-adrenergic antagonist. In animal models of cocaine toxicity, beta-adrenergic antagonists have led to decreased coronary blood flow, increased seizure frequency, and higher fatality rates. As a result of data, the use of beta-adrenergic antagonists for the treatment of cocaine toxicity is *contraindicated*.

Cocaine can directly injure the vascular endothelium and increase platelet aggregation through a variety of pathways increasing the risk of acute MI. As a result, the use of aspirin, heparin, and fibrinolytic agents make theoretical sense in the setting of vascular ischemia. When considering the use of fibrinolytic agents for acute myocardial infarction, you must be aware that there are several case reports that document adverse outcomes following fibrinolytic administration in patients with recent cocaine use, most notably, catastrophic CVAs. Also, patients with cocaine-associated chest pain often have ST-segment elevation in the absence of actual ischemia. Thus, fibrinolytics should never be given to patients with cocaine-associated AMI in the prehospital setting. The use of fibrinolytic agents should be reserved for patients who failed to respond to vasodilator therapy and have low risk for cerebrovascular or other serious bleeding catastrophes. Fibrinolytic agents should be used with caution in the hospital setting.

Cocaine-induced atrial tachydysrhythmias that have not responded to sedative hypnotics may respond to verapamil or diltiazem. The treatment of cocaine-induced ventricular dysrhythmias depends upon the time between cocaine use, dysrhythmia onset, and commencement of treatment. Ventricular dysrhythmias that develop immediately following cocaine use should be presumed to occur from either catecholamine excess or the local anesthetic effects of cocaine on the myocardium. Cocaine-induced wide-complex dysrhythmias may respond to administration of sodium bicarbonate. In patients who present several hours after the last use of cocaine, the ventricular dysrhythmias may be generated by an ischemic myocardium, and standard management for ventricular dysrhythmias (e.g., lidocaine) is indicated.

RETURN TO THE CASE

Medical direction is consulted en route to the hospital. The patient is then treated with intravenous administration of Valium in incremental 5 mg doses with a moderate response. There is a decrease in the degree of agitation but some persistence of chest pain (3 out of 10 pain scale). The blood pressure decreases to 170/90 and the pulse slows to 105 bpm. Paramedics administer 325 mg of aspirin and sublingual nitroglycerin every 5 minutes for 2 doses with complete resolution of pain. Care is transferred to the emergency department staff. The patient receives optimal prehospital treatment incorporating the use of aspirin, nitroglycerin, and a benzodiazepine. The initial ED 12-lead ECG does not show acute ischemia and the patient is subsequently admitted to the hospital to "rule out myocardial infarction." Once ruled out, the patient has a negative stress test and enters a cocaine rehab program.

REFERENCES

Albertson, T. E., A. Dawson, F. de Latorre, R. S. Hoffman, J. E. Hollander, A. Jaeger, W. Kerns II, T. G. Martin, and M. P. Ross. "TOX-ACLS: Toxicologic-Oriented Advanced Cardiac Life Support." *Annals of Emergency Medicine* 37 (April 2001): 578–590.

Bledsoe, Bryan E., Robert S. Porter, and Richard A. Cherry. *Medical Emergencies.* Vol. 3 of *Paramedic Care: Principles & Practice.* Chapter 2, "Cardiology." Upper Saddle River, NJ: Brady/Prentice Hall Health, Pearson Education, 2001.

Hoffman, R. S. and J. E. Hollander. "Evaluation of Chest Pain after Cocaine Use. In S. Curry, (ed)., *Critical Care Clinics of North America* 13, no. 4 (1997): 809–828.

Hollander, J. E. "Management of Cocaine Associated Myocardial Ischemia." *New England Journal of Medicine* 333, no. 19. (1995): 1267–1272.

Jonnathan Busko, MD, MPH, EMT-P

10

CONGESTIVE HEART FAILURE

CASE PRESENTATION

It is another sweltering shift when you and your partner are dispatched for a 68-year-old male with cardiac history who is having difficulty breathing. As you pull up in front of an old apartment building, you realize that you have transported this patient several times for acute exacerbation of congestive heart failure (CHF). You recall that he is hypertensive, diabetic, and has had multiple MIs.

Entering the apartment feels like entering a blast furnace. As you walk into the living room, you find your patient semi-recumbent on an old sofa. Your initial impression is that this is a pale, obese elderly male who is in marked respiratory distress, although not in extremis. You sit him upright, place him on a nonrebreather at 15 L/min, and begin your assessment.

The primary survey reveals a patient with a patent airway who is coughing up pink-tinged sputum. He is tachypneic with supraclavicular retractions, although he is not collapsing the reservoir on the nonrebreather. Auscultation of the lungs reveals crackles and scattered wheezes. Your cardiovascular exam reveals tachycardia with palpable radial pulses and cool, diaphoretic skin.

As you place the patient on the monitor, he tells you (in three-word, gasping phrases) that he was doing well until an hour ago, when he suddenly became short of breath. He states that this feels like his previous CHF exacerbations and denies chest pain, recent illness, fevers or chills, nausea, or vomiting. He states that he takes his antihypertensives, insulin, diuretics, and aspirin as directed and that he has not increased his salt intake, although he has been drinking more fluids because of the heat. Your partner obtains vital signs and finds that the patient has a pulse rate of 114, a blood pressure of 196/112, a respiratory rate of 42, and a pulse ox of 89% on the 15 L/min nonrebreather.

It is clear to you that your patient is in significant congestive heart failure and that respiratory failure is impending. You need to decide how you are going to treat his CHF and prevent complete respiratory failure.

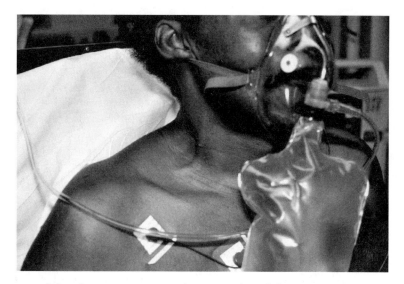

Distended jugular veins in a patient with congestive heart failure (CHF).
Courtesy of Edward T. Dickinson, MD.

QUESTIONS

1. What is the most likely cause of this patient's acute pulmonary edema?
2. Should you intubate this patient immediately?
3. If you elect not to intubate this patient, what are your pharmacological and nonpharmacological treatment options?

DISCUSSION

Congestive heart failure occurs when the heart is unable to adequately pump blood forward. Although the symptoms may be minor (leg edema, mild shortness of breath with heavy exertion, etc.), the severe manifestation of acute pulmonary edema is not uncommon. Of the more than 3 million Americans with CHF, approximately 30% to 40% will be hospitalized each year. The median length of survival after diagnosis is 3.2 years for males and 5.4 years for females. Although these patients typically die from worsening heart failure, as many as 46% will die from sudden cardiac death. The prognosis is significantly worse for patients with diabetes who require insulin therapy.

It is important to recognize that pulmonary edema is not identical to CHF. Pulmonary edema is the collection of fluid in the intraalveolar space and can occur for many reasons. Congestive heart failure (specifically left heart failure) is only one of many causes of pulmonary edema. Conversely, CHF has many manifestations that result from blood "backing up" in the pulmonary and venous circulatory systems; pulmonary edema is just one manifestation of heart failure.

Fluid in the circulatory system is kept inside the blood vessels by a balance of many factors. These include the hydrostatic (fluid) pressure inside and outside the vessels, the presence of large molecules that create an "oncotic" pressure that draws fluids into the vessels, and the degree of "leakiness" of the vessels. The capillaries in the lungs usually do not leak much because the hydrostatic pressure in the vessels is low, the oncotic pressure is high, and the capillary walls have a low degree of leakiness. Fluid that does escape is removed via lymph vessels. For acute pulmonary edema to occur, the pressure in the capillaries must be greatly increased (such as in left heart failure), the oncotic pressure must be low (which can occur in some kidney and liver disease), or the capillaries must become leakier (caused by some drugs, toxic inhalations, infections, etc.). If enough fluid leaks out of the vessels so that the lymph system cannot drain it all, eventually the fluid will enter into the alveoli, causing pulmonary edema.

All that crackles is not CHF. The differential diagnosis for pulmonary edema is broad and although cardiac failure is probably the most common cause, many disease states and toxins can precipitate pulmonary edema as well. These include cocaine and heroin use, infections (pulmonary and systemic), near-drowning and other aspirations, toxic inhalations, liver and some kidney diseases, pulmonary embolus, and other less common causes. EMS providers in high-altitude areas (between 5,000 and 7,500 feet) must consider High Altitude Pulmonary Edema (HAPE) in tourists or people who have very rapidly ascended from a low altitude to the higher altitude.

When evaluating a patient with pulmonary edema, however, remember that common things are common, and congestive heart failure is common. The most common causes of acute CHF are worsening heart failure (26%) and myocardial infarct (26%). Coronary ischemia (21%) with impaired muscle function is also very common. However, a patient can have congestive heart failure without ever having had coronary artery disease (CAD). Other causes include acute dysrythmias (9%) and valvular insufficiency (3%). Interestingly, only 7% of exacerbations can be attributed to medication noncompliance and only 3% can be attributed to dietary causes. The remaining 5% of patients develop CHF from hypertension, cardiomyopathy (heart muscle diseases), congenital heart disease, and inflammatory diseases such as myocarditis and infectious endocarditis. Patients with endocrine disease (e.g., hyperthyroidism) can also develop CHF.

The treatment of congestive heart failure relies on altering the physiology to move fluid out of the alveoli and back into the intravascular space. Patients in congestive heart failure can be classified as having either hypertensive or normotensive CHF, or hypotensive CHF. The management for these states differs in that normotensive and hypertensive patients require fluid redistribution, whereas hypotensive patients require an improvement in their cardiac function (chronotropy, inotropy, and contractility).

For the patient in extremis, aggressive airway management including endotracheal intubation is warranted. However, as will be discussed below, if the patient is not critically ill (profound hypoperfusion and shock or respiratory arrest or agonal respirations), intubation is not usually warranted because these patients' conditions can often be rapidly reversed by other interventions.

For the hypotensive patient, improvement of cardiac output is the target. These patients may be in cardiogenic shock with functional loss of greater than 40% of their myocardial mass. Although a small fluid challenge can be considered, the first-line medication will usually be dopamine. Its effects are dose dependent and cardiac chronotropy and ionotropy occur at 5–15 micrograms per kilogram per minute (mcg/kg/min) with peripheral vasoconstriction occurring at doses >15 mcg/kg/min. Typically, best results will occur in the 5–15 mcg/kg/min range where beta-mediated cardiac effects predominate. Other pressor agents to be considered include norepinephrine and dobutamine (useful if the patient is not profoundly hypotensive). It is important to recognize that patients with CHF and prehospital hypotension have a 50% mortality rate and that patient care may not get past providing for the ABCs.

For hypertensive and normotensive patients in CHF, the focus is on redistribution of fluid from the intraalveolar space to the intravascular space. This is most often accomplished in the prehospital environment with the tools of the L-M-N-O-P mnemonic. This mnemonic stands for Lasix (or any loop diuretic), morphine, nitrates, oxygen, and positive-pressure ventilatory support. These five modalities improve oxygenation and decrease the amount of pulmonary edema. *P* also stands for positioning the patient in an upright position with the legs dangling as this simple intervention can have an extraordinary effect on rapid fluid redistribution and respiratory status.

Lasix (furosemide), a loop diuretic, has two effects on the patient in CHF. Immediately after administration, it acts as a vasodilator, reducing intravascular pressure and promoting movement of fluid back into the intravascular space. This makes Lasix useful even for the CHF patient with renal failure who makes little or no urine. Within 5–10 minutes of administration, loop diuretics promote sodium and water excretion through the kidney, which decreases intravascular volume and "sucks" fluid out of the intraalveolar spaces. Critically, if Lasix is given to patients with other pulmonary pathologies (COPD, pneumonia, asthma, toxic inhalation, etc.), mortality from these conditions may be increased from 8% without Lasix to 14% with it. Therefore, it is important to reserve repeated Lasix dosing for patients in whom the diagnosis of CHF is clear. Identifying Lasix or other diuretics among the patient's prescribed medications is helpful in confirming the prehospital diagnosis of CHF. In the setting of CHF, Lasix should be administered at doses up to 1 milligram per kilogram per dose (mg/kg/dose).

Morphine works in a number of ways. By acting centrally as a sympatholytic, it reduces vascular tone and decreases preload. Other sympatholytic benefits include decreased contractility, decreased myocardial oxygen demand, decreased blood pressure, and decreased heart rate. Furthermore, morphine acts as an anxiolytic, often making the patient much calmer and able to tolerate interventions. Morphine is administered in 2–4 mg IV boluses every 3–5 minutes, titrated to effect.

Nitrates are critical in the prehospital treatment of CHF. At lower doses, nitrates are primarily venodilators and reduce preload. However, at high doses, they are also arteriodilators and reduce afterload, particularly when given intravenously. Through these mechanisms, nitrates decrease myocardial oxygen demand and improve pump function. Sublingual therapy can be initiated before an IV is established. However, it is advised to have an IV in place with repeated nitroglycerin dosing to provide small fluid boluses in the event of hypotension. The onset of action for sublingual nitroglycerin is 2 minutes, with tablets lasting 20 minutes and sprays lasting 2 hours. Typically, if patients have not become hypotensive after the first two to three doses of sublingual nitroglycerin, they will tolerate aggressive redosing every 3 to 5 minutes. It is important to monitor blood pressure after each dose. Transdermal nitroglycerin is not well absorbed in these patients since they have poor peripheral perfusion. Sublingual administration is the best route in the prehospital environment.

Oxygen is an immediate, first-line intervention for these patients. Regardless of the cause, all patients with pulmonary edema will be hypoxic. Provision of supplemental oxygen will improve systemic and myocardial hypoxia. Be aware that some patients in CHF will not be able to tolerate a nonrebreather mask. In these patients, either high-flow blow-by (a nonrebreather held off the face) or light sedation and anxiolysis with vigilant ventilatory monitoring is appropriate.

Another intervention for any CHF patient (regardless of blood pressure) is positive-pressure ventilation. Those with impending respiratory failure will benefit from ventilatory assistance. Traditionally, these patients were often intubated either nasally or under sedation in the prehospital environment. Now, it is much more common to provide positive-pressure ventilatory support, either via bag-valve-mask or through portable continuous positive airway pressure (CPAP) devices. The assisted ventilation reduces the work of breathing and oxygen demand by the respiratory muscles. Additionally, the positive pressure promotes fluid shifting from the intraalveolar spaces to the intravascular spaces. Because the pharmacological interventions listed above will often provide rapid improvement of a patient with CHF, positive-pressure ventilatory support can serve as both a treatment and a bridge to eliminate the need to intubate these patients.

RETURN TO THE CASE

As your partner prepares to provide assisted ventilations, you administer a sublingual nitroglycerin spray. You then establish an IV and repeat vitals. While your partner provides assisted BVM ventilations, you give two more doses of nitroglycerin and the 80 mg IV Lasix allowed by your protocols. At this point you have intervened with positioning, nitroglycerin, Lasix, oxygen, and the ventilatory support and your patient is already showing some improvement. You contact medical command and get orders to administer morphine sulfate 2 mg IV every 5 minutes to a maximum of 10 mg and sublingual nitroglycerine every 5 minutes if the systolic blood pressure is above 110. As you carry the patient in the stair chair down the five flights, you stop at every floor to catch your breath, check the patient's vitals, and administer a dose of morphine and nitroglycerin. By the time you load the patient in the back of the ambulance, he is less diaphoretic, more comfortable, and able to speak in full sentences. Repeat vitals show a blood pressure of 140/70, heart rate of 88, and a respiratory rate of 24 with oxygen saturation (SpO_2) of 95% on the nonrebreather. You hear bilateral crackles in the bases but the upper lungs are clear. You continue therapy and by the time you arrive at the emergency department, your patient's blood pressure is 120/60, heart rate is 76, and respiratory rate as 18 with a SpO_2 of 100% on the nonrebreather.

This patient is presented 1 month later at a run review and your medical director praises your management, telling you that you saved the patient's life. He tells you that the patient was evaluated in the ED and had a chest x-ray consistent with pulmonary edema. His initial ECG showed no ST elevation, although he had ST depression in leads V_2–V_4. Initial cardiac enzymes were negative and the ST-segment changes were resolved in the ED. The patient was admitted and serial cardiac enzymes were drawn. His second set of cardiac enzymes was positive and the patient was started on heparin and a glycoprotein IIb/IIIa inhibitor. He was taken to the cardiac catheterization lab on the third day of his admission and was found to have severe three-vessel coronary artery disease. It was decided, based on his risk factors and comorbidities, that maximizing his medical therapy rather than undergoing bypass surgery would be the best option, and he was discharged to home on day 5.

Eight months later you respond to his apartment when he suffers sudden cardiac death and cannot be resuscitated. You learn from his neighbor that in the 9 months since you last took care of the patient, he had reconciled his differences with his son and developed a relationship with his granddaughter.

REFERENCES

American Heart Association. "Hypotension/Shock/Acute Pulmonary Edema." In *Advanced Cardiac Life Support*. Dallas, TX: American Heart Association, 1997, 1–47.

Bledsoe, Bryan E., Robert S. Porter, and Richard A. Cherry. *Medical Emergencies*. Vol. 3 of *Paramedic Care: Principles & Practice*. Chapter 2, "Cardiology." Upper Saddle River, NJ: Brady/Prentice Hall Health, Pearson Education, 2001.

Grossman, S., and D. F. M. Brown. "Congestive Heart Failure and Pulmonary Edema." *eMedicine Journal* 2, no. 5 (May 16, 2001). Available at http://www.emedicine.com/emerg/topic108.htm.

Eric Ossmann, MD

11

DEHYDRATION

CASE PRESENTATION

You and your partner are providing medical coverage for the final day of a 3-day charity walk. Over the course of 3 days the participants walk approximately 40 kilometers (km) per day. The walkers are of all ages and range in fitness from conditioned athletes to the typically sedentary. The walk has been well organized with excellent support services available to the walkers. It is a beautiful September day with blue skies and a high temperature expected to be in the upper 80s. It is the end of the day and you have seen only a couple of minor problems when you receive a radio call for a "person down" near the finish line of the walk.

As you approach, you notice a large crowd gathered around a middle-aged female lying supine on the ground. As you get closer you see that the patient is talking and making intermittent purposeful movements of all extremities. Bystanders note that the patient seemed to be walking in an erratic fashion and then collapsed. She apparently was unconscious for 30 to 60 seconds before returning to a slightly confused but otherwise normal level of consciousness.

The primary survey reveals that she is speaking and her airway is open. Her respiratory rate is 28 breaths per minute and the depth of her respirations appears normal. Her radial pulse is rapid and weak in quality with an initial rate of 140 to 150 bpm. She is awake, alert, and confused about the events of the last 5 minutes. A brief secondary survey reveals no obvious trauma or extremity deformity with a grossly normal neurological examination. Her skin is warm and moist to touch with a mild flush.

A brief history reveals that prior to her syncopal episode she was feeling extremely weak and dizzy with cramping in her legs and upper extremities. She notes that she has a history of hypertension and takes hydrochlorothiazide for blood pressure control. She has no allergies and ate a light breakfast, but skipped lunch. She recalls that she has been drinking at least one glass of water at every rest stop.

As you attempt to help her to her feet she suddenly becomes very dizzy and nauseated, vomiting once. At this point you elect to place the patient on the monitor and initiate a single large-bore IV.

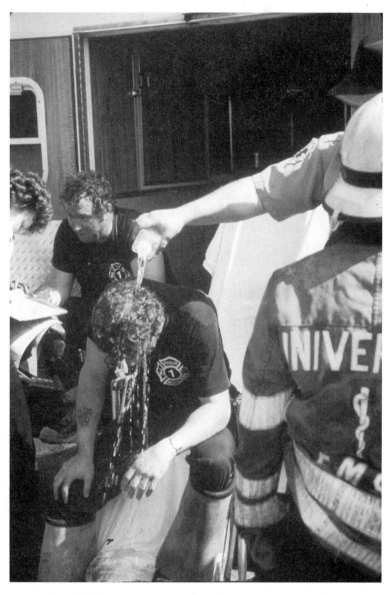

Heat stress and dehydration are common during fire suppression operations.

QUESTIONS

1. How does dehydration induce syncope and the additional symptoms experienced by this patient?
2. Are all patients with suspected heat-related illness suffering from dehydration?
3. Which crystalloid solution is most appropriate for this patient?

DISCUSSION

The body maintains normal volume and osmolarity by balancing water (solvent) and sodium (primary extracellular solute) intake with output. Dehydration occurs when the body moves from a state of euhydration to hypohydration. Dehydration can occur from diminished intake of water and sodium or from an increased loss.

Water input is derived primarily from water consumed as a liquid, with small contributions from the water content of food and water generated during the oxidation of food. The average person ingests and generates approximately 2 to 3.5 L of water per day. Water is lost from the body via four primary routes: insensible losses, sweat, feces, and urine. Insensible losses total 0.8 to 1.0 L per day and occur via expired air and evaporation through the skin. Losses from sweat vary dramatically depending on the ambient temperature, humidity, and degree of exertion. Typical losses can be as little as 0.2 to as great as 10.0 L per day. Fecal loses are usually 0.2 L per day, but can approach as much as 5.0 L in the setting of diarrheal illness. Urine loss can be strictly regulated by the body and averages 1 to 2 L per day, but can range from 0.5 to 20.0 L per day.

Sodium input is directly related to the sodium content in fluids and foods consumed, with the average adult ingesting from 100 to 400 millimole (mmol) per day. Sodium output is primarily regulated by the renal system, varying output from almost nothing to 600 mmol per day. Fecal sodium loss is normally inconsequential, but can approach 1000 mmol per day in the setting of severe diarrheal illness. Sweat losses of sodium depend on the volume of sweat and the degree of individual heat adaptation. Non–heat-adapted individuals lose more sodium via sweat than an acclimatized individual.

Commonly prescribed diuretic drugs primarily work by increasing the amount of sodium and water excreted in the urine. Hydrochlorothiazide (HCTZ) is one of the most popular antihypertensives utilized in the United States and works by inhibiting sodium and chloride reabsorption in the ascending loop of Henle and early distal tubule. This will typically produce a threefold increase in daily urine output for the average adult.

Dehydration is a pathological state that is characterized by water or sodium depletion. A patient suffering primarily from water depletion will typically have an elevated concentration of sodium in the extracellular space (hypernatremia), whereas primary sodium depletion results in a lowered concentration of sodium (hyponatremia). A detailed past medical history and history of present illness will aid in the differentiation and treatment of these subtly different entities.

Characteristic water depletion dehydration tends to occur in acclimatized individuals who are physically exerting themselves in a hot and humid environment while failing to drink an adequate amount of replacement fluids. Most individuals replace only 75% of water losses when exposed to a thermal stress. Consequently, if episodes of exertion are not interrupted by periods of rest and hydration, dehydration will occur. In an acclimatized individual the sodium concentration of the sweat is significantly lower; typically 5 milliequivalents per liter (mEq/L) versus 65 mEq/L in an individual that has not been acclimatized to the heat stress. The classic symptoms of water depletion dehydration are fatigue, weakness, nausea, profound thirst, and mental dullness. Physical signs will depend on the degree of dehydration, but include tachycardia, orthostatic hypotension, poor skin turgor, and dry mucous membranes. The treatment for water depletion dehydration is based on free water replacement. Patients that can tolerate oral fluids should be given water or an oral rehydration solution at a rate of 1 to 2 (L/hr). Individuals who are unable to tolerate oral solutions should receive IV hydration with 0.9% saline at a rate of 1 to 2 L/hr. Rapid rehydration with a hypotonic solution such as 0.45% saline or 5% dextrose should be avoided. Large amounts of hypotonic fluid can drop the extracellular sodium levels too quickly, possibly resulting in cerebral edema and seizures.

Primary sodium depletion dehydration typically occurs in a person who has a pre-existing sodium deficit or is not acclimatized. Individuals who are taking diuretics such as hydrochlorothiazide are at particular risk to develop sodium depletion dehydration. Sodium depletion dehydration can also occur with protracted periods of exertion, adequate water intake, and inadequate electrolyte or food intake. With sodium depletion dehydration, patients experience fatigue, weakness, and mental dullness but typically do not have an intense thirst and are subject to much more severe nausea and vomiting. These patients will also tend to experience significant muscle cramping. Physical signs of tachycardia, orthostatic hypotension, poor skin turgor, and dry mucous membranes are similar to patients with water depletion dehydration. Because of severe nausea and vomiting, treatment of sodium depletion dehydration will often require IV rehydration with 0.9% saline at 1 L/hr. The use of antiemetics such as compazine to treat associated nausea and vomiting is indicated when dehydration is not encountered in conjunction with heat illness. Patient with heat exhaustion and sodium depletion dehydration will usually experience relief from nausea and vomiting with repletion of sodium. The anticholinergic effect of many of the antiemetics may actually worsen heat illness by interfering with sweat production.

Dehydration is frequently encountered in conjunction with heat illness; however, both conditions can exist independently of one another. Dehydration increases basal metabolic rate leading to an elevation in body temperature. Dehydration can also be seen in isolation of heat illness when water and or sodium output exceeds input. Patients with severe diarrheal illness or those who cannot voluntarily gain access to water can suffer severe dehydration in the absence of heat illness.

RETURN TO THE CASE

After initiation of a large-bore IV, 0.9% saline is infused at a rate of 1 L/hr. The patient is placed on the cot and moved to the ambulance. She is placed on a heart monitor, which displays a normal sinus rhythm at a rate of 140. Vital signs at this point reveal a correlating pulse rate of 140 bpm and supine blood pressure of 110/80. The patient is still unable to sit up secondary to dizziness and nausea. After 500 ml of 0.9% normal saline, the patient is feeling subjectively better and her heart rate has dropped to 110 bpm. On arrival in the emergency department the patient exhibits mild orthostatic hypotension, but is feeling dramatically improved. After 1.5 L of 0.9% saline the patient's symptoms and orthostatic hypotension have completely resolved. An electrolyte panel is remarkable for a slightly low sodium level. After 2 hours in the emergency room (ER) the patient is discharged without complication.

REFERENCES

Bledsoe, Bryan E., Robert S. Porter, and Richard A. Cherry. *Medical Emergencies*. Vol. 3 of *Paramedic Care: Principles & Practice*. Chapter 10, "Environmental Emergencies." Upper Saddle River, NJ: Brady/Prentice Hall Health, Pearson Education, 2001.

Crouse, B., and K. Beattie. "Marathon Medical Services: Strategies to Reduce Runner Morbidity." *Medicine & Science in Sports & Exercise* 28, no. 9 (1996): 1093–1096.

Howard Greller, MD

12

Diabetic AMS

CASE PRESENTATION

You receive a call for an unconscious female. As you arrive at the house, the patient's father comes running from the front door. As you and your partner gather your equipment, the father tells you that his daughter has been acting strangely for the last day, and now is barely responding to him. This morning he found her in the bathtub, babbling incomprehensibly. He is concerned that she may be using drugs.

As you mount the top of the stairs, you see the patient through the bathroom door. She is a young female, in her late teens, lying fully clothed in a partially filled freestanding bathtub. She appears intoxicated. She looks pale, and has an arm and a leg hanging over the edge of the tub. The bathroom smells like ripe fruit. There is no evidence of illicit drug-related paraphernalia. There are a bottle of insulin and a syringe on the counter, which the father informs you is his (he was headed to administer his dose when he found his daughter in the bathroom). She is moaning softly, and responds slightly when her name is called loudly.

Your primary survey reveals that her airway is patent. The patient is making regular, rapid, deep respirations at a rate of approximately 30, without evidence of snoring or wheezing. Auscultation reveals equal breath sounds bilaterally. The patient's left arm (the one hanging out of the tub) is cool and dry, with a bounding radial pulse at a rate approaching 140. There are no obvious signs of external hemorrhage or other trauma.

You and your partner carefully extract the patient from the bathtub and logroll her onto a backboard. While your partner establishes a large-bore peripheral IV, you obtain the remainder of her vital signs and place her on high-flow oxygen by mask.

You perform an assessment of the patient's blood glucose using the portable glucometer. Your partner speaks with the father and obtains a SAMPLE history. He has known insulin-dependent diabetes mellitus, but the daughter has never been evaluated for this, nor does she have any other known medical history or take any medications. The father believes that she ate dinner last night, and says she ate a muffin for breakfast. Over the last day, she

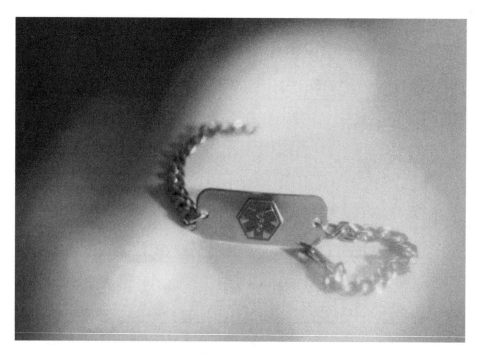

MedicAlert® bracelet commonly worn by patients with diabetes.

has been complaining of extreme thirst, and that she has been urinating very often. She also has been feeling run-down, and has been complaining of discomfort when she urinates.

You double-check the calibration of the machine. Twice the reading has returned as HI. You are concerned that this patient may be suffering from diabetic ketoacidosis (DKA).

QUESTIONS

1. What is an important evaluation that should be performed at this time?
2. What are the common causes of altered mental status in diabetic patients?
3. What other information should you gather at this time?
4. What interventions should be initiated at this point?

DISCUSSION

The primary survey is one of the most important aspects of all emergency care. It rapidly defines and directs caretakers to the important, immediate threats to life and limb. It is commonly remembered by the mnemonic A-B-C-D-E. In this case, the A (airway), B (breathing), and C (circulation) have already been assessed and addressed by the paramedics. That brings us to the D of the primary survey. The D, or disability, is a rapid assessment of the neurologic status of the patient. D can also be thought of as dextrose (sugar), to remind us of one of the more common causes of altered mental status. A common assessment of disability includes the AVPU scale (*a*lert, responds to *v*erbal stimuli, responds to *p*ainful stimuli, *u*nresponsive), which is rapidly applied to both pediatric and adult patients. Readily available in most communities, assessment of a patient's serum glucose level with rapid reagent strips or portable glucometers helps define whether or not the patient is having a problem with blood sugar.

The final component of the primary survey is *E*, or environment and exposure. Often, patients are encountered in situations where their surroundings or situation places them at risk for considerable harm from temperature, or other local factors (fire, chemical spills, animal bites or envenomations, ice, etc.). Patients near or in water, regardless of depth, are at risk for multiple problems including hyper- or hypothermia, burns, and near-drowning. In all cases, attempts should be made to remove the patient from this environment (e.g., removing the patient from the bathtub), and also remove whatever remains in contact with the patient (removing what wet clothing you can).

Altered mental status is a common presentation to EMS for patients who have diabetes mellitus. Both hypoglycemia (low blood sugar) and hyperglycemia (high blood sugar) may result in an alteration of a diabetic patient's normal mental status.

Hypoglycemia is a more common cause of altered mental status than is hyperglycemia. Hypoglycemia in diabetics is almost always caused by an imbalance of too much medication (either injected insulin or oral hypoglycemic inducing agents) and too little dietary intake of carbohydrates that provide the body with sugar. Acute hypoglycemia (sometimes referred to as "insulin shock") is normally rapid in onset and results in the classic presentation of altered mental status, ranging from confusion to complete unresponsiveness, and diaphoretic skin.

Although the presentation of a diabetic with hypoglycemia may be very dramatic, hypoglycemia is relatively easy to treat prehospital with equally dramatic results. The mainstay of treatment is the administration of exogenous simple sugar. In diabetics with only mildly altered mental status who have an intact gag reflex and can swallow, orange juice sweetened with sugar packets can be administered. In unresponsive patients, IV 50% dextrose or IM glucagon (in patients in whom an IV cannot be established) are the mainstays of treatment to return the patient's serum glucose to normal.

Hypoglycemic patients, especially insulin-dependent diabetics, will frequently refuse transport and further EMS treatment once their hypoglycemia has been reversed. Such practices are usually safe in experienced insulin-dependent diabetics, but are very problematic in patients who have taken too much oral hypoglycemic because these medications' effects can last many hours as opposed to the relatively short half-life of insulin. In such cases, follow local protocols in regard to the refusal, but always ensure that such patients immediately eat starchy foods (rich in complex carbohydrates) to help prevent recurrent hypoglycemia.

Diabetic ketoacidosis is an acute, life-threatening complication of diabetes mellitus. Although its onset is less sudden and immediately less obvious, it is a far more life-threatening condition than hypoglycemia The majority of cases occur in those with Type I or insulin-dependent diabetes mellitus, although it is also described in Type II or non-insulin-dependent diabetes mellitus. DKA occurs in approximately 25% of new onset diabetics, and is the initial presentation in many of these.

> *Water, water, everywhere,*
> *Nor any drop to drink.*
>
> —The Ancient Mariner, by Samuel Taylor Coleridge

Insulin is the key hormone responsible for the body's ability to utilize fuel. It is an anabolic (growth) hormone. It enables the body to metabolize, store, and utilize the food we eat. In diabetics, there is a relative insulin deficiency (either a lack of insulin, or a resistance to the effects of insulin). DKA is an ironic disease process: The body is being bathed in fuel (glucose) rich blood, but the organs that need that fuel (muscle, brain, etc.) can't get it or use it because the key (insulin) is lacking. Without the effects of insulin, the body is unable to utilize the circulating glucose. Thus, the above quote could be rewritten "Sugar, sugar, everywhere, nor any drop to use."

DKA is the body's response to starvation at the level of the cell. Essentially, all of the problems of DKA are related to three primary problems: hyperglycemia, dehydration, and acidosis, which in turn are all related to the relative lack of insulin.

When the body senses that it doesn't have enough glucose, it sets off a cascade of mechanisms designed to correct this. The liver begins to synthesize new glucose, as well as break down stored glycogen into useable glucose. Additionally, the liver converts free fatty acids to the ketone bodies beta-hydroxybutyric acid and acetoacetic acid, as an alternative fuel source.

The relative lack of insulin also leads to the inability of the body to utilize and store these sources of energy. This leads to hyperglycemia and ketonemia (high glucose and high ketones in the blood). The elevated glucose in the intravascular space draws water into this space. The extra fluid and osmotic load lead to a diuresis. Diuresis is an increased production of urine by the kidneys. In DKA, the kidneys are trying to get rid of the large amount of glucose in the body. In order to get rid of it, they make more urine, depleting water from the body. This diuresis leads to the initial symptoms of DKA, polyuria (production of large volumes of urine), and polydipsia (abnormally intense thirst).

The osmotic diuresis also leads to the loss of many important electrolytes including sodium, chloride, potassium, phosphorous, calcium, and magnesium. The excessive ketones (which are acids) lead to a metabolic acidosis, which is worsened by the kidney's efforts to excrete these ketones, leading to a loss of bicarbonate (a buffer for acid). The lungs are stimulated by the increasing acidosis to blow off extra carbon dioxide to help compensate. This leads to the characteristic respirations of DKA, called Kussmaul's respirations, which are rapid and deep. Acetone (a breakdown product of acetoacetic acid) gives the characteristic "fruity" odor to the breath of people with DKA.

The initial management of patients with DKA is focused on making the correct diagnosis and correcting the volume losses that patients have already sustained prior to presentation. Rapid fluid administration is the single most important intervention that can be made prehospital. IV fluid helps restore the volume lost, helps restore to normal the osmolarity of the serum, helps perfuse vital organs, and helps lower the serum glucose and ketones. Paying meticulous attention to the ABCs, as well as addressing environmental factors and other potential causes of change in mental status, is also very important.

RETURN TO THE CASE

The patient is started on a normal saline infusion, and is placed into the warm ambulance with plenty of blankets. A rhythm strip is obtained, showing sinus tachycardia. Naloxone is administered, and the patient shows no change in her clinical picture. She maintains her airway throughout the transport, and is delivered to the waiting emergency department staff.

In the emergency department, the patient is found to be in diabetic ketoacidosis, and in addition to the fluid infusion that was started, begins to receive insulin. Her initial serum glucose is found to be 561, and she has an initial serum pH of 6.99 (normal 7.35–7.45). She is also found to have a urinary tract infection, thought to be the trigger of this episode. She is admitted to the intensive care unit, where over the course of the next few days her metabolic derangements are corrected and she slowly returns to her baseline mental status. On day 7 of her hospitalization, she is transferred to a general-care floor and 1 day later, after intensive diabetic instruction and education, is discharged home on a regimen of insulin.

REFERENCES

Bledsoe, Bryan E., Robert S. Porter, and Richard A. Cherry. *Medical Emergencies*. Vol. 3 of *Paramedic Care: Principles & Practice*. Chapter 4, "Endocrinology." Upper Saddle River, NJ: Brady/Prentice Hall Health, Pearson Education, 2001.

Murphy, P., and C. Colwell. "Prehospital Management of Diabetes." *Emergency Medical Services* 29, no. 10 (October 2000): 78–85, quiz 95.

Tintinalli, J. E., G. D. Kelen, and J. S. Stapczynski. *Emergency Medicine: A Comprehensive Study Guide*. 5th ed. Dallas, TX: American College of Emergency Physicians, 2000.

Patrick Hinfey, MD
Edward T. Dickinson, MD

13

CHRONIC RENAL FAILURE

CASE PRESENTATION

You are working the Sunday night shift when you are dispatched to a house for a patient with difficulty breathing. You arrive to find an elderly woman with labored breathing sitting on the couch. A young woman standing next to the couch identifies herself as the patient's daughter. The patient is unable to speak due to difficulty breathing, but the daughter gives the history. The patient is 65 years old with a past medical history of renal failure and hypertension. She undergoes hemodialysis at a nearby facility but has missed her last two dialysis sessions because she was not feeling well. She has no allergies and her medications include extended-release nifedipine and clonidine. The patient had gone to bed at 11:00 P.M. and was feeling well but awoke at 1:00 A.M. with trouble breathing. She has no chest pain.

On initial assessment the patient is awake and alert and appears to be in severe respiratory distress with diaphoresis and accessory muscle use. Her blood pressure is 240/130, respiratory rate is 36, and heart rate is 120 and regular. Room air oxygen saturation is 91%. Physical exam reveals a patent airway, jugular-venous distention, a midline trachea, and rales in all lung fields. There is no peripheral edema. An arteriovenous (AV) fistula is present in her right arm and a palpable thrill is present.

You administer oxygen by nonrebreather mask and her oxygen saturation rises to 97%. The cardiac monitor reveals a narrow complex tachycardia with slightly peaked T waves. As your partner searches her left arm for a suitable IV site, the daughter comments that IV access is always difficult in her mother.

QUESTIONS

1. What are some of the common complications encountered by paramedics in patients who are on dialysis?
2. What is the best way to treat this patient's respiratory distress, and does it differ from the treatment of pulmonary edema in a nondialysis patient?

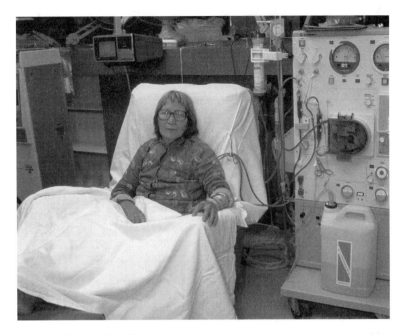

Patient undergoing hemodialysis.
Courtesy of David Young-Wolff and PhotoEdit.

DISCUSSION

Patients in chronic renal failure who are on dialysis can present unique assessment and treatment challenges to paramedics. Many diseases result in chronic renal failure that eventually leads to the loss of kidney function. Uncontrolled and untreated hypertension is the most common cause of chronic renal failure, also referred to as end-stage renal disease (ESRD). Other causes include diabetes, and autoimmune and hereditary diseases. Although patients with progressive renal failure are initially treated with medications and diet modification, eventually they often require being placed on intermittent dialysis as the kidneys can no longer provide adequate filtration of the blood.

There are two types of dialysis: hemodialysis (HD) and peritoneal dialysis (PD). Patients on HD have their blood filtered by having their blood stream accessed via a dialysis catheter placed in a central vein or by a surgically created subcutaneous AV fistula on an extremity. Once the circulation is accessed, the patient is placed on a dialysis machine that circulates the blood through filters. The dialysis machine not only filters the blood but also removes excessive water. Patients on PD use large volumes of dialysis fluid placed in the peritoneal cavity through an implanted catheter as a means of filtering their blood volume. Once the fluid is instilled in the peritoneal cavity it is left in place for an extended period and then subsequently trained by gravity. Unlike HD that is done exclusively in hospitals and outpatient dialysis centers by trained personnel, PD is done by the patients themselves at home.

Patients on dialysis are prone to certain medical emergencies for which advanced life support (ALS) may be called. Most of these conditions are common both to HD and PD patients. However, certain emergencies are unique to the type of dialysis the patient uses.

PROBLEMS COMMON TO DIALYSIS PATIENTS IN GENERAL

Hyperkalemia (high serum potassium)—One of the crucial balances that the kidneys are responsible for is the regulation and excretion of electrolytes. Patients with ESRD will develop hyperkalemia if they miss their dialysis treatments. This can result in cardiac arrhythmias and even sudden death. On the EKG, hyperkalemia may produce peaked T waves or widened QRS complexes. Prehospital treatment includes the administration of intravenous sodium bicarbonate and intravenous calcium chloride. Many clinicians automatically administer both empirically at the outset of cardiac arrest management of dialysis patients under the presumption that hyperkalemia was the cause of the arrest.

Fluid Overload—In addition to the filtration of waste products from the blood, the kidneys also excrete excessive water from the body. Patients who miss dialysis treatments will accumulate bodywide fluid. Pulmonary edema is frequently encountered in these patients.

Because many ESRD patients have both hypertension and chronic congestive heart failure as well, missed dialysis (especially missed HD) can be a trigger to life-threatening CHF/pulmonary edema as has occurred in the patient in this case study.

PROBLEMS ASSOCIATED WITH HEMODIALYSIS PATIENTS

Bleeding from the Fistula Site—Patients receive heparin during dialysis and severe bleeding can occur from the site on the fistula where the dialysis needle was inserted. This bleeding can be life threatening since the fistula is directly connected to the radial artery or other artery. The bleeding is controlled by standard measures of direct pressure, elevation, and so on.

Infection at the Fistula Site—These patients may exhibit redness and tenderness of the skin over the fistula site, or may have altered mental status and shock if the infection has resulted in bacteremia (bacteria in the blood) and sepsis. The prehospital care is supportive measures.

Hypotension after Dialysis—Because HD dialysis removes pounds of water from the patient's body, it is possible that too much fluid is removed during dialysis resulting in hypovolemia and hypotension. Postdialysis hypotension is treated with boluses of IV normal saline.

PROBLEMS ASSOCIATED WITH PERITONEAL DIALYSIS PATIENTS

Peritonitis—Bacteria may contaminate the catheter or the fluid within the peritoneal space of the abdomen. This can result in infection of the peritoneal space known as peritonitis. PD patients with peritonitis will complain of abdominal pain and generally report that the PD fluid they have withdrawn has become cloudy in color rather than the usual clear color. On physical examination these patients will usually have a tender abdomen to palpation.

The patient appears to have acute cardiogenic pulmonary edema. This condition has multiple etiologies, but the final result is movement of fluid from the pulmonary capillary to the alveolar space in the lungs. In cases of pulmonary edema in ESRD patients, fluid overload is often more severe as the kidneys have lost the ability to diurese excessive fluid in the body, further increasing preload on the heart.

The major problem in cardiogenic pulmonary edema is that the heart is unable to pump enough blood in a forward direction, such that pressure backs up into the pulmonary circulation and causes fluid to move into the alveoli. Treatment must be aimed at decreasing preload or afterload, increasing contractility, or restoring a normal rhythm to the heart.

Treatment of pulmonary edema begins with ensuring a patent airway. Most patients with pulmonary edema do not require endotracheal intubation as long as treatment is timely. Intubation should be considered for patients who are unable to maintain adequate oxygenation despite supplemental oxygen, who develop lethargy, or whose pulse or respiratory rate decline in the absence of clinical improvement.

Next, breathing and circulation must be addressed. It is critical to ensure that patients with pulmonary edema are adequately oxygenated and ventilated. All patients with pulmonary edema should be treated initially with high-flow oxygen by nonrebreather mask. Patients with pulmonary edema have increased work of breathing and without treatment will tire of breathing and suffer respiratory arrest. One method to assist patients in breathing is the use of noninvasive ventilation. Noninvasive ventilation has been used in hospitals for the treatment of pulmonary edema and appears to decrease the need for endotracheal intubation and intensive care unit admission. Two forms of noninvasive ventilation are in common use: continuous positive airway pressure (CPAP), and bi-level positive airway pressure (Bi-PAP). Assisted ventilation with a bag-valve-mask device is essentially a manual way of delivering CPAP ventilation, and is readily available and familiar to paramedics. In some ALS systems CPAP is being used in the prehospital setting.

Treatment of the cause of the pulmonary edema will address the breathing and circulation, and several agents are typically available to paramedics. Nitroglycerin is the first-line agent for the treatment of pulmonary edema. Nitroglycerin causes smooth muscle in the walls of arteries and veins to relax, leading to vasodilation. This results in decreased preload and afterload. At doses typically used, nitroglycerin causes much less dilation of arteries than of veins, hence, it decreases preload much more than afterload. Nitroglycerin can be given sublingually, transdermally, and intravenously. In the prehospital environment, the sublingual and transdermal routes are advantageous because patients with pulmonary edema can be rapidly treated even if vascular access is difficult or impossible. This is especially true in ESRD patients on HD. The typical dose is 0.4 mg of nitroglycerin sublingually by spray or tablet. The dose should be repeated every 3 to 5 minutes as long as hypertension or respiratory distress remain.

Furosemide has been used for years in the treatment of pulmonary edema. A diuretic, furosemide has two actions that are beneficial in patients with pulmonary edema. First, furosemide causes venodilation and reduces preload. This effect occurs within 5 minutes of administration. Second, furosemide decreases fluid reabsorption by the kidney and causes a decrease in total body fluid volume by increased urine excretion, a process that takes approximately 30 minutes. Edematous patients benefit from the diuretic effects that occur later, but even patients with renal failure (who produce no urine) benefit from furosemide due to the initial preload reduction. Note that the preload reduction from nitroglycerin is greater than that from furosemide, thus furosemide should be used after nitroglycerin. A typical dose for furosemide is 1 mg/kg, slow IV push.

Morphine sulfate is another drug used extensively in the treatment of pulmonary edema. It, too, works primarily by reducing preload via release of histamine from mast cells. The histamine causes vasodilation mainly in veins. Morphine has been studied in the treatment of pulmonary edema in a prehospital environment and it was found that patients given morphine did worse than patients not given morphine. Morphine doses typically used in the treatment of pulmonary edema are 2 to 4 mg IV. Both nitroglycerin and furosemide are more potent preload reducers than morphine. Morphine is a third-line agent for the treatment of pulmonary edema.

In the case above, IV access was noted to be difficult. Patients with renal failure who receive hemodialysis may have an indwelling catheter or a surgically created AV fistula. This fistula is typically placed in the arm. The function of the fistula can be checked by palpation of a thrill or auscultation of a bruit at the site. Because the fistula is used for life-sustaining dialysis treatments, the arm with the fistula should never be used for routine IV access or blood pressure measurements. Percutaneous dialysis catheters should also not be used for routine vascular access. Alternate treatment routes, such as the sublingual route, or alternate IV sites, such as the external jugular vein, should be chosen. Patients with pulmonary edema often have jugular venous distension, making it much easier than normal to access the external jugular vein. In situations where cardiac arrest is imminent or present, obtain IV access by the most expedient route.

RETURN TO THE CASE

The patient receives 3 doses of nitroglycerin en route to the hospital. Per protocol, vascular access is obtained with an 18-gauge catheter placed in the right external jugular vein. Furosemide, 70 mg, is given intravenously. The patient is improved somewhat by the time she is transferred to an ED stretcher. She is started on a nitroglycerin infusion and noninvasive ventilation by CPAP is initiated. After 30 minutes, she is markedly improved and is weaned off CPAP. She undergoes hemodialysis later in the morning and is discharged to home afterward. Her medications are adjusted and she experiences no recurrences over the next year.

REFERENCES

Bledsoe, Bryan E., Robert S. Porter, and Richard A. Cherry. *Essentials of Paramedic Care*. Upper Saddle River, NJ: Prentice Hall, 2003.

Bledsoe, Bryan E., Robert S. Porter, and Richard A. Cherry. *Medical Emergencies*. Vol. 3 of *Paramedic Care: Principles & Practice*. Chapter 7, "Urology and Nephrology." Upper Saddle River, NJ: Brady/Prentice Hall Health, Pearson Education, 2001.

Maloney, G., H. Wehrum, and W. Fraser. "Kidney Complications." *Journal of Emergency Medical Services* (July 2000): 51–66.

Richard Levitan, MD

14

DIFFICULT INTUBATION

CASE PRESENTATION

You and your partner have responded to a cardiac arrest call involving a 40-year-old morbidly obese woman who collapsed at her home. Family members had called 911 and two police officers were the first responders on the scene. An automated external defibrillator (AED) has been applied but the patient was found to be asystolic and CPR was initiated. The patient lies supine on the floor and is confirmed to be asystolic.

As the police officers continue to do compressions, your partner initiates mask ventilation while you prepare for intubation. It is very difficult to ventilate the patient even after a properly sized oral airway has been inserted. Your partner states the patient has full dentition and a large tongue relative to the size of her mouth. When you attempt to insert the laryngoscope the handle of the laryngoscope bangs into the patient's chest wall. By turning the handle toward the patient's right shoulder you are able to insert the laryngoscope blade, but neither the epiglottis nor any laryngeal structures can be visualized.

QUESTIONS

1. What anatomic features contribute to difficult ventilation and difficult intubation?
2. What techniques can be used to effectively ventilate and intubate patients with difficult airways?

DISCUSSION

Creating an effective mask seal for ventilation can be more difficult by lack of teeth, the presence of facial hair, and numerous other problems (e.g., burns, wounds, vomit, etc.). Ventilation can be impeded by any problem affecting the soft tissues of the upper airway.

Obesity and a large tongue-to-pharynx ratio contribute to obstructive sleep apnea, a condition where patients have trouble maintaining a patent airway during sleep. This also makes mask ventilation challenging. The facial soft tissues and hypopharyngeal tissues can collapse and occlude the airway even if an oral airway is properly placed.

Effective mask ventilation is best achieved by a combination of three things: a correctly placed oral airway, proper patient positioning, and elevation of the mandible and submandibular tissues. The oral airway should fit around the curvature of the tongue and not push the tongue downward. It is best inserted either following the curvature of the tongue or with use of a tongue blade or laryngoscope blade. The historical practice of inserting it upside down and rotating it can cause trauma to the palate and does not necessarily ensure proper placement. To appreciate the patient positioning that maximizes effective ventilation it is helpful to envision how they position themselves when faced with respiratory distress. This involves sitting upright and leaning forward. Sitting upright improves the mechanics of the lungs and diaphragm, and leaning the head forward (i.e., flexing the neck) maximizes the dimensions of the upper airway. Unless contraindicated by cervical spine precautions, the ideal position for mask ventilation is with the head elevated so that the neck is flexed. Exaggerated atlanto-occipital extension, or cranking the head backward, increases the difficulty of ventilation because it pushes the tongue and soft tissues of the hypopharynx backward onto the pharyngeal wall. The amount of head elevation necessary to provide effective ventilation varies depending upon body habitus, although a rough guide is that the head and shoulders should be elevated until the ear canal is at the level of the sternum. For a thin person a few inches of head elevation may achieve proper alignment, whereas a morbidly obese patient may require several feet of head elevation to create proper alignment.

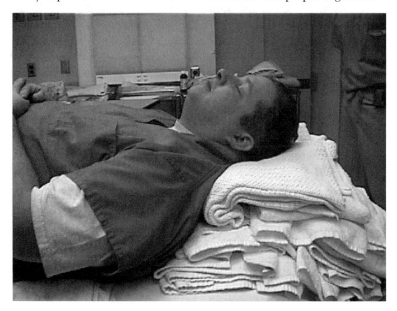

Optimal positioning of the patient is crucial to overcoming the challenges of a potentially difficult intubation.
Courtesy of Richard Levitan, MD.

The same position that facilitates ventilation is also the optimal position for laryngoscopy. It is important to remember during laryngoscopy that head elevation (i.e., more neck flexion relative to the chest) improves laryngeal view. It is a mistake to attempt increasing atlanto-occipital extension of the neck as a means to improve laryngeal view. This maneuver drives the tissues of the tongue and mandible into and against the laryngoscope blade. By lifting the head further (i.e., flexing the neck on the chest) it becomes easier to distract the mandible and submandibular tissues, improving laryngeal exposure. Such maneuvers, however, cannot be used in cases of cervical spine immobilization with in-line stabilization.

Obstruction of the upper airway during cardiac arrest and unconsciousness is due to collapse of the soft tissues of the hypopharynx and epiglottis as well as the tongue. For this reason, placement of an oral airway may not always result in a patent airway and easy mask ventilation. Elevating the mandible and soft tissues beneath the mandible are an important aspect of mask ventilation. The top of the mask should be firmly pressed downward onto the bridge of the nose, but the lower portion of the mask should be held tightly to the face and not in a manner that causes the mandible and lower face to be pushed downward. This is best achieved by using an "E-C" grip, where the center of the mask fits within the "C" created by the thumb and first finger, and the "E" represents the third, fourth, and fifth digits that hold the lower mask to the face and at the same time lift upward at the angle of the mandible. If an assistant is available to help, he or she can elevate the mandible directly or provide a jaw thrust maneuver. When difficulty is encountered with mask ventilation, forceful compression of the bag will likely cause gastric distention. Efforts instead should be directed at improving patency of the upper airway by repositioning the head, mandible, and oral airway. The American Heart Association ACLS 2001 guidelines recommend lower volumes (6–7 cubic centimeters per kilogram [cc/kg]) and slower inflation times (1–2 seconds) to decrease the risk of aspiration, while at the same time providing adequate oxygenation.

Anatomic features that make laryngoscopy difficult can be broken down into the four Ds: disproportion, distortion, dentition, and dysmobility.

Common examples of disproportion include morbid obesity, patients with a short, thick neck, and those with a short distance between the thyroid cartilage and the chin. This space, also called the displacement space, is where the tongue is pushed during laryngoscopy. A short thyromental distance (the distance between the superior part of the thyroid cartilage and the inferior surface of the anterior mandible) is less than three finger breadths wide. This is frequently referred to as an *anterior larynx*, although this is a misnomer because the larynx is not truly anterior, rather the mandible is less prominent.

A large tongue-to-pharynx ratio also makes laryngoscopy difficult. This is referred to as the Mallampati score, named after the anesthesiologist who devised a scoring system based upon the visibility of pharyngeal structures when patients maximally open their mouths and protrude their tongues. Practically speaking, patients in emergency settings who are being intubated rarely can cooperate to achieve proper Mallampati grading. The details of the score are less important than an awareness of the concept. Macroglossia, or an enlarged tongue, can be due to pathologic processes, but it is also common among certain groups of patients, such as those with Down's syndrome.

Distortion of the tongue, mandible, or upper aerodigestive tract can make laryngoscopy difficult by obstructing or obscuring landmarks, and by making the mandible and tongue more difficult to control. Examples include massive lower facial trauma, angioedema (swelling of the tongue due to an allergic response), or abscesses in the floor of the mouth (Ludwig's angina). Less commonly seen emergency situations are neoplasms (cancers) affecting the tongue and larynx.

Direct trauma to the larynx and trachea can cause distortion of structures, even though visualization of the vocal cords may be possible. Laryngeal fractures or tracheal injuries can create false passages or laryngotracheal disruption. In such situations a tracheal tube may pass through the vocal cords but not into the trachea. These injuries are categorized by wounds to the neck, subcutaneous emphysema, stridor, and hemoptysis.

Dentition can make laryngoscopy difficult by restricting visualization and by restricting manipulation of the laryngoscope. Specifically, a full set of prominent upper teeth may restrict the view. When there are large gaps in the upper teeth this can catch the flange of a Macintosh blade, causing difficulty in sweeping the tongue to the left. If patients have false teeth they should always be removed for laryngoscopy. In general, no teeth means "no problem" when it comes to laryngoscopy, although lack of teeth may make establishing a face seal for mask ventilation more difficult.

There are three regions of mobility relevant to laryngoscopy: the temporomandibular joint (opening the mouth), neck flexion (lifting the head upward), and atlanto-occipital extension (tilting the head backward). Processes that encumber these movements can make laryngoscopy more challenging. This is most commonly encountered with cervical spine precautions. Arthritis of the neck, marked cervical kyphosis, and other processes that affect the cervical vertebrae can severely limit neck mobility. Fractures of the mandible involving the temporomandibular joint can mechanically prevent mouth opening, and wire fixation of the mandible (used to treat mandible fractures) prevents mouth opening.

A cervical collar when tightly applied prevents mouth opening as well as limiting neck flexion and atlanto-occipital extension. For this reason the front of a cervical collar should always be removed prior to laryngoscopy to allow for distraction of the mandible and effective mouth opening. Laryngoscopy should be done gently with in-line stabilization and avoidance of neck flexion or atlanto-occipital extension in patients with suspected cervical spine injuries.

Given this patient's body habitus, large tongue, and small mouth, it is not surprising she is both difficult to ventilate and intubate. Proper positioning, namely massive support of the head and shoulders, is critical for both procedures.

Successfully intubating this patient also requires strict attention to the details of laryngoscopy. The redundant tissue of her upper airway, large tongue, and small mouth mandate a careful progressive exposure of landmarks. On a manikin, plunging the laryngoscope blade fully into the mouth and then slowly withdrawing often works well to expose the larynx. This technique should never be done on real patients. It can easily traumatize the upper airway and cause perforation of the posterior pharyngeal wall and hypopharynx. Additionally, it is very easy to become lost in the "pink mush" of the upper airway and esophagus, especially in this type of patient. Because the epiglottis is reliably located at the base of the tongue, it should become visible by progressively marching down the tongue as the curved blade is rotated down into position. Occasionally the epiglottis sits on the posterior pharyngeal wall and its edge cannot be seen distinctly. If the blade tip is gently directed downward (i.e., pushing the mandible downward) as it is inserted over the tongue, the epiglottis will be lifted upward off the posterior pharyngeal wall and allow for its proper visualization. Following introduction of the curved blade on the right side of the mouth, the blade should be directed slightly leftward. This permits the large flange of the curved blade to direct the tongue to the left side of the mouth, opening up the right aspect of the mouth for laryngeal visualization and tube placement.

A long, curved blade will sometimes allow the laryngoscopist to directly lift the epiglottis, but the curved blade is designed to indirectly lift the epiglottis. This is done by pressure on the hyoepiglottic ligament, beneath the valecutla where the base of the epiglottis and the tongue meet. Pressure on the hyoepiglottic ligament is created by directing the handle of the laryngoscope in a 45-degree vector, not by cranking backward and upward. Cranking backward on the laryngoscope can cause injury to the upper teeth, in addition to causing the tip to slip out of proper position.

A simple means of properly seating the curved blade tip into the valecutla is by using bimanual laryngoscopy and external laryngeal manipulation. This is done by the operator, using the right hand to press externally on the thyroid cartilage while the left hand holds the laryngoscope. This technique causes the tip of the curved blade to wedge into proper position at the valecutla. External laryngeal manipulation also improves laryngeal view because the vocal cords are attached anteriorly at the thyroid cartilage, and by directing the larynx backward it improves the line of sight from the operator to the target. After laryngeal view has been optimized, an assistant can take over external laryngeal manipulation (ELM) at the same location, freeing the operator's right hand to place the tracheal tube.

ELM is distinct from cricoid pressure and also distinct from backward upper rightward pressure (BURP). Cricoid pressure is done not to improve laryngeal view but to prevent gastric distention during ventilation and also regurgitation during laryngoscopy. BURP is manipulation of the thyroid cartilage by an assistant, moving the thyroid cartilage in specific direction and amounts. ELM, by contrast, allows the operator to fine tune the movements of the right hand on the neck with direct visualization of the resultant laryngeal view. Theoretically, there is a risk that release of cricoid pressure, in order to perform ELM, will permit regurgitation. By improving laryngeal view, and permitting first-pass success with intubation, ELM may avoid the need for repeat episodes of bagging which carries a definite risk for gastric distention and subsequent aspiration. It is recommended that laryngoscopy always be done with cricoid pressure initially, and then, if the view is inadequate, to employ operator directed ELM with release of cricoid pressure under direct view and with suction immediately available.

It is important to note that in some cases only the posterior aspect of the larynx may be visualized. The landmarks of the posterior cartilages and the interarytenoid notch are critical to recognize when the true vocal cords cannot be seen. Frequently the vocal cords and glottic opening are dark or completely shadowed because the epiglottis hangs down between the light source on a curved blade and the inner aspect of the larynx. The interarytenoid notch is of particular significance because it serves as the divide between the larynx and esophagus. It is the most posterior and inferior aspect of the laryngeal inlet, a ring of structures that surround the entrance of the larynx. Superiorly, this is defined by the epiglottis. The paired aryepiglottic folds come down from the epiglottis on each side, to the posterior cartilages on each side. The interarytenoid notch is between the paired posterior cartilages. Above, or anterior, to the interarytenoid notch during laryngoscopy is the entrance into the larynx and the glottic opening. Beneath, or posterior, to the interarytenoid notch is the esophagus.

It is the author's practice to reserve use of a straight blade for situations when intubation cannot be achieved using a large curved blade, proper patient positioning, and external laryngeal manipulation. Straight blades generally have a smaller flange, and because they do not have a natural fit with the tongue they are generally more challenging to hold in position. The smaller flange, particularly of the Miller blade, makes control of the tongue much more difficult and creates a very small working area for tube placement. Because of its smaller flange the straight blade requires a different technique than the curved blade. It should not be used to try to sweep the tongue to the left, but instead it should be placed in a paraglossal manner, staying fully to the right side of the tongue. Progressive visualization of landmarks, namely finding the epiglottis first before trying to expose the larynx, is critical. After the epiglottis is seen the blade is directed very slightly posteriorly and advanced a centimeter or two to directly lift the epiglottis. At this point the tip of the straight blade is directed at the posterior wall of the hypopharynx. This is an area particularly vulnerable to perforation and trauma if care is not used to gently advance the blade. If adequate laryngeal visualization is not achieved after elevating the epiglottis directly, ELM can be tried to bring the larynx into better alignment. Additionally, the patient's head can be elevated further, which will lessen the force of the tongue against the blade and allow better laryngeal exposure with less force.

Once the target is exposed, it is often difficult to place the tracheal tube within the narrow working area created by the small flange of the Miller blade. The trick is not to try to pass the tube down the barrel of the blade. A standard 7.0 or 8.0 mm tracheal tube will not fit down the barrel, and if attempted will completely obscure the view of the target. Instead, the styletted tracheal tube should be directed beneath the tongue and should come at the larynx from below, keeping the lumen of the blade open to permit observation.

Whether using straight or curved blade, successful placement of the tracheal tube will be greatly facilitated by correctly shaping the tracheal tube and stylet. The tube (and stylet) should be perfectly straight down from the back end of the tube to the cuff and then should bend upward at an angle of approximately 45–60 degrees. This creates a narrow profile to the tube when viewed down its long axis. If the tube is given a broad gentle arc, the midsection of the tube will block the operator's line of sight during placement. By creating a narrower profile, up-down and side-to-side maneuverability with the mouth is dramatically increased. If only the epiglottis edge is seen, the tube tip can be rotated under the epiglottis edge and advanced blindly toward the larynx. The sharp upturned distal bend will help direct the tube tip into the larynx.

RETURN TO THE CASE

With the assistance of the police officers, blankets and towels are wedged under the patient's head and neck. Two-person mask ventilation is achieved with use of an oral airway and upward force on the mandible and submandibular tissues. Laryngoscopy using external laryngeal manipulation permits visualization of posterior structures only. Despite the fact that neither the glottic opening nor vocal cords are seen, you are able to place the tube having carefully shaped the stylet and watching the tube tip pass anterior to (above) the interarytenoid notch. Proper tube placement is then confirmed by a colorimetric end-tidal CO_2 detector and the presence of bilateral breath sounds. Following intubation and ACLS medications down the tube, the patient regains pulses. Though she does not survive to hospital discharge, the family consents to organ donation and they subsequently express their appreciation for your efforts.

REFERENCES

Bledsoe, Bryan E., Robert S. Porter, and Richard A. Cherry. *Introduction to Advanced Prehospital Care*. Vol. 1 of *Paramedic Care: Principles & Practice*. Chapter 13, "Airway Management and Ventilation." Upper Saddle River, NJ: Brady/Prentice Hall Health, Pearson Education, 2000.

Levitan, R. M. "Rescuing Intubation: Simple Techniques to Improve Airway Visualization." *Journal of Emergency Medical Services* 26 (2001): 37–54.

Levitan, R. M., and A. E. Ochroch. "Airway Management and Direct Laryngoscopy: A Review and Update. *Critical Care Clinics of North America*, 16 (2000): 373–388.

Edward T. Dickinson, MD

15

FACILITATED INTUBATION

CASE PRESENTATION

You are working a stand-by detail at a steeplechase horse race. You watch as one of the horses stumbles and falls during a landing, rolling on top of its rider. The mishap is within walking distance of where you are standing. You and your partner ensure that all the other horses have completed the jump, await the OK from the steward, and slide under the rail onto the track.

As you approach the patient, your initial impression is that she is a female in her 20s who is severely injured as evidenced by cyanosis of the face, a stream of blood coming out of her left nostril, and a fixed gaze to the left.

The primary survey reveals her airway is tenuous with snoring respirations through tightly clenched teeth. A jaw thrust minimally reduces the snoring, but her teeth remain clenched. Her breathing is irregular and shallow at a rate of 6 to 8, and there are decreased breath sounds on the right. Your paramedic partner begins to ventilate the patient with a BVM. There is a palpable radial pulse present with no signs of significant external bleeding.

You radio your dispatch center and request a medical helicopter to the scene. An ETA of 12 minutes is advised.

You have been on the scene 2 minutes as the second paramedic crew onboard the ambulance arrives at the patient. While your partner continues to bag the patient you and the two other paramedics apply a collar, logroll the patient onto a backboard, and establish a large-bore IV.

The ETA of the helicopter is now 9 minutes. You know that the patient's airway must be secured prior to flight.

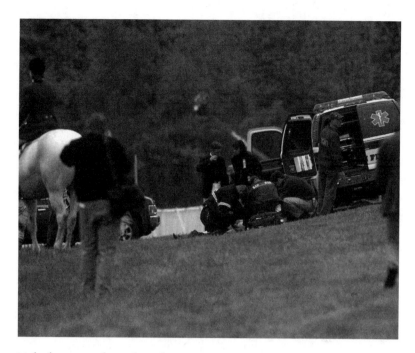

Medical team attends to a downed equestrian.
Courtesy of Pete Bannan/Main Line Life.

QUESTIONS

1. What are the various options available to the paramedic to secure the airway of a conscious or unconscious patient with clenched teeth?
2. How will you control and secure this patient's airway?

DISCUSSION

Control of a patient's airway is the most important component of emergency care. *Airway* is the "A" of the ABCs taught at all levels of care. No matter what other interventions you provide, without an open and patent airway the patient will die. Without an adequate airway the patient will eventually become hypoxic and hypercarbic leading to anaerobic metabolism, acidosis, and cellular death.

In the vast majority of patients treated by EMS the airway is not an issue per se. Most patients are awake and alert with an open, unobstructed airway. On the other extreme are patients in cardiac arrest who are in immediate need of endotracheal intubation. Yet, even in the arrested patient, airway control by direct oral laryngoscopy and endotracheal intubation is a relatively simple task because the patient is flaccid. The patient in this case study has neither an open unobstructed airway nor is she flaccid as to permit simple oral endotracheal intubation. Yet, it is clear that this patient requires intubation both for airway control and because prehospital intubation results in improved long-term neurological outcome in head-injured patients.

The definitive airway is the placement of a cuffed (uncuffed in children less than 8 years of age) endotracheal tube in the trachea inferior to the vocal cords. There are three routes to the trachea: oral, nasal, and percutaneously through the skin overlying the anterior neck. No matter what route is used to secure the airway, tube placement must be confirmed not only by the presence of breath sounds and the absence of epigastric sounds but also by an objective measure such as end-tidal CO_2 or esophageal aspiration device.

Nasal intubation is an important advanced airway skill for paramedics. Nasal tracheal intubation has become less commonly performed in emergency medicine in recent years with the increased availability of rapidly acting drugs to facilitate oral intubation. Indeed, the procedure is now far more common prehospital than in the ER or other hospital settings.

Nasal intubation has been traditionally discouraged in the setting of head and maxillofacial trauma due to the perceived risk of the endotracheal tube passing through fractures into the sinuses or even the cranial vault. The reality is that there is little in the medical literature to support this relative contraindication to the procedure and for many patients with severe head and facial injuries, nasal intubation by paramedics has been life-saving. Because of the midface trauma and the fact that the paramedics in this scenario are credentialed and trained in the use of drugs to facilitate oral intubation, the nasal route would not be the first-line approach to control this patient's airway.

Standard oral tracheal intubation is not an immediate option in this patient as her teeth are tightly clenched. The use of pharmacologic agents to relax the patient, unclenching the teeth and allowing direct oral visualization of the vocal cords to facilitate intubation is a viable option in this patient. Indeed, in EMS systems where pharmacologically assisted intubation is approved, it would represent the method of choice for the control of the airway in the patient described in this case. There are two general classes of drugs used in "facilitated intubation." There are *induction agents* that render the patient transiently unconscious and *paralytic agents* that prevent the patient from using skeletal muscles. Numerous studies have demonstrated that the use of induction agents alone or the combination of induction and paralytic drugs are safe and effective in facilitating endotracheal intubation in conscious and semiconscious patients.

The induction agents most often used in EMS and emergency medicine include midazolam, a benzodiazepine, and Etomidate, a nonbarbiturate, nonbenzodiazepine hypnotic. As induction agents, these drugs render the patient unconscious and neurologically "relaxed." Both drugs appear safe for prehospital use, but transient hypotension has been reported when higher doses of midazolam have been used for intubation. Many EMS systems utilize induction agents alone to facilitate oral intubation. When induction agents are used alone (without paralytic agents) there is reported to be an approximate 85% success rate to accomplish intubation of patients who could not have been otherwise intubated.

When an induction agent is followed by a paralytic agent that renders the unconscious patient skeletally paralyzed, the procedure is considered a full "rapid sequence intubation" (RSI). The most commonly used paralytic agent in out-of-hospital use is succinylcholine. Succinylcholine is a rapid onset paralytic agent that depolarizes the body's muscle endplates prior to paralysis. This depolarizing results in the characteristic bodywide fasciculations or muscle twitching associated with the onset of paralysis. There are other nondepolarizing paralytic agents that can be used in RSI. Nondepolarizing agents including vecuronium do not cause the patient to fasciculate prior to paralysis. Fasciculation is to be avoided in some patients because it results in transient increases in intracranial and intraocular pressures. The fasciculations associated with the onset of succinylcholine paralysis can be attenuated by the use of small "priming" doses of either succinylcholine or a nondepolarizing agent like vecuronium given about a minute prior to the full dose of succinylcholine. In addition, succinylcholine is usually avoided in patients with high serum potassium levels (such as renal dialysis patients) because it may further raise the serum potassium resulting in cardiac arrhythmias.

Some EMS systems that have induction and paralytic agents available utilize a "step RSI" where the paramedic is taught to evaluate the ability to orally intubate the patient after the induction agent and then intubate the patient. If the patient is not ready, then the paramedic gives the paralytic agent to render the patient completely flaccid.

Once intubated by an induction agent alone or RSI, patients may require additional doses of drugs to maintain the paralysis or achieve adequate sedation. Because its paralytic effects last only a few minutes, patients who were RSI'd with succinylcholine should be reparalyzed with a longer acting agent, most commonly vecuronium. Similarly, because the half-life of Etomidate is very short, and it offers no persistent sedation or amnestic effects, a dose of a benzodiazepine such as midazolam is indicated.

If all other methods of intubation fail, and the patient has an inadequate and unmaintainable airway, then the patient will require a cricothyrotomy. A cricothyrotomy can be accomplished using a variety of commercially available and makeshift devices. Although some EMS systems prefer the use of small catheter cricothyrotomy with transtracheal jet insufflation, many progressive EMS systems have moved to larger lumen tubes that can be ventilated with a standard bag-valve device. Cricothyrotomy should be considered as a final step in a failed airway algorithm only when the patient can neither be successfully intubated nor effectively ventilated.

RETURN TO THE CASE

While your partner continues BVM ventilations, you place the patient on a cardiac monitor and pulse ox. You then apply anterior cricoid pressure (the Sellick maneuver) and cervical stabilization while the patient is given a sequence of paralytic agents (Etomidate, 15 mg), a defasciculating dose of vecuronium (1 mg), and then succinylcholine (120 mg) by the third paramedic. Once the patient is flaccid, the paramedic who had been providing BVM ventilations performs direct laryngoscopy and is able to pass a 7.5 mm endotracheal tube through the vocal cords. Tube placement is confirmed by direct visualization, a colorimetric end-tidal monitor, and by the presence of bilateral breath sounds. Once the tube is secured by a commercially available Velcro and vise devise, the patient receives an additional paralytic dose of vecuronium (8 mg) and a dose of midazolam (2 mg). The patient is then transitioned to the arriving flight crew with a verbal report of the medications used in the RSI.

The patient is then flown to the regional trauma center. During her initial resuscitation a chest x-ray reveals multiple rib fractures and a 20% pneumothorax on the right, which is treated by the placement of a right chest tube. An unenhanced CT scan of the patient's brain reveals a small left frontal subdural hematoma that is managed conservatively by neurosurgery and gradually resolved without operative intervention. The patient is extubated on the third day after admission and the chest tube is removed the following day. Eventually the patient is discharged to a rehabilitation facility specializing in head-injured patients. One year later, she is once again riding, with rare episodes of double vision as her only persistent symptom.

REFERENCES

Bledsoe, Bryan E., Robert S. Porter, and Richard A. Cherry. *Introduction to Advanced Prehospital Care*. Vol. 1 of *Paramedic Care: Principles & Practice*. Chapter 13, "Airway Management and Ventilation." Upper Saddle River, NJ: Brady/Prentice Hall Health, Pearson Education, 2000.

Dickinson, E. T., J. E. Cohen, and C. C. Mechem. "The Effectiveness of Midazolam as a Single Pharmacologic Agent to Facilitate Endotracheal Intubation by Paramedics." *Prehospital Emergency Care* 3 (1999): 191–193.

Wayne, M. A., and E. Friedland. "Prehospital Use of Succinylcholine: A 20-Year Review." *Prehospital Emergency Care* 3 (1999): 107–109.

Dan Mayer, MD

16

Hypertensive Crisis

CASE PRESENTATION

You are dispatched to the home of a 72-year-old man. His wife had called because she said "he just didn't seem to be right" and she was worried that he might be having a stroke.

The patient states that his vision has felt a little funny for a few days and that today he doesn't feel quite like himself. He can't put his finger on the exact sensation he is experiencing. He denies any chest pain, shortness of breath, lightheadedness or dizziness, abdominal pain, numbness or tingling of his arms or legs, or any other focal symptom.

On examination he is found to be alert and oriented times three. His pulse is 78 and regular, and his blood pressure in the right arm is 230/170. His respiratory rate is 16, regular and nonlabored. You decide to repeat the blood pressure because you are not sure about the reading. You get the same value and then take a blood pressure in the left arm, which is only 5 mmHg less than the right.

Secondary survey reveals pupils to be equal and reactive, lungs clear, heart regular, abdomen soft and nontender, and his extremities with good capillary refill and distal pulses. Due to distance and traffic, your ETA to the hospital is 25 minutes. You are concerned that his blood pressure is too high and you must lower it prior to getting to the hospital.

QUESTIONS

1. What are the different types of hypertensive emergencies?
2. When should blood pressure be controlled and lowered?
3. What are the various options for lowering blood pressure in prehospital care?

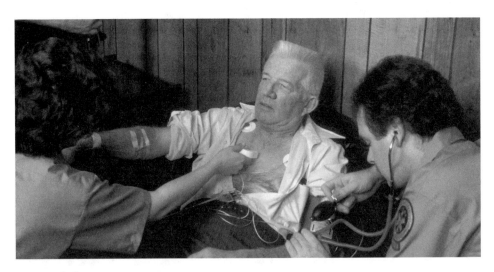

Assessing the hypertensive patient.

DISCUSSION

Hypertension is a chronic disease of the cardiovascular system. The causes of hypertension are varied but the most common is "essential hypertension," which has no specific known cause. It is one of the most common diseases of modern life. There are several issues that are important in the prehospital treatment of the hypertensive patient.

A "hypertensive emergency" is present when a patient presents with an elevated blood pressure that is causing or capable of causing end organ dysfunction. The most commonly affected end organs are the heart, brain, and kidneys. This is also called malignant hypertension or hypertensive crisis. Rapid blood pressure reduction and control is required to prevent irreversible end organ damage. The common presentations of a patient with a hypertensive emergency may include altered mental status or a focal neurological deficit (stroke), headache, shortness of breath (congestive heart failure), or chest pain. Specific syndromes seen in the setting of a hypertensive emergency are hypertensive encephalopathy, intracranial hemorrhage, acute myocardial infarction, acute left ventricular failure with pulmonary edema, dissecting aortic aneurysm, acute renal failure, and (in the setting of pregnancy) eclampsia. All these conditions must be treated emergently.

"Hypertensive urgencies" are defined as a diastolic blood pressure over 130 mmHg without signs or symptoms of end organ dysfunction. Although the patient must be treated soon, the treatment does not need to be done in an emergent manner and rarely will require prehospital intervention other than careful monitoring. The blood pressure should be controlled within about 24 hours.

Simple elevated blood pressure is defined when the blood pressure is above 130/90 but below 130 diastolic. These patients do not require immediate treatment for their elevated blood pressure. When simple hypertension is first detected, treatment is required, but is often begun only after a full medical evaluation by a primary care physician.

If a patient has a true hypertensive emergency, blood pressure control should be initiated immediately in the prehospital setting. There are relatively few prehospital options available in an ALS system for the treatment of elevated blood pressure. Nitroglycerin given sublingually or transcutaneously (with nitropaste) is a vasodilator and can be given for several doses until a lower blood pressure is reached. This is especially useful for patients with congestive heart failure or chest pain who may also be having an acute MI. Correction of blood pressure should not occur too rapidly. The most rapid rate recommended for decreasing blood pressure is 20% of the systolic or diastolic pressure over 30 minutes. In general, the prehospital goal should be to decrease the diastolic blood pressure to the 120 mm Hg range. Too rapid a correction could result in a hypoperfusion-induced stroke in a system used to operating at high pressures.

Other potential drugs in the prehospital arena include metoprolol, a beta-adrenergic blocker. This drug can be given intravenously in 5 mg doses. It is a rapidly acting drug that can effectively reduce blood pressure in a fairly short period. Metoprolol is becoming more widely carried by ALS units, as it has become a mainstay of rate control in the tachycardic patient with cardiac ischemia or infarction. Labetalol, another fast-acting IV beta blocker, is also used in some progressive EMS systems specifically as a parenteral agent for blood pressure control. Labetalol is usually administered with an initial slow IV bolus of either 10 or 20 mg. Contraindications to the use of IV beta blockers would include overt congestive heart failure, moderate to severe asthma, and hypertension secondary to sympathomimetic substances (such as cocaine in all its forms).

Nitroprusside may be available for prehospital use. It is a very rapid acting vasodilator that requires special expertise to use. The bags must be wrapped in foil to avoid exposure to light as that causes degradation of the medication. Advanced paramedics would most likely give this drug in an aeromedical or interfaculty transport system.

Popular a decade ago in emergency medical services, sublingual nifedipine *should not* be used to acutely lower blood pressure. Its effect is unpredictable and uncontrollable. It can cause sudden severe drops in the pressure. It can also take a long time to begin to lower the blood pressure. If other drugs are later given to lower the pressure, the result can be catastrophic, causing a stroke from low pressure.

Other priorities in treating patients with elevated blood pressure include cardiac monitoring and frequent repeat vital signs. Continuous reassurance helps calm the patient and will also help reduce the blood pressure. Morphine sulfate can be used both to lower pressure and to treat sources of pain. A patient with an elevated blood pressure as a result of a painful injury or associated with congestive heart failure or chest pain, will respond to narcotic treatment.

Patients can have elevated blood pressure as a result of taking stimulant medications such as cocaine or amphetamines. In these cases a beta-adrenergic blocker such as metoprolol should not be given. This would result in unopposed alpha-adrenergic activity and intense vasoconstriction, actually making the patient worse. The preferred drug for that situation is a benzodiazepine such as diazepam (Valium) or midazolam (Versed). Diazepam is given intravenously in a 5–10 mg bolus, whereas midazolam is given intravenously in 1–5 mg doses.

RETURN TO THE CASE

Medical direction is contacted and the base station physician orders one and a half inches of nitropaste be applied to the patient's anterior chest wall and begin transport. The physician explains that he is concerned that any agent may lower the blood pressure too quickly and at least the nitropaste can be readily removed if this occurs. During transport you carefully monitor the patient's vital signs and note a mild decrease in the patient's blood pressure.

Upon ED arrival the patient's initial blood pressure is 198/140. The emergency medicine physician opts to administer a 20 mg bolus of IV labetalol slowly. Shortly after the initial dose of labetalol the blood pressure is noted to be 170/119. The patient is begun on a labetalol drip and admitted to the intermediate ICU. His blood work subsequently shows moderate renal insufficiency as a result of his hypertension. He is discharged home on the fourth hospital day with two different antihypertensive medications.

REFERENCES

Bledsoe, Bryan E., Robert S. Porter, and Richard A. Cherry. *Essentials of Paramedic Care*. Upper Saddle River, NJ: Prentice Hall, 2003.

Bledsoe, Bryan E., Robert S. Porter, and Richard A. Cherry. *Medical Emergencies*. Vol. 3 of *Paramedic Care: Principles & Practice*. Chapter 2, "Cardiology." Upper Saddle River, NJ: Brady/Prentice Hall Health, Pearson Education, 2001.

Zavarella, M. S. "190/120 and Rising: Understanding and Managing Hypertensive Emergencies." *Journal of Emergency Medical Services* 25, no. 10 (October 2000): 50–61.

Michael Dailey, MD

17

HYPOTHERMIA WITH ALTERED MENTAL STATUS

CASE PRESENTATION

In mid-December, somewhere in the Northeast, crew members of a freight train passing through a ravine just outside of the city see a person lying in an icy puddle by the side of the tracks, not moving, and contact railway police. Railway police, EMS, and Rescue are dispatched. At that time train traffic along that section of track is suspended until rescue operations are completed.

First arriving units access the patient after walking approximately one-half mile through deep snow along the railroad tracks. They discover an unconscious male who appears to be in his forties. He is at the bottom of an approximately 50-foot, 45- to 60-degree ravine, which slopes up to a major road. He is not dressed appropriately for the weather, wearing only a pair of jeans, sneakers, and a sweatshirt. His clothing is wet, and he feels very cold. There are several empty beer cans near him. There are no tracks leading to him along the rail bed; however, there is a trail in the snow down from the top of the ravine. He is unresponsive and has a Glasgow Coma Scale of 3. His respiratory rate is 6; his heart rate is 30.

Rescue operations are set up at the top of the hill, arrangements are made to transfer the patient up the hill, and additional manpower and equipment are brought down the hill to him. At this time he is administered warm oxygen from the ambulance. He is placed on a long board with a collar, wrapped in blankets, and packaged for the trip up the hill. The extrication is done slowly and gently.

When the patient reaches the top of the hill his vital signs are unchanged. He is placed in a warm ambulance where his clothes are removed. He is transferred to a dry backboard, wrapped in blankets, placed on a cardiac monitor, and two IVs are started. At that time he is noted to have an abrasion on his forehead, but no other external signs of injury. Because of the patient's level of consciousness, the decision is made to secure his airway via endotracheal intubation. The patient is intubated with trauma precautions,

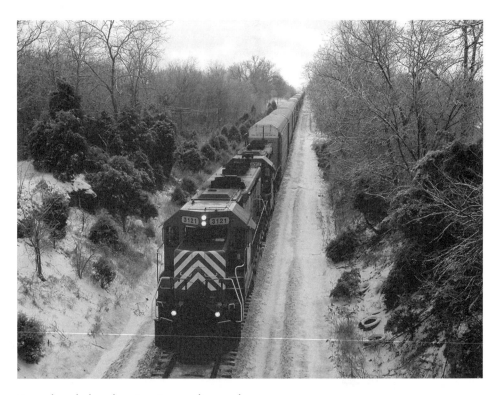

Scene where the hypothermic patient was discovered.
Courtesy of David Snyder and Michael Dailey, MD.

but without medications, and is noted to not have a gag reflex. The ETT placement is confirmed by direct visualization, as well as a waveform on the CO_2 capnography.

Shortly after intubation, the patient is noted to have no spontaneous respirations and no pulse. Rhythm is wide complex bradycardia at 20 complexes per minute. Tube placement is reconfirmed, and CPR is begun. One round of medications—epinephrine 1 mg, and atropine 1 mg—are administered IV, the patient is given a 1 L fluid bolus, and is transferred to a trauma center. During the ride, warm packs are placed in his axilla and at his neck and his groin. CPR is ongoing.

QUESTIONS

1. What considerations must be taken to treat this patient with clinical hypothermia, bradycardia, and decreased responsiveness?
2. With decreased responsiveness and hypoventilation, do you attempt to control the patient's airway on the scene?
3. How does treatment of cardiac arrest change in the hypothermic patient?

DISCUSSION

Hypothermia is a complex series of events, which can easily be thought of as a process of the body slowing down. This patient was demonstrating many of these with a decreased mental status, decreased heart rate, and decreased respiratory effort. The most serious potential problem for patients with hypothermia is cardiac arrhythmias. This is both primarily from the hypothermia, as well as cardiac response to profound bradycardia as the ventricular cells can create their own escape beats. In addition, increasing metabolic acidosis in hypothermic patients is also arrhythmogenic. The attempt should be made to do everything possible for these patients in as gentle a manner as possible, whether transporting or intubating or starting intravenous lines.

If the patient is to be intubated, the most senior or experienced person should perform the intubation to minimize trauma to the posterior pharynx and the potential for cardiac arrhythmias. Stimulation of the vagus nerve can cause acute bradydysrhythmias, and pressure in the hypopharynx can cause this stimulation. Indeed, this patient suffered cardiac arrest shortly after successful intubation. Whether the cause was tube manipulation during BVM ventilation or continued progression of his bradycardia will never be known.

Another consideration in the hypothermic patient is that pulse checks must be made for a longer period of time as the patient may have a very slow heart rate. A heart rate of 20 may be minimally perfusing, yet be missed on a cursory pulse check. Was this patient in pulseless electrical activity (PEA)? We don't know.

Prior to arrest, cardiac medications should be avoided because many do not work well below normal body temperature. In this patient, the bradycardia was initially left untreated, as it is a normal physiologic response. Following arrest, treatment falls to cardiac arrest protocols. However, it is important to realize that while ACLS guidelines suggest epinephrine and atropine as first-line medications for asystole or pulseless electrical activity, there is no documented proof of their efficacy in hypothermic patients. Medical control requested that multiple rounds of medication not be given, as the metabolism of the medications is decreased.

If this patient were in ventricular fibrillation, amiodarone would seem to be the current drug of choice. Lidocaine is metabolized poorly in the hypothermic setting, and bretylium tosylate—the previous drug of choice, based upon multiple dog model studies—is no longer available. There are no research studies that demonstrate any pharmacological treatment of hypothermic human cardiac arrest, so all treatment is based upon anecdotal success.

For the patient who is not in cardiac arrest, primary prehospital treatment of hypothermia is comprised of passive rewarming techniques, including removing wet clothing, wrapping the patient in warm blankets, utilizing warm fluids and oxygen if possible, and minimizing handling trauma. There are now warming blankets available to EMS agencies as well. In the colder months, care should be taken in all cases to prevent iatrogenic (rescuer-caused) hypothermia, caused by stripping trauma patients and leaving them exposed to the elements. In the hospital, rewarming by active techniques—including hemodialysis, heart bypass machines, or lavage of the chest or the abdomen—has been done. The best results seem to be from heart bypass and dialysis, which can warm the blood rapidly and continually cycle warm blood into the body.

Note the caveat that "no patient is cold and dead." There are case reports of people who have been in cardiac arrest for extended periods and have been successfully resuscitated using active rewarming techniques. This is particularly true for children.

RETURN TO THE CASE

On arrival at the trauma center the patient is noted to be in cardiac arrest and rectal temperature is 76 degrees Fahrenheit (°F)/24.5 degrees Celsius (°C). He has two IVs in his bilateral antecubital fossae and heart rhythm is noted to be sinus bradycardia, with prominent Osborne waves and very slow cardiac activity noted by ultrasound. The patient is placed on warmed humidified oxygen via ventilator, and a warming blanket is placed on him. A Foley catheter is placed and warm saline irrigation is begun. The patient is given a large femoral dual lumen line and is placed on dialysis for purposes of rewarming.

Following active rewarming, the patient awakes. Although he does have a period of amnesia, he remembers he had been walking along the highway coming from a party, but he remembers little else. He has sustained significant trauma to his hands and feet from frostbite; however, he is discharged to rehabilitation and ultimately does well.

REFERENCES

American College of Surgeons. *ATLS—Advanced Trauma Life Support for Doctors*. 6th ed. Student Course Manual. Chicago: American College of Surgeons, 1997.

Bledsoe, Bryan E., Robert S. Porter, and Richard A. Cherry. *Medical Emergencies*. Vol. 3 of *Paramedic Care: Principles & Practice*. Chapter 10, "Environmental Emergencies." Upper Saddle River, NJ: Brady/Prentice Hall Health, Pearson Education, 2001.

Letsou, G. V., G. S. Kopf, J. A. Elefteriades, J. E. Carter, J. C. Baldwin, and G. L. Hammond. "Is Cardiopulmonary Bypass Effective for Treatment of Hypothermic Arrest Due to Drowning or Exposure?" *Archives of Surgery* 127, no. 5 (May 1992) 525–528.

Limmer, Daniel, Michael F. O'Keefe, Harvey D. Grant, Robert H. Murray, J. David Bergeron, Beth Lothrop Adams, and Edward T. Dickinson, eds. *Emergency Care*. 9th ed. Upper Saddle River, NJ: Prentice Hall, 2000.

Orts, A., C. Alcaraz, K. A. Delaney, L. R. Goldfrank, H. Turndorf, and M. M. Puig. "Bretylium Tosylate and Electrically Induced Cardiac Arrhythmias during Hypothermia in Dogs." *American Journal of Emergency Medicine* 10, no. 4 (July 1992): 311–316.

Rankin, A. C., and A. P. Rae. "Cardiac Arrhythmias during Rewarming of Patients with Accidental Hypothermia. *British Medical Journal* 289, no. 6449 (October 6, 1984): 874–877.

Wollenek, G., N. Honarwar, J. Golej, and M. Marx. "Cold Water Submersion and Cardiac Arrest in Treatment of Severe Hypothermia with Cardiopulmonary Bypass." *Resuscitation* 52, no. 3 (March 2002): 255–263.

Kevin Curtis, MD

18

MENINGITIS

CASE PRESENTATION

You are responding to a call at a home involving a 30-year-old male with decreased mental status. On arrival, you are met by the patient's tearful wife. "My husband is really sick! When I left the house awhile ago, he had a fever to 104 and a really bad headache. I just got home and found him on the couch. I can't seem to wake him up."

As you approach the patient, he is in the fetal position on the couch. He is breathing spontaneously, but at a rate of only 6 with some gurgling. He fails to respond to his name or to being shaken. Your paramedic partner places the patient supine on the floor and notes that he has nuchal rigidity. Despite repositioning and jaw thrust, there is no significant improvement in his airway. His blood pressure is 90/palp, heart rate 140, pulse oximetry 88% on room air, and he has a high tactile temperature. His lungs are clear bilaterally and he is in sinus tachycardia on the monitor. His pupils are 4 mm and reactive bilaterally and there is no evidence of trauma. He responds to noxious stimuli with movement of all four extremities.

Your partner ventilates the patient with a BVM while you establish a large-bore IV. Fingerstick glucose is 95. The patient is orotracheally intubated with an 8.0 mm ET tube without difficulty. Correct placement is confirmed by bilateral breath sounds and by an end-tidal CO_2 device. During transport to the hospital you administer a 500 cc IV normal saline, with improvement in his blood pressure to 100/60.

QUESTIONS

1. What initial precautions would decrease the risk of transmission of meningitis from the patient to you and your partner?
2. What is unique about the clinical presentation of bacterial meningitis (a) in neonates and (b) in elderly people?

3. Should you take antibiotics to decrease your chance of contracting meningococcal meningitis?

DISCUSSION

Meningitis is defined as infection of the membranes that surround the brain and spinal cord to form the subarachnoid space. It is generally classified as either bacterial or aseptic (nonbacterial). Whereas aseptic meningitis is a relatively benign process with no substantial complications, bacterial meningitis has the potential for significant morbidity and mortality.

Approximately 25,000 cases of bacterial meningitis occur annually in the United States, with two-thirds of cases occurring in children. The epidemiology has changed drastically since the introduction of the *Haemophilus influenzae* (H. flu) vaccine in 1981, with H. flu once being a leading cause of meningitis and now being relatively uncommon. In addition, since H. flu was the most common cause of bacterial meningitis in children, with its near eradication, the median age of patients with bacterial meningitis has increased from 15 months to 25 years. Currently, approximately three-fourths of cases of bacterial meningitis are caused by either *Streptococcus pneumoniae* or *Neisseria meningitides (meningococcus)*.

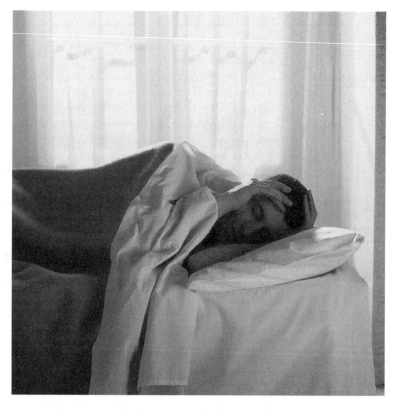

Patients with meningitis will often appear acutely ill with severe headache and neck stiffness. Courtesy of Dorling Kindersley.

S. pneumoniae is the most common agent in adults, with *N. meningitides* being most frequently noted in children. The most common cause of aseptic meningitis is viral, particularly enterovirus. Other etiologies include tuberculosis, fungus, syphilis, and malignancy.

Patients with meningitis generally present with either several days of insidious symptoms or, conversely, several hours of an acute fulminant course. The classic triad of meningitis is fever, headache, and stiff neck. Headache may be quite severe, and is most often frontal or retroorbital. The classic triad may be accompanied by photophobia, nausea, vomiting, drowsiness, and generalized malaise. The patient presenting with high fever and severe headache, with or without neck stiffness, should be presumed to have meningitis until proven otherwise. However, it is important to note that up to 20% of cases of meningitis may present in an atypical fashion.

Although bacterial meningitis has a markedly different prognosis than aseptic meningitis, on initial clinical presentation, it is often impossible to distinguish the two entities. Thus, paramedics should never attempt to distinguish between them and always presume that the patient has the more serious bacterial form of the disease. Bacterial meningitis is a true neurologic emergency. Patients may be very ill, and, in some cases, may lapse into stupor or coma within hours. Untreated, bacterial meningitis carries a mortality of greater than 90%. Even with appropriate treatment, the mortality is 25% and has not decreased significantly in the last 15 years. The long-term complication rate after bacterial meningitis is 25–50%, with sequelae including hearing loss, seizure disorder, cognitive deficits, and hydrocephalus.

Although 80% of patients with meningitis do present with the classic triad of symptoms, clinical features may differ based on the age of the host. Infants, and especially neonates, often lack the usual signs and symptoms of meningitis. They tend to appear septic rather than displaying obvious features of central nervous system (CNS) involvement. Typical symptoms can include listlessness, vomiting, irritability, or poor feeding. A stiff neck is a very unusual finding. Elderly patients with meningitis are also more likely to present with an atypical symptom complex. Symptoms often consist of fever, which is frequently low grade, and a change in mental status. Classic headache and nuchal rigidity may not be prominent.

Two classic clinical signs of meningeal irritation are Brudzinski's sign and Kernig's sign. Brudzinski's sign is present if flexing the patient's neck results in flexion of the hips and knees. Kernig's sign is present if extending the patient's knee with the hip flexed causes pain in the hamstring and back. Although concerning when present, Kernig's and Brudzinski's signs are commonly absent in adult patients with meningitis and are actually rare in infants.

Other findings can include (1) acute rash (petechiae and purpura), particularly in cases of meningococcal meningitis; (2) seizures in up to 30% of patients with bacterial meningitis; and (3) focal neurologic findings in 25% of cases.

Particularly in light of the fact that acute bacterial meningitis can rapidly progress to coma, initial attention to the ABCs is essential. In the most severe cases, intubation may be necessary. Initial evaluation should also include vitals signs, assessment of peripheral perfusion, pulse oximetry, and mental status. Supplemental oxygen and cardiac monitoring should be instituted for any patients with signs of respiratory or cardiovascular compromise. For patients with altered mental status, seizures, or shock, a large-bore intravenous line is indicated. Dehydration and shock are treated with normal saline. For patients with altered mental status, a rapid blood glucose determination should be made and 50% glucose given only if hypoglycemia is documented.

Meningococcus and H. flu are transmitted via respiratory droplets. Mouth-to-mask ventilation, intubation, and suctioning put paramedics at risk for disease transmission. Therefore, health care providers should institute universal precautions as soon as the possibility of meningitis is even considered. In particular, the application of masks on yourself and/or the patient with possible meningitis will protect you from transmission.

Due to the increased risk of infection after possible exposure to respiratory and oral secretions, the Centers for Disease Control and Prevention (CDC) currently recommends that paramedics who have had "intensive" contact with a patient who is diagnosed with bacterial meningitis due to *meningococcus* take prophylactic antibiotics. Intensive contact includes mouth-to-mask ventilation, endotracheal intubation, suctioning, and close examination of the oropharynx. Antibiotic prophylaxis can prevent infection in health care workers who have had these high-risk exposures to patients with *meningococcal* meningitis. Prophylaxis should begin within 24 hours of exposure. In those cases in which *meningococcal* meningitis is strongly suspected, but not yet confirmed within 24 hours, antibiotics are also appropriate.

Options for antibiotic prophylaxis include the following:

Rifampin	600 mg orally every 12 hours for 2 days
Ciprofloxacin	500 mg orally; one dose only
Ceftriaxone	250 mg by intramuscular injection; one dose only

Despite antibiotic prophylaxis, development of symptoms requires urgent evaluation. Based on a significantly lower risk of transmission, prophylactic antibiotics are not recommended for exposure to patients with bacterial meningitis that is not *meningococcus*.

RETURN TO THE CASE

After arrival in the emergency department, intravenous antibiotics are administered for presumed bacterial meningitis. A lumbar puncture is performed with a cell count that supports the diagnosis and a gram stain revealing *Neiserria meningitides*. The patient is admitted to the medical ICU, with gradual improvement. He is discharged on day 20 at his baseline, with the exception of some minimal residual neurologic deficits.

REFERENCES

Bledsoe, Bryan E., Robert S. Porter, and Richard A. Cherry. *Medical Emergencies*, Vol. 3 of *Paramedic Care: Principles & Practice*. Chapter 11, "Infectious Diseases." Upper Saddle River, NJ: Brady/Prentice Hall Health, Pearson Education, 2001.

Centers for Disease Control and Prevention. "Prevention and Control of *Meningococcal* Disease and *Meningococcal* Diseases and College Students; Recommendations of the Advisory Committee on Immunization Practices (ACIP)." *MMWR Morbidity and Mortality Weekly Report* 49, no. RR07 (2000): 1–10.

Coyle, P. K. "Overview of Acute and Chronic Meningitis." *Neurologic Clinics* 17 (1999): 691–700.

Susan A. O'Malley, MD
Jeanmarie Perrone, MD

19

Overdose

CASE PRESENTATION

You and your partner are summoned to the scene of an adult male who is unconscious.

You arrive at a private home to find a young woman stating that she can't wake her husband. You grab your equipment and follow her into the house. As you enter the residence, you note a well-kept home. You are escorted to an upstairs bedroom where you find your patient lying supine on the bed, half dressed, with a belt around his arm. You quickly notice in your survey of the scene a bent spoon and syringe on the bedside table along with an empty bottle of a prescription medication, Elavil. There are empty beer bottles strewn around the room.

As you approach the patient to begin your primary survey, you note that he is snoring. You quickly use the head-tilt, chin-lift method to open the airway and the snoring stops. His respirations are shallow at a rate of 8–10 per minute. Your partner begins ventilating the patient with a bag-valve-mask as you listen for breath sounds. You note he has breath sounds that are equal and clear bilaterally. The rest of your primary survey reveals a radial pulse, no gross bleeding, and pinpoint pupils that are equal and responsive to light. The patient groans when a sternal rub is applied. The secondary survey is remarkable for fresh needlesticks in his left antecubital fossa. As you begin to take his vital signs, your partner continues ventilating the patient and obtains further information from the wife.

The wife reports the patient has no allergies. He has a history of alcohol and intravenous drug abuse, but has been clean and sober for the past 6 months. He takes no medications. She states that after dinner the previous night the patient went to a Narcotics Anonymous® meeting. He came home late smelling of alcohol. They had an argument and she went to a friend's house for the night. She tried calling her husband this morning and got no response. When she returned home around noon she found her husband in his current condition and was unable to arouse him.

You record the patient's vital signs—heart rate 120, respiratory rate 10, blood pressure 90/70 and oxygen saturation 100%—and then start a large-bore IV in his right AC and determine a blood glucose of 120 mg/dl by AccuCheck. An ECG strip reveals sinus

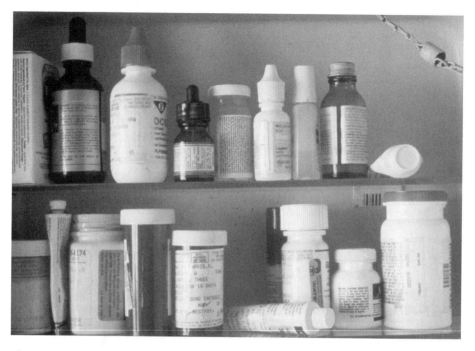

The presence of multiple medications on the scene of an overdose may make it difficult to determine exactly what was ingested.

tachycardia at a rate of 120 bpm, PR interval 20 msec, and a QRS of 100 msec. (See Figure 19-1). You correctly decide to treat this patient for an opioid overdose as he has a depressed level of consciousness, hypoventilation, and pinpoint pupils.

QUESTIONS

1. How do you manage an opioid overdose?
2. What should the abnormal ECG alert you to?

DISCUSSION

Initial management of the overdose patient involves the ABCs—oxygen, IV, and monitor. Prehospital "supportive care" for overdoses may include securing the airway with intubation, providing BVM ventilation, and stabilizing the blood pressure with intravenous fluids. Only a small percentage of overdoses have true "antidotes" or definitive prehospital interventions beyond supportive care. These include narcotics, cyclic antidepressants, cyanide, and, in a limited number of cases, benzodiazepines.

In the case presented, the patient has two potential overdoses that have viable ALS prehospital interventions that may stabilize the situation. The most important aspect of this patient's assessment is the adequacy of ventilation. Once the initial management has

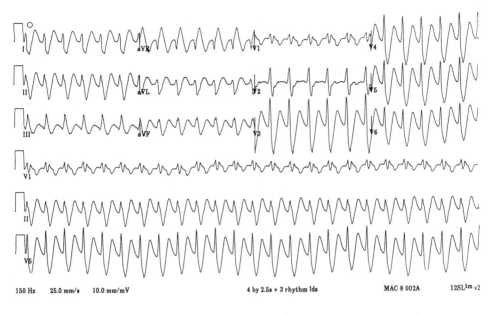

150 Hz   25.0 mm/s   10.0 mm/mV   4 by 2.5s + 3 rhythm lds   MAC 8 002A   12SL^tm v2

Figure 19-1 Widened QRS complexes, typical of an ECG with a cyclic antidepressant overdose.

been addressed, the next step would be to administer naloxone in a patient with inadequate respirations. Opioid overdoses rarely require intubation because the respiratory depressant effects are readily reversible with naloxone.

Naloxone (Narcan) is a competitive antagonist that binds to opioid receptors. Although it binds the opioid receptors, it does not activate them, thereby reversing the respiratory depression and altered mental status associated with opioid toxicity. It has a rapid onset of action within 1–2 minutes after administration. It can be administered intravenously, intramuscularly, sublingually, or via an endotracheal tube. The only absolute contraindication is known hypersensitivity to Narcan. Extra caution should be used in reversing opioid intoxication in a chronic opioid user to prevent precipitation of severe withdrawal. Complications are rare but include severe agitation, nausea and vomiting, which can lead to aspiration in patients who are opioid dependent. Therefore, the recommended initial dose is 0.4 mg IV. The endotracheal dose is 2–2.5 times the IV dose diluted in normal saline to provide 10 ml of fluid. If there is no response or an inadequate response 3–5 minutes after the initial dose, then a 1–2 mg IV should be administered every 3–5 minutes. If there is no response after 10 mg, another cause for the patient's symptoms should be sought. Some opioid overdoses will require much higher doses of naloxone—up to 10 mg—to achieve the desired therapeutic effect. This may be required in overdoses of agonist-antagonist opioids or occasionally with drugs such as clonidine with partial effects at the opioid receptor. The goal of naloxone therapy is *not* complete reversal of the opioid intoxication but resumption of adequate respirations. The patient should be easily arousable with adequate respirations but not fully awake. Intermittent titrated doses will minimize the possibility of producing unwanted withdrawal symptoms.

A review of the ECG findings raises concern for a concomitant cyclic antidepressant (CA) overdose (See Figure 19-1). Antidepressants are the second most common cause of fatal poisonings. Older first-generation cyclic antidepressants such as amitryptiline (Elavil) are very effective pharmacotherapy for the treatment of depression and are often prescribed for the depression that accompanies substance abuse. However, these drugs are being used less often due to their toxicity, and due to the availability of newer, less toxic drug class of selective serotonin reuptake inhibitors (SSRIs)—Prozac, for example.

Knowledge of the pathophysiology of CAs aids in understanding the signs and symptoms of a CA overdose. Cyclic antidepressants have a multitude of receptor effects. These drugs block the reuptake of norepinephrine, dopamine, and serotonin in the brain. This may account for their antidepressant efficacy by increasing synaptic catecholamines. In overdose, initial release of these catecholamines can induce transient tachycardia and hypertension followed by catecholamine depletion and relative hypotension. Central anticholinergic effects may lead to agitation, lethargy, hallucinations, ataxia, seizures, and coma whereas peripheral effects include tachycardia, dilated pupils, dry, flushed skin, decreased bowel sounds, and urinary retention. The most important toxic effects of cyclic antidepressants are due to the inhibition of myocardial sodium channels. Inhibition of fast sodium channels prolongs phase zero of myocardial depolarization, causing delayed conduction. This can be evidenced by ECG changes: prolongation of the QRS and the QTc, and classic "wide complex dysrhythmias." Negative inotropic effects and alpha-adrenergic blockade contribute to subsequent hypotension. Bradycardia is usually a terminal event. A QRS greater than or equal to ($\geq$) 100 ms in a suspected CA ingestion is cause for concern. QRS prolongation correlates with clinical effects: A QRS greater than (>) 100 ms is associated with seizures; >160 ms is associated with ventricular dysrhythmias. Whereas most fatalities associated with CAs occur early in the overdose, these overdoses are treatable when early recognition and therapy occur. A QRS $\geq$100 ms, hypotension, seizure, or dysrhythmia in a suspected CA overdose should be treated immediately.

The principal therapy of CA poisoning is sodium bicarbonate. It is effective by two mechanisms. First, it causes an alkalemia which decreases the binding affinity of the CA to the myocardium. Second, by increasing sodium concentration it increases the gradient for sodium across the membrane, decreasing fast sodium channel blockade and increasing conduction. An initial bolus of 1 milliequivalent per kilogram (mEq/kg) is given IV followed by an IV drip. The drip is made by adding 3 ampules (amps) of sodium bicarbonate to a liter of 5% dextrose in water (D$_5$W). The drip is then infused at a rate of 2–3 cubic centimeters per kilogram per hour (cc/kg/hr). The aim of this therapy is reversal of hypotension and narrowing of the QRS complex. Medical command needs to be contacted for a specific order to administer sodium bicarbonate therapy.

RETURN TO THE CASE

Naloxone 0.4 mg is administered IV and the patient regains adequate respirations. Medical command is contacted and an order for sodium bicarbonate is requested and you are instructed to give 2 amps IV and follow it with a drip at a rate of 2 cc/kg/hr. The patient is transported to the ED. En route your reassessment reveals a decreased respiratory rate and you administer an additional 0.4 mg of naloxone with good effect. The rest of the transport is uneventful. The sodium bicarbonate drip is continued and the ED physician congratulates you on recognizing the importance of the widened QRS and beginning appropriate therapy in the field. A toxicology screen is positive for opioids, amitriptyline, nicotine, and alcohol. The patient is admitted to the intensive care unit for close observation and continued therapy. The next day, the patient is alert and oriented, has normal respirations, and his ECG changes have resolved. He is transferred to the psychiatric unit to undergo definitive treatment of his depression and substance abuse.

REFERENCES

Bledsoe, Bryan E., Robert S. Porter, and Bruce R. Shade. *Paramedic Emergency Care*. 3rd ed. Upper Saddle River, NJ: Prentice Hall, 1997.

Bledsoe, Bryan E., Robert S. Porter, and Richard A. Cherry. *Medical Emergencies* Vol. 3 of *Paramedic Care: Principles & Practice*, Chapter 8, "Toxicology and Substance Abuse." Upper Saddle River, NJ: Brady/Prentice Hall Health, Pearson Education, 2001.

Sporer, K. A. "Acute Heroin Overdose." *Annals of Internal Medicine* 130, no. 7 (1999): 584–590.

Alexander P. Isakov, MD, MPH

20

PAIN MANAGEMENT

CASE PRESENTATION

As the sun sets over Atlanta, you are dispatched to a downtown construction site to respond for a construction worker who has had a fall. When you and your partner arrive, you are told that one of the work party has sustained an injury after the fall. He is still on top of the construction site on the 25th floor. You are escorted to the patient by taking the construction elevator to the 21st floor and climbing the remaining four stories on narrow construction ladders in the structure. As you arrive on the roof of the building, you see that the construction crew has been able to extract the patient from the arm of the crane where he had apparently slipped and fallen—not any great distance, but into the steel frame of the crane.

He appears to be in his 30s. He is yelling loudly that his right leg hurts and that he is very much in need of assistance. The primary survey reveals that his airway is intact, he is adequately ventilating, he has good peripheral pulses, and his capillary refill is less than 2 seconds. He is completely awake and lucid, has a GCS of 15, and has a noticeable blood stain on his right pant leg. After assessing the ABCs and finding them intact, you cut the pant leg to better assess the wound. You find a deformity of the right lower leg with an open fracture of the patient's tibia/fibula with minimal but active bleeding. You immediately apply a dressing and direct pressure to the wound to stop the bleeding. The leg has brisk distal pulses, the skin color is good, sensation is intact, and the patient can move his ankle and toes but complains of severe pain. You quickly splint the leg while the patient complains again of pain, and upon application of the splint, reassess the neurovascular status of the leg, which is intact. The remainder of the secondary survey is unremarkable. Specifically, he has no head trauma or neck pain, his lungs are clear, his abdomen is soft, nontender, and without guarding. His pelvis is nontender and stable, and his back is without injury. The patient states he was walking on the arm of the crane when he lost his footing. As he started to fall, his leg got caught in the crane's frame, causing the fracture

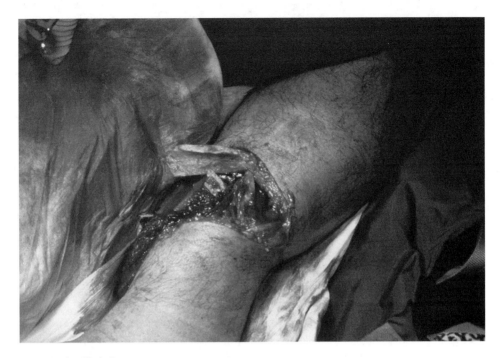

An open tibia/fibula fracture.

of the leg but resulting in no other injury. He is currently taking no medications and has no allergies.

You radio to dispatch that the patient is approximately 220 pounds, nonambulatory, and that it will be nearly impossible to navigate him down the four stories of ladders that lead to the construction elevator below. You determine that the crane is available to hoist him down but you don't have the equipment to properly secure him for the ride. The fire department is dispatched and the high-angle rescue team is being sent to assist you. The patient is crying out in pain. You know it will take at least 10 minutes for the fire crew to arrive and then perhaps another 30 minutes for them to get their gear upstairs and properly secure the patient for the descent.

QUESTIONS

1. How can you assist your distressed patient while you wait for assistance from the fire crew?

2. What are the risks associated with administering analgesics to patients in the prehospital setting and what are your considerations before giving a drug?

DISCUSSION

Acute pain is one of the most common complaints emergency providers will encounter. Remarkably it is also one of the most underrecognized and undertreated complaints managed by prehospital providers and emergency medicine clinicians alike. White and his fellow researchers showed that of 1,000 patients managed by EMS with suspected extremity fractures, only 18 (1.8%) received analgesics in the prehospital setting, even with standing orders allowing their administration. Another study of analgesic administration in the emergency department showed that only 30% of 401 patients who presented with acute fractures were given any pain medication in the ED. "Oligoanalgesia," or the lack of adequate pain control, has recently come under greater scrutiny and study with the purpose of exposing the issue and giving us tools to improve our management of acute pain.

For prehospital and emergency health care providers, the recognition and timely management of pain should be of great importance. Pain is commonly encountered by paramedics. We have tools to assist our patients in the management of their suffering, and there is evidence that prolonged exposure to pain may in fact make patients increasingly sensitive to painful stimuli. Timely interventions in pain management can potentially decrease subsequent perception of pain and pain medication requirements. It has even been suggested that poorly treated acute pain may trigger functional and structural changes of the central nervous system, contributing to chronic pain.

Morphine has been shown to be a safe drug for administration in the prehospital setting and is likely the most commonly available prehospital analgesic drug. Some services might include the nonsteroidal anti-inflammatory drug (NSAID) ketorolac (Toradol). Fentanyl may also be seen, but more likely on critical care transport and air ambulance services.

Morphine has many favorable qualities. It can be given intravenously, intramuscularly, or sublingually. Its onset of action when given intravenously is a few short minutes. The cardiovascular effects are minimal. The drug is metabolized in the liver, so renal failure does not affect the half-life, though renal failure patients do appear to have an increased sensitivity to the drug. Morphine does, however, release histamine that can cause peripheral venodilation. This decrease in preload to the heart may result in hypotension, especially in a patient who is volume depleted, say from hemorrhage. This histamine release may also result in urticaria and bronchspasm. Morphine also produces moderate respiratory depression and has the potential to cause sedation.

Ketorolac is an NSAID like ibuprofen and is carried by some EMS agencies because it has been shown to be effective in the treatment of renal colic and offers a nonnarcotic alternative for pain management. The inhibition of prostaglandins is thought to decrease smooth muscle tone in the ureters, decreasing intraluminal pressure and peristalsis. Ketorolac as a musculoskeletal analgesic, however, has been shown to be no more effective than 800 mg of ibuprofen given by mouth. Like the other NSAIDs, ketorolac has the potential to exacerbate gastrointestinal bleeding, inhibit platelets and thus increase bleeding time, and precipitate renal insufficiency or failure.

Fentanyl offers the advantage of a short duration of action, no histamine release, and no decrease of cardiac output. It does, however, have a recognized side effect of sometimes inducing muscular rigidity which has resulted in respiratory compromise.

Considerations for the treatment of pain in the prehospital setting include drug allergies, respiratory compromise, likelihood of hemodynamic instability, route of delivery, and severity of the pain.

It is very important to determine a patient's drug allergies and reactions before giving any medication to any patient. Morphine, like many drugs, can result in serious allergic reactions, including anaphylaxis and death if given to patients with a known allergy.

The next two considerations often result in prehospital protocols for narcotic analgesia in trauma being limited to isolated extremity injuries. Because morphine and other narcotic analgesics can produce moderate respiratory depression, patients who are exhibiting signs of respiratory compromise and may proceed to respiratory failure are often not considered good candidates for the drug. Although the likelihood of respiratory failure after an appropriate dose of a narcotic alone is rare, one should always be prepared to manage a patient's airway if narcotic analgesics are given.

Patients who are already hypotensive or have the potential to become hemodynamically unstable, for example, from an occult intracavitary hemorrhage, have also not been considered good candidates for prehospital narcotic analgesia. The histamine release may precipitate hypotension. One should always be aware of a patient's hemodynamic status and be prepared to support a patient's blood pressure with IV normal saline or lactated Ringer's solution when administering morphine for pain.

The ideal route for delivery of morphine is IV. This allows for rapid onset of action as well as an ability to titrate the drug to effect. The IM or SQ administration of the drug can certainly be considered, especially in the absence of the ability to gain IV access. However, the IM and SQ routes have some disadvantages. The onset of action is delayed and not reliable. The patient may not experience any relief for 20–30 minutes. It is also difficult to titrate the drug to effect.

Pain severity is very subjective, but must be taken into account when managing someone's pain. Having some means for the patient to estimate the level of discomfort will be helpful for two reasons. One, it may help document improvement in the patient's outcome with regard to management of his pain. Perhaps more importantly it will bring the issue of pain to the forefront of the initial patient evaluation and help prevent pain management from being overlooked in the treatment of the patient. Many are advocating a pain scale be included as the sixth vital sign after heart rate, blood pressure, respiratory rate, temperature and oxygen saturation, to focus attention on the importance of this issue in the management of our patients.

There are many factors that contribute to oligoanalgesia that have been described. They include (1) concerns that pain medication might obscure the proper evaluation of the patient by the emergency physician or specialist, (2) concerns about side effects of the medications, (3) concerns that patients may be rendered incompetent to give informed consent for evaluation or for special procedures if given narcotic analgesics, (4) miscommunication between the patient and the health care provider about the severity of the patient's pain, (5) age bias, (6) gender bias, (7) racial bias, and (8) health care provider indifference.

As emergency health care providers, we must strive to properly evaluate our patients, recognize their discomfort, and provide adequate analgesia, per protocol. Studies show that morphine can be given safely in the prehospital setting. Studies in the ER, especially with regard to the evaluation of abdominal pain, show that pain medications do not interfere with the physician's ability to accurately make a diagnosis or determine a disposition. The concept that patients would lose their ability to participate in informed consent because of excessive analgesia has not been demonstrated in the literature and according to Gabbay and Dickinson has been "largely debunked in the legal and ethics literature." The issue of achieving better communication between the patient and the provider might be accomplished by establishing a protocol that mandates the evaluation of pain, and incorporates the use of a visual analog score or a verbal rating score to measure pain. With regard to age, gender, and racial bias, we must all continue to be vigilant in our efforts to provide a uniform level of care and continue to read the literature that studies these biases for guidance in eliminating this problem.

RETURN TO THE CASE

You have determined that the patient is still a long way from arriving at the ED and appears quite uncomfortable. You ask the patient to tell you on a scale from 0 to 10, with 10 being the worst pain he could imagine and 0 being no pain at all, how he currently rates his pain. He tells you emphatically that his pain is a 10. From the primary and secondary survey you have determined that the patient has not suffered a head injury and has a GCS of 15. His respiratory status is intact, and the patient has a blood pressure of 150/80 with a heart rate of 98, indicating no apparent hemodynamic compromise. He repeats that he has no drug allergies. After considering these issues you determine that this patient meets criteria for your acute pain management protocol. As you start an IV, you contact medical control on the radio for orders. You relay the vitals and the condition of the patient over the radio to the medical control physician and request an order for morphine. The medical control physician concurs and asks how much you want to give him. You state that given his weight of 220 pounds and the recommended dose being about 0.1 mg/kg, you would like to give him a test dose of 2 mg morphine IV to ensure no significant side effects and then titrate up to 10 mg of IV morphine until he states he has some relief. The physician agrees with your plan. The patient is given the 2 mg of morphine IV. He denies any rash or difficulty breathing, and his blood pressure remains 152/80. He stills complains his pain is a 10/10. You now dose him with an additional 4 mg of morphine. After 5 minutes, the patient reports that he is somewhat improved, but still in pain. He now reports his pain to be approximately a 6/10. He is still lucid, his blood pressure is now 146/76, and his pulse rate is 92. Respirations are still adequate. You give the patient an additional 4 mg of IV morphine—total is now 10 mg. The patient feels much improved. He is still alert and oriented but much more comfortable. He reports his pain to be a 3/10, but states it is now quite manageable. He thanks you for your help. Shortly thereafter, the high-angle rescue team arrives and prepares the patient to be lowered the 25 stories in a stokes basket. Without difficulty, the patient is transported to the ED for further evaluation and management.

REFERENCES

Bledsoe, Bryan E., Robert S. Porter, and Richard A. Cherry. *Medical Emergencies*. Vol. 3 of *Paramedic Care: Principles & Practice*. Chapter 2, "Cardiology," Chapter 3, "Neurology," Chapter 6, "Gastroenterology," Chapter 7, "Urology and Nephrology." Upper Saddle River, NJ: Brady/Prentice Hall Health, Pearson Education, 2001.

Gabbay, D. S., and E. T. Dickinson. "Refusal of Base Station Physicians to Authorize Narcotic Analgesia. *Prehospital Emergency Care* 5, no. 3 (July–September 2001): 293–295.

White, L. J., J. D. Cooper, R. M. Chambers, and R. E. Gradisek. "Prehospital Use of Analgesia for Suspected Extremity Fracture." *Prehospital Emergency Care* 4 (2000): 205–208.

Zack Meisel, MD
Francis DeRoos, MD

21

POISONING

CASE PRESENTATION

You are dispatched to the home of a man and woman who have been caring for their 2-year-old grandson for a week while his parents are on vacation in the Caribbean. Upon arrival to their rural farmhouse, you are greeted by a worried-appearing woman who reports that her grandchild "is very sleepy and not breathing right." She thinks that the child may have "gotten into his grandfather's heart medications." She hands you a pill box with various unlabeled tablets. The woman does not know the names of her husband's medicines; she states that she thinks "some of the pills are missing." As the woman leads you to the child, you instruct her to collect all pill bottles that the child could have gotten into.

Upon approaching the child, you note a toddler lying prone on the sofa. He is unconscious, but arouses with vigorous stimulation, opening his eyes and emitting a loud cry. Upon discontinuing the stimulation, he falls asleep again, with shallow breathing at approximately 8 breaths per minute. You immediately roll the patient onto his back and begin a careful assessment. Breath sounds are equal bilaterally. His pulse, measured at the brachial artery, is 50 bpm. You place a bag-valve-mask on the child in anticipation of initiating assisted ventilation, but again he wakes, shaking off the mask. His heart rate increases to a rate of 100 bpm and respiratory rate to 30. His systolic blood pressure ranges from 100 mmHg while awake, to 60 mmHg while somnolent.

You place a pediatric-sized 100% nonrebreather mask on the patient, establish a 20-gauge IV, place the patient on a cardiac monitor, and move him to the ambulance. A finger stick is performed for blood glucose measurement: it measures 90 mg/dl. En route to the hospital, you continue your secondary survey of the patient. You note the following: pinpoint pupils minimally reactive to light; the skin is cool but pink and dry; mucous membranes are normal; temperature is 95 degrees Fahrenheit; and bowel sounds are normal.

Further questioning of the grandmother and an inspection of the pill bottles gathered reveals that the only medications in the home are blood pressure pills for her husband. The label shows the pills to be clonidine.

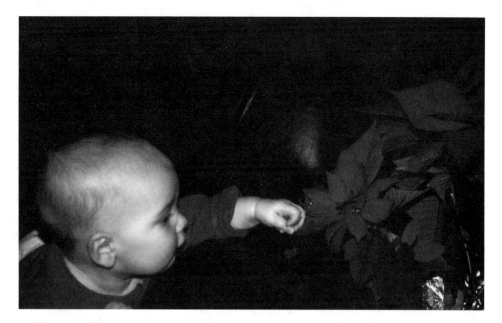

Toddlers have a high incidence of accidental poisoning.
Courtesy of Francis DeRoos, MD.

QUESTIONS

1. What is the approach and management for prehospital care of poisoned patients? How does pediatric poisoning differ from that of adults?
2. How do the patient's clinical signs and symptoms indicate the presence of a toxidrome associated with common poisonings and ingestions?

DISCUSSION

The initial management of a poisoned patient is no different from that of other patients. Airway, breathing, and circulation should be addressed first. Once the patient has been stabilized, IV access obtained, and transport to the nearest emergency department begun, a focused clinical exam should be initiated to elicit the presence of a toxidrome. A *toxidrome* is defined as the constellation of signs and symptoms typically displayed by patients with a specific type of poisoning (see Table 21-1).

Poisoned patients differ from other critically ill patients in certain key ways. One of the primary issues when approaching the management of the poisoned patient is the need for decontamination. Decontamination is essential both to rescuer safety and to abate the exposure of the patient to further toxins. The chemical should be removed from the patient's skin, clothes, and eyes using primary decontamination techniques: this includes removing the patient's clothes and irrigating the exposed area with water. Also, to avoid exposure, the health care workers must use protective equipment and provide adequate ventilation if poisonous gases or cutaneously absorbable chemicals (insecticides) are suspected.

Children are frequently unintentionally exposed to medicines or chemicals. Often children will reach for, sip, or spill a household chemical (such as a liquid or powder cleanser or bleach). The peak incidence for childhood poisoning is toddler age (between 1 and 3 years). Exposed toddlers often have ingested a single agent, often in very small quantities and without suicidal intent. Exposures to toxins are not only more common in children but also can be significantly more dangerous, with serious physiologic effects seen at relatively small exposure doses as compared to adults. Additionally, because children may not be able to verbalize their symptoms or their exposures, the prehospital provider will be instrumental in the "detective work" that is necessary to determine the cause of the illness and to establish an appropriate treatment plan. In addition to questioning household occupants and collecting possible sources of poisoning such as pill bottles, chemical containers, or space heaters, identifying the signs and symptoms that define a "toxidrome" is essential in diagnosing and treating these patients.

Vital signs (including temperature and oxygen saturation) are an important component in the focused exam of a poisoned patient. Poisons, which by definition may have serious physiologic effects, will often cause consistent changes in vital signs depending on the nature and extent of the exposure. Cardiac medicines (especially antihypertensives), narcotics, sedatives, and insecticides are ingestions that can be most lethal to children. Many of these poisonings will demonstrate classic combinations of vital sign abnormalities and symptoms that can be recognized as toxidromes (see Table 21-1).

Antidotes *may* be appropriate for use in the prehospital setting. ALS units will have different protocols and access to antidotal agents. Naloxone and atropine are universally carried ALS drugs and are effective antidotes for narcotic overdose and organophosphate poisoning, respectively. The use of antidotes in the prehospital setting is not without controversy. Remember, it is essential to address the airway, breathing, and circulation for critically ill patients prior to attempting to diagnose and treat a potential poisoning. Similarly, prehospital decontamination of the patient's gastrointestinal tract (using activated charcoal or, rarely, orogastric lavage) is also controversial. It may be best to reserve these treatments for the hospital setting because naso- and orogastric intubation may induce emesis and compromise an already tenuous airway. Prehospital use of syrup of ipecac to induce vomiting is not recommended except in rare cases. If the transit time to a hospital is expected to be prolonged, then orders for the administration of activated charcoal or the induction of vomiting with ipecac can be considered in consultation with the receiving hospital or medical direction.

RETURN TO THE CASE

Based on the patient's symptoms (change in mental status, hypotension, depressed respirations, and pinpoint pupils) you identify an opioid-type toxidrome. However, because the history pointed to a cardiac medication exposure, you also suspect a clonidine exposure. Clonidine, a centrally acting blood pressure medication, often presents with central nervous system and cardiovascular effects identical to opioid intoxication. Clonidine is available in tablets as well as transdermal patches. Full body inspection for a dermally adhered patch should be initiated if exposure to a patch is suspected. Children can develop

TABLE 21-1

TOXIDROME TYPES AND SYMPTOMS

Sympathomimetic Toxidrome

Causes: *cocaine, amphetamines, methylphenidate (Ritalin)*

- Blood pressure: elevated
- Heart rate: fast
- Respiratory rate: fast
- Body temperature: elevated
- Pupils: dilated
- Skin: moist
- Bowel sounds: hyperactive
- Behavior: restless, agitated, tremors, psychosis, and seizures

Anticholinergic Toxidrome

Causes: *antihistamines, cold preparations, scopolamine (contaminant in heroin), tricyclic antidepressants, muscle relaxants such as cyclobenzaprine (Flexeril), plants such as Jimson Weed (smoked for recreational consciousness-altering purposes)*

- Blood pressure: elevated
- Heart rate: fast
- Respiratory rate: fast
- Body temperature: elevated
- Pupils: dilated
- Skin: dry*
- Bowel sounds: diminished*
- Neuro: lethargic, blurred vision, psychosis*

*These characteristics distinguish this syndrome from Sympathomimetic toxidrome.

Anticholinesterase (or Cholinergic) Toxidrome

Causes: *organophosphate insecticides (contact or ingestion), carbamate insecticides (contact or ingestion)*

- SLUDGE
    - Salivation
    - Lacrimation (tears)
    - Urination
    - Diarrhea
    - Gastrointestinal emesis
- Bronchorrhea (fluid in airway)
- Skin: wet
- Neuro: tremors, weakness, fasciculations, coma, seizures

Opioid Toxidrome

Causes: *prescription analgesics (OxyContin, Percocet, oxycodone, morphine, methadone), illegal narcotics (heroin)*

- Blood pressure: low (rarely)
- Heart rate: slow
- Respiratory rate: slow and shallow (common)

- Pupils: pinpoint (common)
- Bowel sounds: diminished
- Neuro: depressed

Note: Clonidine overdose or poisoning may have similar symptoms, especially in children.

Sedative-Hypnotic Syndrome

Causes: *benzodiazepines (Valium, Xanax, Ativan, Klonopin, etc.), barbiturates (Seconal, etc.), ethanol*

- Blood pressure: low
- Temperature: low
- Respiratory rate: slow and shallow (common)
- Pupils: unchanged
- Neuro: depressed, slurred speech, ataxia; occasionally, paradoxical agitation

---

severe symptoms with minimal exposure to clonidine tablets or patches. Toddlers have been known to "teethe" on the patches as a means of poisoning.

Organophosphate-insecticide exposure was also considered in this case as the patient was staying on a farm and presented with bradycardia and small pupils. However, the patient's grandmother noted that this was an organic farm and no insecticides were present in the home. In the absence of any other symptoms of organophosphate poisoning (e.g., SLUDGE—see Table 21-1), you make the appropriate decision not to decontaminate the patient's skin; however, you use basic contact precautions when handling the child.

As the ambulance approaches the hospital, the patient continues to remain intermittently drowsy, but awakes with stimulation. Airway, breathing, and circulation are closely monitored throughout the transit by one paramedic who remains at the child's head. Because the patient is easily aroused with stimulation and his vital signs remain stable throughout the transit to the hospital, the decision to intubate the child's airway is deferred. Remember, it is appropriate to have a low threshold for endotracheal intubation in these patients.

After contacting medical command and identifying the child as a case of clonidine versus opioid poisoning, a trial of naloxone is agreed upon. Naloxone, an opioid antagonist, may have very limited and transient effects on alertness, respiratory efforts, heart rate, and blood pressure in clonidine poisoning when administered in high doses. But the primary clinical indication for naloxone is in opioid-intoxicated patients. The patient receives 1.0 mg of naloxone (0.1 mg/kg) by IV push and a saline flush. No changes in the patient's mental status or vital signs are noted. Supplemental oxygen and continuous cardiac and saturation monitoring are continued.

In the emergency department, oxygen monitoring is continued. A nasogastric tube is placed and activated charcoal/sorbitol administered. The pills in the box are identified as clonidine after the local poison center identifies the numbers stamped on the tablets. The boy is admitted for observation for 2 days, but remains stable in the hospital without further intervention. He returns home on day 3 with no persistent symptoms or deficits.

REFERENCES

Anderson, R. J., G. R. Hart, C. P. Crumpler, and M. J. Lerman. *"Clonidine Overdose: Report of Six Cases and Review of the Literature."* Annals of Emergency Medicine 10, no. 2 (February 1981): 107–112.

Bledsoe, Bryan E., Robert S. Porter, and Richard A. Cherry. *Medical Emergencies.* Vol. 3 of *Paramedic Care: Principles & Practice.* Chapter 8, "Toxicology and Substance Abuse." Upper Saddle River, NJ: Brady/Prentice Hall Health, Pearson Education, 2001.

Shamai A. Grossman, MD, MS

22

POST-CABG SURGERY

CASE PRESENTATION

You receive a call about a patient in a posh downtown restaurant. You arrive on the scene and find a man who appears to be in his early 50s lying on a bench with sweat pouring from his face. The patient's wife tells you he was released from the hospital this morning after having emergency bypass surgery 5 days ago, and had been feeling great. But now, his wife states, "he just doesn't look right."

As you approach the patient you find he is warm and diaphoretic, but easily aroused. As you wake him he tells you that he feels fine and wants to go home and relax after his surgery. You check his pulse and it is rapid and irregular, his blood pressure 88/50. Your partner promptly starts an 18-gauge IV and hangs a bag of saline, while you place the patient on a monitor.

The patient's wife peers over your shoulder and tells you that her husband had been complaining of palpitations, shortness of breath, and a little chest pain right after eating dinner, but notes that he was able to eat a hearty meal of beef tenderloin, spinach, and french fries.

QUESTIONS

1. What is the most likely rhythm to occur in this patient, and why does the patient have this rhythm now?
2. What are the various therapeutic options for this patient and in what scenarios would one be preferred over another?

DISCUSSION

Following coronary artery bypass graft (CABG) there are two peaks in the incidence of arrhythmias. The first occurs in the operating room, and the second between the second and fifth postoperative days. The underlying mechanisms of perioperative arrhythmias are incompletely understood, but are likely related to a combination of the effects of circulating catecholamines, alterations in autonomic nervous system tone, transient electrolyte imbalance, myocardial ischemia or infarction, and mechanical irritation of the heart.

Several factors may predispose to the development of arrhythmias, including fever, hypokalemia, hypomagnesemia, hypocalcemia, anemia, myocardial ischemia, low cardiac output and reflex increase in sympathetic tone, hypertension, pericardial inflammation, and deleterious effects of medications such as digitalis toxicity, or bradycardia induced by diltiazem.

Although atrial fibrillation (AF) is an extremely common arrhythmia following cardiac surgery, optimal management strategy has not been established. Even after prophylactic therapy with beta-blockers, transient symptomatic AF occurs in at least 25% to 30% of patients after CABG.

The two fundamental methods for treating postoperative AF in the prehospital setting are the same as those employed for other patients with rapid AF regardless of etiology.

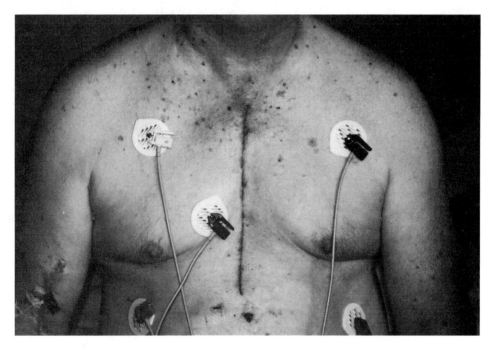

Sternal scar of the post-CABG sugery patient.
Courtesy of Kerry Reilly, PA-C.

In hemodynamically stable patients, this would be rate control with either a calcium channel blocker (e.g., 5 mg bolus of verapamil every 5 to 10 minutes for three or four doses; or 0.25–0.35 mg/kg bolus of diltiazem over a period of 2 minutes) or a beta-blocker such as metoprolol (5 mg every 5 minutes for up to three doses).

Medications eliminate the need for anesthesia (used for cardioversion), and reduce anxiety for the patient. However, in the hemodynamically unstable patient (systolic blood pressure under 90 mmHg) direct synchronized current cardioversion is the treatment of choice, starting at 50 joules (J) and utilizing Valium, Versed, or morphine sulfate for sedation, if blood pressure will tolerate it.

Supraventricular and ventricular arrhythmias are also common and can be ascribed to the same mechanisms as atrial fibrillation. Sinus bradycardia or sinus arrest may be seen postoperatively and are associated with advanced age, hypothermia, drug effects, preoperative sinus node dysfunction, intraoperative trauma to the sinus node, and postoperative elevation in vagal tone. Although new conduction defects may develop in up to 45% of patients following cardiac surgery, the majority are usually transient and related to the extensive use of cold cardioplegia, hypothermia, perioperative electrolyte shifts, or surgical trauma.

Other common postoperative complications include myocardial ischemia or infarction, pericardial effusion and tamponade, infection of both the chest incision site (i.e., the mediastinitis) and of the leg harvest site, vascular complications, renal failure, and neurologic deficits.

Cardiac ischemia frequently occurs during CABG, with a 5% to 15% chance of occurrence of perioperative myocardial infarction. Potential causes of myocardial ischemia in the perioperative period include incomplete revascularization; diffuse atherosclerotic disease of the distal coronary arteries; spasm, embolism, or thrombosis of the native coronary vessels or bypass grafts; technical problems with graft anastomoses; inadequate myocardial preservation intraoperatively; increased myocardial oxygen needs. Hemodynamic derangements in the postoperative period such as hypotension, hypertension, and tachycardia can also result in perioperative myocardial infarction.

Almost all patients have a pericardial effusion after cardiac surgery. These effusions may develop into cardiac tamponade postoperatively and must be considered in patients with diminished heart sounds, jugular-vein distension (JVD), pulsus paradoxus (inspirational changes in systolic blood pressure), or hypotension.

Postoperatively, patients may have an elevated temperature for up to 6 days. In the absence of infection, early fevers may be caused by alterations in blood components after cardiopulmonary bypass. In addition to infectious causes, fevers that occur beyond 6 days may be due to drug reactions, phlebitis at the site of intravenous lines, atelectasis, pulmonary emboli, or the postpericardiotomy syndrome. Infections of the leg wound are typically manifested by fever, induration, pain, erythema, local warmth, and drainage from the suture line.

Mediastinitis occurs in about 2% of patients who undergo median sternotomy. Most cases of mediastinitis occur within 2 weeks after sternotomy and are seen in patients with fevers greater than 101°F/38.3°C beyond the fourth postoperative day. These patients may demonstrate leukocytosis, bacteremia, and a purulent discharge from the sternal wound.

Mediastinitis should be suspected in patients who are persistently febrile late into the first week after surgery and who have no other obvious focus of infection, such as pneumonia or urinary tract infection. Risk factors for the development of mediastinitis include prolonged cardiopulmonary bypass time, excessive postoperative bleeding with reexploration for control of hemorrhage, and diminished cardiac output in the postoperative period. The incidence of mediastinitis is increased when both internal mammary arteries are mobilized bilaterally for use as bypass conduits. Therefore, many surgeons prefer to use only the left internal mammary artery, particularly in elderly diabetic patients, who may already be predisposed to delayed sternal wound healing. Definitive diagnosis requires exploration of the wound and culture of suspicious areas.

Most adults who undergo cardiac surgery, especially coronary revascularization, have atherosclerosis of the peripheral vasculature (e.g., ileofemoral system) and may experience lower extremity ischemia after surgery because of low flow in the perioperative period with in situ thrombosis, embolism from the heart or aorta, or vascular compromise from an intraaortic balloon pump catheter. Asymptomatic deep venous thrombosis of the calf can develop in about one-third to one-half of patients who receive saphenous vein bypass grafts. Occasionally, these thrombi propagate to the proximal leg veins, but rarely do they cause massive pulmonary embolism.

Most cases of acute renal failure after cardiac surgery result from renal ischemia and, if severe or prolonged, can induce acute tubular necrosis. Other causes include sepsis, nephrotoxic drugs, radiocontrast material injection, cholesterol plaque embolization in the renal circulation, increased urine-free hemoglobin levels from hemolysis while undergoing cardiopulmonary bypass, and the effects of angiotensin-converting enzyme (ACE) inhibitors on glomerular capillary pressure.

Neurological complications after cardiac surgery are common, and can include short-term memory loss, lack of concentration, and depression. More serious neurological complications such as stroke occur in 1% to 5% of patients, but some neurologic deficit may be seen in as many as 10% of patients older than 65.

RETURN TO THE CASE

The rhythm strip demonstrates atrial fibrillation with a rapid ventricular response of 170. After administering 1 mg of Versed IV, synchronized cardioversion is performed with 50 J. Subsequent rhythm strips show sinus rhythm at 80 bpm. Repeat blood pressure is 130/70. Minutes later the patient shakes your hand and says, "Thank you; you saved my life."

On arrival at the hospital, the patient is in sinus rhythm and is noted to have a temperature of 102°F/38.8°C. The sternal incision site is erythematous and purulent. After blood cultures are obtained, the patient is promptly started on IV antibiotics and taken to the operating room later that day for irrigation and debridement. The patient remains in sinus rhythm following surgery and is discharged home 2 days later after a nutrition consult and on an oral antibiotic. Blood cultures grew *Staphylococcus aureus*. Discharge diagnosis is mediastinitis with prehospital atrial fibrillation.

REFERENCES

Bledsoe, Bryan E., Robert S. Porter, and Richard A. Cherry. *Medical Emergencies*. Vol. 3 of *Paramedic Care: Principles & Practice*. Chapter 2, "Cardiology." Upper Saddle River, NJ: Brady/Prentice Hall Health, Pearson Education, 2001.

Humphries, J. O. "Unexpected Instant Death Following Successful Coronary Artery Bypass Graft Surgery (and Other Clinical Settings): Atrial Fibrillation, Quinidine, Procainamide, et cetera, and Instant Death." *Clinical Cardiology* 21 (October 1998): 711–718.

Kahn, J. K. "Caring for Patients after Coronary Bypass Surgery: Follow-up Tips for Primary Care Physicians." *Journal of Postgraduate Medicine* 93 (1993): 249.

Owen Lander, MD

23

SEIZURE

CASE PRESENTATION

Dispatch sends you and your partner to the local mall for "a seizure." You and your partner arrive to find a young female at the base of an escalator. She is supine and actively seizing, with generalized rhythmic motions of all four extremities. Primary survey shows her airway to be patent, although her jaw is clenched shut and she has a moderate amount of secretions being expressed from her mouth with respirations. Her breathing is shallow and forceful at a rate of 16–20 breaths per minute. Lungs are clear. Chest is symmetric with even rise. Her pulse is 120 by palpation of a strong radial pulse.

The patient's oxygen saturation is 89% and her blood pressure is 164/68. You complete a secondary survey while your partner administers oxygen with a nonrebreather mask and maintains in-line cervical immobilization. Your secondary survey finds a 3 cm laceration to her right temple with moderate bleeding. Her abdomen is soft and her extremities are warm and well perfused with no evident deformity or injury. On brief neurologic exam, the patient is actively seizing with rhythmic flexion/extension of all four limbs, pupils are reactive, and she is unresponsive to voice or stimulation.

Her oxygen saturation has improved to 96% with oxygen therapy. You apply a rigid cervical collar, a pressure dressing to her bleeding laceration, and logroll her onto a long board. A companion at the scene states that she has a history of seizures and rarely has them "as long as she takes her Dilantin." At this point the patient's seizure resolves, although she remains lethargic and only minimally responsive to voice. You obtain IV access and prepare for transport to the nearest emergency department which is 16 minutes away. One minute into transport, the patient begins to actively seize again.

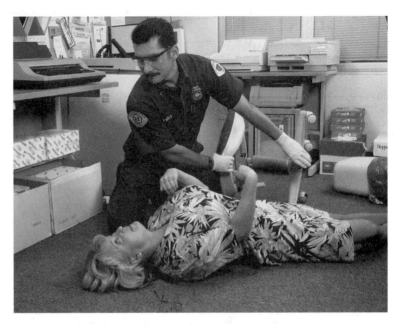

Protecting a patient from further injury during a seizure.
Courtesy of Michal Heron and Prentice Hall, Inc.

QUESTIONS

1. What are the primary prehospital concerns in treating a seizure patient?
2. What are the indications for prehospital pharmacological treatment of generalized seizures and what options are available?
3. What is the basic pathophysiology of seizures and why should they be treated emergently?

DISCUSSION

There are numerous types and gradations of seizures. They are generally categorized by whether they alter consciousness only (as in subtle "staring spells" that last only a few seconds); affect motor function only (as in simple repetitive motions of an arm or leg); or affect both motor function and consciousness. However, they are all produced by abnormal, repetitive electrical activity in the brain. The extreme form of this is the generalized tonic-clonic seizure, which reflects an "electrical storm" involving both sides of a patient's brain, producing both a loss of consciousness and generalized motor activity.

Although all new or prolonged seizures should be evaluated, the generalized form is the one which most often invokes the EMS system and requires most immediate care. Generalized seizures can either begin spontaneously or progress to such from a partial, localized seizure. More than 85% of generalized seizures terminate spontaneously in less than 2 minutes. The term *status epilepticus* (SE) refers to a patient who either sustains a prolonged seizure or has multiple seizures without a return to a normal state of consciousness. Previously, the definition of SE was a duration of 20–30 minutes. However, more recent research supports a much shorter duration of 5 minutes or longer as qualifying as SE and being an indication for treatment. This is supported by several facts. First, the vast majority of seizures are less than this in duration. Secondly, there is a direct correlation between the duration of a generalized seizure and how difficult it is to terminate. In short, the longer it lasts, the harder it is to stop. Finally, there is evidence that after a duration greater than 10–15 minutes, permanent changes may occur in the patient's brain that both alter later function and make the patient more prone to seizures in the future.

Seizures may have multiple causes. Structural lesions in the brain, traumatic injury, hypoglycemia, metabolic disturbances, hypoxia, and alcohol or sedative withdrawal can all precipitate seizures. The majority, however, have no known specific cause. Regardless of the cause, generalized seizures are treated the same way in the prehospital setting.

Special note should be made of pediatric febrile seizures. These usually occur in children less than 6 years old in the setting of a febrile illness. Most are self-limited and can be prevented by controlling the patient's temperature in the setting of illness.

After a seizure, patients typically have a depressed level of consciousness that slowly resolves over time. This is known as the postictal state. The longer and more intense the seizure, the longer the postictal state. Patients may also have a residual specific motor deficit after a seizure, which is known as Todd's paralysis. In the prehospital setting it can be difficult to distinguish this from a stroke, particularly if the seizure is unwitnessed. Patients who suffer generalized seizures are frequently incontinent of urine and stool. These signs should be specifically looked for or inquired about when evaluating a patient with altered mental status or focal motor deficit.

Specific concerns regarding generalized seizures in the prehospital setting include the following:

1. If there is any possibility of associated trauma, either as a precipitating cause or consequence of the seizure, the patient must be treated with standard traumatic precautions including cervical spine and long board protection of the spinal column. Patients may also suffer direct trauma from the strength of muscle contractions such as posterior shoulder dislocations, falls, oral trauma, and traumatic injury from surrounding objects.

2. Respiratory compromise is a concern. Most patients will maintain adequate oxygenation, particularly if the seizure is less than 2 to 4 minutes in duration. However, blood from oral trauma, secretions, and hypoventilation from inadequate respiratory effort during a generalized seizure may all contribute to respiratory compromise.

3. It is extremely helpful to subsequent care to ask companions or family members about seizure history and current medications.

TREATMENT

All actively seizing patients should receive general supportive care including moving furniture and potentially harmful objects away from the patient, suctioning the airway, and providing supplemental oxygen. IV access should be obtained as feasible, but transport should not be significantly delayed for this purpose. Overly aggressive attempts to suction the airway, place oral airways, or insert "bite blocks" should be avoided in the setting of severely clenched jaws. Doing so frequently results in intraoral or dental trauma, which can lead to worsening airway compromise.

Because sustained seizure activity almost always results in airway or respiratory compromise, treatment should primarily be directed at controlling the seizure. However, all the usual indications for intubation apply. These include frank respiratory failure, postseizure obtundation and inability to protect the airway, as well as the rare case of significant respiratory depression following the successful pharmacological treatment of seizures. It is critical to note that if a patient is intubated using RSI (rapid sequence intubation) protocols, continued cortical electrical seizure activity will be masked by the use of a paralytic agent.

Indications for pharmacological treatment of generalized seizures include (1) respiratory compromise or hypoxia; and (2) status epilepticus, as defined by sustained seizure activity of longer than 5 minutes, or multiple seizures without an intervening return to normal cognitive activity.

Benzodiazapines are the initial treatment of choice for all types of sustained seizures in the prehospital setting. The particular drug and route of administration will be dictated by local medical treatment protocol, but a general discussion of the three most common agents follows.

Diazepam—May be administered intravenously, orally, or rectally. Oral routes are generally not feasible in seizing patients secondary to airway concerns. A rectal gel formulation of diazepam (Diastat, 0.2–0.5 mg/kg) is extremely effective and does not require intravenous access which can be difficult to obtain in an actively seizing patient, particularly a child. If intravenous access is present, this route is even more effective. However, it does carry a slightly higher risk of subsequent respiratory suppression. The dose is 0.1–0.3 mg/kg. It is also less effective at preventing subsequent seizures due to the pharmacokinectics of intravenous versus rectal absorption. Of note, this drug may be administered via an endotracheal tube as well.

Lorazepam—This drug has been a standard in emergency department therapy of SE. Like diazepam, it may be administered intravenously, rectally, or orally (0.1 mg/kg). It has a longer duration of action than diazepam, and is associated with a lower incidence of respiratory suppression. However, it has not been as well studied as diazepam in the prehospital setting and is less commonly available. Its use is limited in the prehospital setting by the need for refrigeration. One randomized trial comparing lorazepam (2 mg) versus diazepam (5 mg) intravenously versus placebo in the prehospital setting for seizures longer than 5 minutes found a success rate of 55%, 43%, and 21%, respectively. The rates of respiratory or circulatory compromise were 10.6% (lorazepam), 10.3% (diazepam), and 22.5% (placebo). Although this is only one such study, it suggests that withholding benzodiazepine therapy for concern of respiratory suppression is not justified.

Midazolam—This is a unique benzodiazepine in that it is water soluble, and may be administered intramuscularly as well as by the intravenous, sublingual, and intranasal routes. A prospective emergency department study found intramuscular midazolam (0.15–0.30 mg/kg) to be as effective as intravenous lorazepam in the termination of seizure activity with no increase in side effects. The intramuscular route is attractive given the frequent difficulty in obtaining intravenous access in the seizing patient and social concerns over rectal administration. Another prospective study found that liquid midazolam (10 mg) applied to the buccal surface was 75% effective versus 59% with rectal diazepam. However, there have been no formal studies of this drug in the prehospital setting for status epilepticus.

In summary, benzodiazepines are the standard of care for status epilepticus. All three formulations and the different routes of administration discussed above are effective. The particular choice of agent and route will be dictated by clinical circumstances and local protocol. Regardless of the agent and route, it is imperative to be prepared for respiratory suppression and the need for respiratory support, including intubation, prior to the administration of these agents.

KEY POINTS

1. The need for primary protection of airway, breathing, and circulation is the same in the seizing patient as in others.
2. Provide general support and supplemental oxygen, and protect the seizing patient from further harm to herself.
3. Always consider prior and subsequent traumatic injuries in the seizure patient and treat appropriately.
4. Generalized seizures that are causing respiratory compromise, last longer than 5 minutes, or recur require urgent attempts at pharmacological therapy without delaying transport.
5. Always consider a postictal state for a patient with altered mental status and unknown history.

RETURN TO THE CASE

The patient's oxygen saturation falls to 88% on full nonrebreather support and she is actively seizing. You administer 0.2 mg/kg of diazepam. The patient's seizure resolves in 2 minutes. She continues to breathe spontaneously at a rate of 14/min and maintains her airway with an oxygen saturation of 96%. Upon arrival at the emergency room, the patient's phenytoin level is found to be markedly subtherapeutic. She is loaded with an IV dose of phenytoin. Her laceration is repaired, and subsequent evaluation reveals no other significant injury. She returns to a normal mental status after a period of observation. Further history reveals that she had "run out" of her medication 3 days prior. The patient is given her normal oral dose in the emergency department and is discharged to home with a prescription for oral phenytoin and a follow-up appointment with her neurologist the next day.

REFERENCES

Alldredge B. K., A. M. Gelb, S. M. Isaacs, M. D. Corry, N. O'Neil, M. D. Gottwald, S. K. Ulrich, J. M. Neuhaus, M. R. Segal, and D. H. Lowenstein. "A Comparison of Lorazepam, Diazepam, and Placebo for the Treatment of Out-of-Hospital Status Epilepticus." *New England Journal of Medicine* 345 (2001): 631–637.

Bledsoe, Bryan E., Robert S. Porter, and Richard A. Cherry. *Medical Emergencies* Vol. 3 of *Paramedic Care: Principles & Practice*. Chapter 3, "Neurology." Upper Saddle River, NJ: Brady/Prentice Hall Health, Pearson Education, 2001.

Smith, B. "Epilepsy: Treatment of Status Epilepticus." *Neurologic Clinics* 19, no. 2 (May 2001).

Warden, C. R., J. Zibulewsky, S. Mace, C. Gold, and M. Gausche-Hill. "Evaluation and Management of Febrile Seizures in the Out-of-Hospital and Emergency Department Settings." *Annals of Emergency Medicine* 41, no. 2 (February 2003).

Roger D. White, MD, FACC

24

SUDDEN-ONSET TACHYCARDIA

CASE PRESENTATION

Transport team paramedics are called to attend a 26-year-old male who had experienced sudden onset of a "fast heart rate" accompanied by a mild substernal tightness. The tachycardia began several hours earlier and because it persisted the patient went to a community hospital where he was given IV diltiazem 20 mg, then 30 mg, without effect. EMS was then called by the community hospital to transfer the patient to another medical care facility. Upon EMS arrival, the patient is noted to be alert and oriented and still describes the same discomfort in the chest and the sensation that his heart is "racing." He has no known medical history, is on no medications, and has no allergies. He had a similar episode about 1 month prior to this event with similar chest tightness and lightheadedness. After about 30 minutes it resolved spontaneously.

Physical examination is completely normal except for the very fast heart rate. The systemic blood pressure is 118 mmHg by palpation. A 3-lead ECG monitor is attached and reveals the cardiac rhythm shown in Figures 24-1 and 24-2.

QUESTIONS

1. How would you describe the rhythm shown in Figures 24-1 and 24-2 in terms of rate, regularity, and QRS morphology?
2. What is the likely origin of the normal-appearing QRS complex seen in Figure 24-2?
3. What is the probable diagnosis?
4. What syndrome should be considered in the diagnosis in this setting?
5. What therapy is appropriate, and what therapy might lead to serious problems?

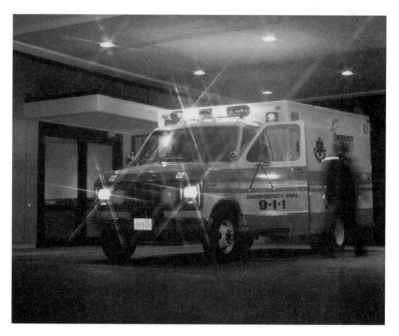

Interfacility transfer of a patient with uncontrolled tachycardia.
Courtesy of Corbis Digital Stock.

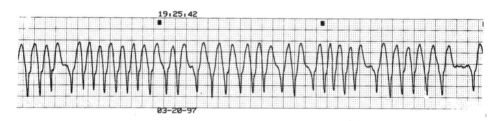

Figure 24-1 Initial ECG rhythm strip.
Courtesy of Roger D. White, MD.

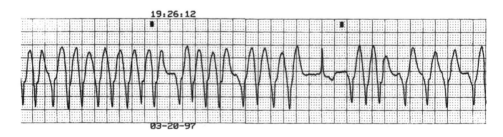

Figure 24-2 Initial ECG rhythm strip (cont'd).
Courtesy of Roger D. White, MD.

DISCUSSION

This patient presents challenging problems both diagnostically and therapeutically. Fortunately, despite the very rapid rate, the patient is hemodynamically stable and complaining of very minimal symptoms. This most likely is related to the fact that he is young and has no underlying structural heart disease with ventricular dysfunction that would lead to hemodynamic intolerance of such a rapid tachycardia. The challenge, then, is to attempt to make a diagnosis of the tachycardia and consider which therapy might be both safe and effective if intervention is needed.

A close inspection of the ECG in Figures 24-1 and 24-2 is revealing. The tachycardia is noted to be very rapid, approximately 220–230 bpm, and irregular. The QRS complex is variably widened from beat to beat. Toward the end of the tracing in Figure 24-1, baseline undulations are noted. In Figure 24-2, along with the other QRS features noted in Figure 24-1, a normal-appearing QRS complex makes a brief, "cameolike" appearance on the ECG stage, then departs. The irregularly irregular appearance of the tachycardia, along with the baseline undulations (which are fibrillatory waves) leads to a diagnosis of atrial fibrillation (AF) with rapid ventricular response. Left to be explained, however, are the variably widened QRS complexes and the totally normal QRS complex in Figure 24-2. Both of these are strongly suggestive of the presence of an accessory pathway for atrioventricular conduction. The variability in the QRS morphology from beat to beat represents variable conduction through the accessory pathway and AV anteriovenous node, and the normal QRS complex reflects conduction exclusively through the AV node.

The differential diagnosis here might include paroxysmal AF with aberrant conduction. The variability in QRS morphology and the isolated normal QRS complex would make that diagnosis less likely, however. One might consider ventricular tachycardia also; the normal QRS complex might lead one to interpret this as a capture beat, but fusion/capture beats occur early in the R-R cycle, when the supraventricular complex is able to capture the ventricle before the ectopic ventricular focus does so. This complex does not demonstrate early activation. Although ventricular tachycardia can be irregular, it is uncommon and would be very unlikely to demonstrate such beat-to-beat variation in QRS morphology and yet remain monomorphic. Collectively, all of the ECG characteristics observed here are suggestive of the presence of an accessory pathway, as in Wolff-Parkinson-White (WPW) syndrome.

In the absence of a history of WPW syndrome, the diagnosis of AF with rapid antero-grade conduction through the accessory pathway should be suspected when ECG features such as those seen here are present. The most common tachyarrhythmia in patients with this syndrome is orthodromic (propagation of the electrical impulse in the normal physiologic direction) AV reciprocating tachycardia, which is the typical very fast, regular, narrow-complex tachycardia, usually without visible atrial activity. These tachycardias conduct antegradely into the ventricles through the AV nodal pathway. Antidromic (reverse propagation of the electrical impulse) AV reciprocating tachycardia occurs much less commonly, and is characterized by wide QRS complexes occurring at a regular rapid rate. The wide QRS complex results from conduction antegradely into the ventricles through the accessory pathway. Antidromic tachycardia can be very difficult to differentiate from ventricular tachycardia.

Atrial fibrillation is the tachycardia of greatest concern in the presence of WPW syndrome because of the risk of degeneration into ventricular fibrillation if conduction into the ventricles through the accessory pathway is very rapid. This is likely to occur when the refractory period of the accessory pathway is very short, permitting ventricular rates of 250 bpm or greater.

In hemodynamically stable patients who are asymptomatic or only minimally symptomatic, as in this case, no urgent treatment is needed and such patients can be transported with continuous observation for any changes in the cardiac rate or rhythm.

Drug therapy can be problematic, because any drug that possesses AV nodal blocking properties can result in an acceleration of the ventricular response and the risk of rapid degeneration into ventricular fibrillation. Several case reports of this often fatal transition appeared after the introduction of verapamil for clinical use. Calcium channel blockers such as diltiazem and beta-blocking drugs such as esmolol are contraindicated. Even though the AV nodal blocking actions of adenosine are short-lived, adenosine is best avoided in this situation as well. Though apparently rare, both alarming acceleration of the ventricular rate and ventricular fibrillation have been reported after administration of adenosine to patients with WPW syndrome in atrial fibrillation with rapid ventricular response. In fact, only procainamide and amiodarone are safe and effective drugs for intravenous administration in this setting. If urgent intervention is required for hemodynamic or symptomatic reasons, cardioversion, rather than drug therapy, is the treatment of choice. Otherwise, it is reasonable to transport and monitor for any rhythm changes.

RETURN TO THE CASE

Prior to initiating the interfacility transport, the transport paramedics consult their medical control physician who recommends that 6 mg adenosine be administered. The attending emergency physician at the community hospital concurs with a trial of adenosine to see if it affects the tachycardia. The drug is injected rapidly with no change observed on the monitor. The patient is then transferred to a university medical center hospital, where the 12-lead ECG shown in Figure 24-3 is obtained. This ECG supports the diagnosis of atrial fibrillation with antegrade conduction over an accessory pathway, consistent with what was seen initially. The patient is electively cardioverted, after which the 12-lead ECG reveals the typical features of WPW syndrome, with a short PR interval and an obvious delta wave (Figure 24-4). The patient undergoes an electrophysiologic study that confirms the presence of an atrioventricular accessory pathway with both anterograde and retrograde conduction properties. This pathway is ablated and the subsequent 12-lead ECG shows a normal PR interval and absence of the previous delta wave.

In retrospect, given the ECG evidence available, atrial fibrillation with rapid ventricular response over an accessory pathway might have been strongly considered and adenosine avoided. Likewise, at the community hospital, diltiazem also would not have been used. Fortunately, in this patient, there were no adverse effects despite the inherent risk. The patient was not a candidate for emergent cardioversion, and there was no urgency to initiate additional pharmacologic therapy.

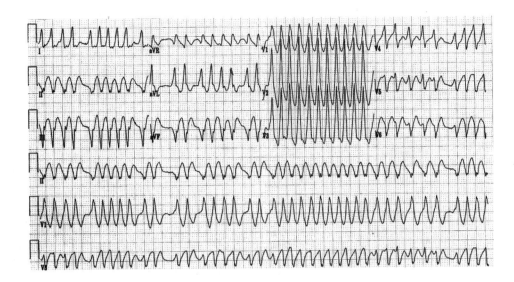

Figure 24-3 ECG upon arrival at university medical center is consistent with atrial fibillation.
Courtesy of Roger D. White, MD.

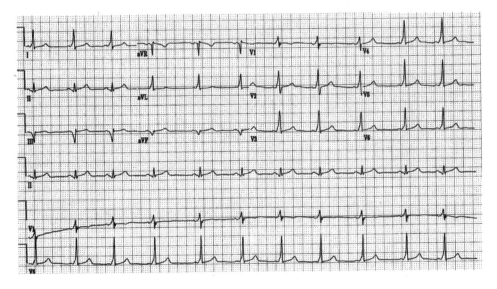

Figure 24-4 ECG after cardioversion shows Wolfe-Parkinson-White (WPW) syndrome. Note short PR interval and delta waves.
Courtesy of Roger D. White, MD.

25

Steve Larson, MD

SYNCOPE

CASE PRESENTATION

You and your partner are returning to the station following a run to the local hospital. As you pass the town park, a young woman flags you down. She excitedly points to a nearby crowd that has gathered around a figure lying on the ground. You stop your rig, get out, and approach the crowd to assess the situation.

On the ground you discover an elderly female resting against the curb. She appears dazed, but makes purposeful movements as she attempts to sit upright. There is a visible abrasion to her forehead and the bridge of her nose. She seems to favor her right shoulder. As you kneel down beside her, you overhear voices in the crowd describing the incident. A witness describes the patient as falling from a standing position, although it is unclear whether she tripped on the uneven curb. The patient made no effort to protect herself as she fell, thereby striking her face and upper torso against the curb. There was a loss of consciousness for approximately 1 minute and seizure-like activity described by the witness as a jerking movement of her body that lasted several seconds. The patient was incontinent of urine. As she regained consciousness, she appeared to answer questions slowly, but appropriately.

You proceed with your primary survey, noting a patent airway with unlabored, spontaneous breathing and a respiratory rate of 16. The patient's heart rate is 96 and there is good capillary refill with bounding peripheral pulses. She has bilateral breath sounds on auscultation and a cardiac exam that is unrevealing. She favors her right shoulder but moves all four extremities on command. Other than the visible facial trauma, she has no other evidence of trauma.

You convince the patient to remain supine while you complete your evaluation. You confirm a blood pressure of 145/90 and sinus rhythm on the monitor. Her pulse oximeter reads 98%. Her finger stick is 143.

As you near the end of your evaluation, an individual steps from the crowd and introduces herself as the patient's daughter. Following a discussion with the patient, the daughter announces that her mother is okay and that she has just had another "spell." Apparently

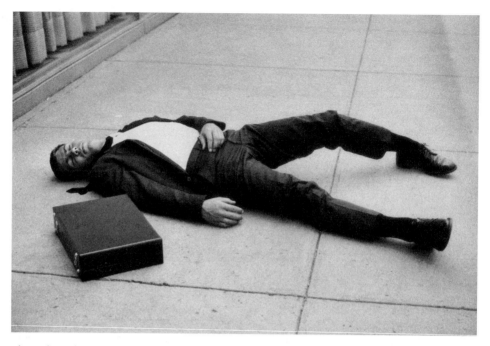

The etiology of syncope can be difficult to ascertain, particularly in the field.
Courtesy of Getty Images–Image Bank and Archive Holdings, Inc.

the patient, who is a diabetic, had taken her insulin earlier that day and not eaten her lunch. The daughter reports recent similar falls that she attributes to "low" sugars. "I'll be okay," the patient offers. "I will contact my family doctor and let him know to check up on my sugars."

You are clearly uncomfortable with this clinical scenario. Your gut instinct tells you something is wrong, but the patient's family appears unconvinced and does not wish to stay for further evaluation.

QUESTIONS

1. Why should this patient and her family be concerned about her unexplained fall?
2. What immediate management concerns should you address?

DISCUSSION

This patient's presentation is typical of syncope. Syncope is defined as the sudden loss of consciousness associated with loss of postural tone. It represents the final clinical pathway for a wide range of pathophysiologic processes ranging from cardiac disease to seizures to dehydration (see Table 25-1). Oftentimes, the etiology of syncope can be difficult to ascertain, particularly in the field. The morbidity and mortality associated with syncope is in part related

TABLE 25-1

CAUSES OF SYNCOPE

Cardiac:
>   Ischemic heart disease
>   Valvular heart disease
>   Arrhythmias

Neurologic:
>   Seizures
>   Subarachnoid hemorrhage
>   Cerebral ischemia

Vasovagal

Orthostatic hypotension
>   Dehydration
>   Blood loss
>   Autonomic insufficiency

Medications

Psychiatric

Miscellaneous

to the underlying cause. Formulating a worst-case scenario upon initial contact with a patient with possible syncope is the best way to avoid minimizing the symptoms and events.

Syncope that is the result of a primary cardiac cause is a particularly ominous event associated with a high subsequent one-year mortality rate and warrants clear consideration for a detailed hospital evaluation. Cardiac causes of syncope include rhythm disturbances, valvular disease, and ischemic heart disease. Cardiac syncope is typically abrupt in onset. Patients who survive the initial event often have rapid resolution of their symptoms. There may be myoclonic motor activity erroneously interpreted by witnesses as a seizure. Patients are not postictal with cardiac syncope. Underlying cardiac risk factors for ischemic heart disease (age, gender, family history, tobacco use, hypertension, elevated cholesterol, and diabetes) may be important clues to the presence of an occult cardiac process. Additionally, a history of chest pain, shortness of breath, or palpitations should raise concern for syncope secondary to heart disease. Concern for a cardiac cause of syncope should be raised in all individuals over the age of 45, particularly with a history of coronary artery disease, congestive heart failure, or valvular heart disease.

Seizures are a frequent neurologic cause of syncope. Patients with seizure-related syncope demonstrate confusion or disorientation with a slow return to their baseline mental status that is defined as the postictal phase. Witnesses frequently describe generalized tonic-clonic motor activity; however, genuine seizure activity can be difficult to distinguish from the myoclonic motor activity seen with cardiac syncope. Syncope may rarely be related with cerebral ischemia or transient ischemic attacks, particularly when they involve the posterior (vertebrobasilar) circulation of the brain responsible for providing blood flow to the reticular activating system. Ataxia (unsteady gait), diplopia (double vision), and speech disturbances may indicate underlying vertebrobasilar insufficiency. An acute subarachnoid hemorrhage may also present with the sudden loss of consciousness, but it is frequently associated with headache, nausea, and nuchal rigidity.

The most common cause of syncope is vasovagal syncope. The classic example of this form of syncope is the individual who passes out at the sight of blood. Stress, fear, pain, or injury may precipitate vasovagal syncope. Susceptible individuals develop paradoxical nausea, pallor, hypotension, and bradycardia in the setting of increased sympathetic activity.

Orthostatic hypotension may also be a cause of syncope. This may be encountered in situations of profound volume loss, such as in the setting of an acute bleed or severe dehydration. It can also be seen with patients on a variety of antihypertensives ranging from beta-blockers to diuretics. These medications may either blunt the body's response to position changes or predispose the patient to volume depletion. Diabetics or patients with peripheral neuropathies may also demonstrate an impaired ability to regulate autonomic function, manifested by orthostatic hypotension.

A variety of drugs (including antiarrhythmics and antidepressants) may precipitate syncope through the development of arrhythmias. Finally, other miscellaneous causes for syncope include hypoglycemia, hyperventilation, and psychiatric illnesses.

The prehospital management of syncope involves close attention to the ABCs of resuscitation. Elderly people, in particular, are vulnerable to falls and subsequent trauma. In this patient, the presence of visible head and upper torso trauma mandates close attention to cervical spine stabilization as a part of the initial ABCs. This patient should be placed on a long board and collared to protect from possible C-spine injury. As you establish the patency of her airway and the presence of adequate circulation, keep in mind the possibility of an occult cardiac process precipitating the event. All patients suspected of syncope should be placed on a cardiac monitor and have intravenous access established. If available, pulse oximetry and a finger stick blood sugar should be documented. Supplemental oxygen via nasal cannula also may be applied.

In spite of the fact that the patient now appears at baseline, the underlying cause of her syncopal episode remains undefined. In the setting of her age, cardiac risks, and visible inability to protect herself from the fall, this patient is at risk for a bad outcome. Prompt transfer should be performed without delay. Although often an inconvenience for patient and family, unexplained syncope must be evaluated further in an emergency department setting. Understanding the pathophysiology and the potential life-threatening causes of syncope enables you to ensure that the family and patient make a well-informed decision regarding further care.

RETURN TO THE CASE

With much convincing, the patient's family reluctantly agrees to an evaluation in the local emergency department. Enroute to the hospital she remains asymptomatic. On arrival in the emergency department the patient has a blood pressure of 148/96; her monitor demonstrates sinus rhythm. An ECG obtained on arrival to the department indicates normal sinus rhythm without evidence of active ischemia. She has no additional complaints. Following her initial evaluation in the emergency department, the superficial facial injuries are cleaned and dressed. While awaiting x-rays of her right shoulder, the sudden appearance of a high-grade AV block is picked up on the cardiac monitor. The patient's blood pressure drops markedly and she becomes symptomatic, requiring external pacemaker placement. She is stabilized in the emergency department and subsequently admitted to the CCU where she is ruled out for a myocardial infarction. Later in the day she has a permanent pacemaker placed and undergoes an uneventful hospital stay. She is discharged home 2 days later.

REFERENCES

Bledsoe, Bryan E., Robert S. Porter, and Richard A. Cherry. *Medical Emergencies*. Vol. 3 of *Paramedic Care: Principles & Practice*, Chapter 3, "Neurology." Upper Saddle River, NJ: Brady/Prentice Hall Health, Pearson Education, 2001.

Kapoor, W. "Evaluation and Management of the Patient with Syncope." *Journal of the American Medical Association* 18 (1992): 2553.

Linzer, Mark, Eric H. Yang, N. A. Mark Estes III, Paul Wang, Vicken R. Vorperian, and Wishwa N. Kapoor. "Clinical Guideline: Diagnosing Syncope." *Annals of Internal Medicine* 126 (June 1997): 989–996.

PART 2

TRAUMA AND SURGICAL EMERGENCIES

Thomas Rahilly, PhD, EMT-CC

26

AMPUTATION

CASE PRESENTATION

You are assigned to an ambulance in a suburban town during its annual 2-day street festival. At approximately 9:30 P.M. when all of the first day's activities have concluded, you receive a call for a motorcycle accident on one of the winding roads that lead out of the town. Approximately one mile from town you encounter the accident scene and observe that two police officers are already on scene motioning the ambulance for immediate assistance.

As you approach the police officers you notice a badly damaged motorcycle lying at the side of the road. There is no fire or any other apparent threat to the safety of you or your partner. One officer is providing in-line stabilization for the accident victim. The second officer tells you that the motorcyclist apparently failed to negotiate a curve in the road and sideswiped a utility pole. He will ensure that vehicle traffic is not an issue for you and your patient. A fire-rescue unit has also been requested to respond.

The initial assessment of the patient reveals that he is conscious and is experiencing a great deal of pain. He is lying supine in the road with his helmet on, his airway is patent, and the officer has control of the cervical spine. The patient's breathing is regular, although shallow and labored. He has obvious blunt trauma to his right chest. Your partner begins administration of oxygen via nonrebreather mask at 12 L/min. His pulse is regular but weak and there is external hemorrhage at the site of a traumatic amputation of the right leg just below the knee. Direct pressure is applied to the amputation site over a large trauma dressing. This maneuver controls the bleeding. Vital signs are obtained and pulse is 126 bpm, respirations are 26 and shallow, blood pressure is 94 by palpation. The patient is alert and oriented to person, place, and time; pupils are round and reactive to light. His upper and left lower extremities are neurologically intact with weak peripheral pulses. Further examination of the patient reveals soft-tissue trauma to the right shoulder and arm.

At the completion of the initial assessment, you and your partner perform a helmet removal and apply a cervical collar to the patient. The police officer maintains C-spine stabilization.

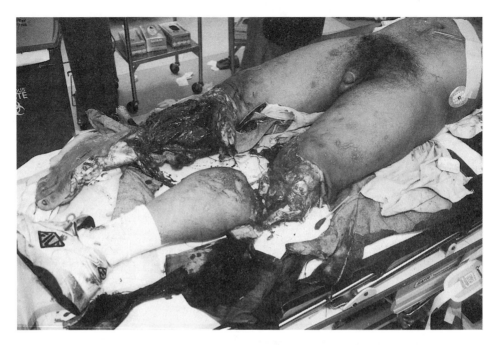

Lower extremity amputations.
Courtesy of Edward T. Dickinson, MD.

Your partner informs you that he contacted dispatch for a medical helicopter, but the only helicopter in service at this time is on an assignment and its ETA is 30 minutes to your location.

A fire-rescue crew is now on scene and advises you that they have located the severed leg of the patient.

The patient is placed on a backboard and a large-bore IV is established.

QUESTIONS

1. What are the on-scene priorities for this patient?
2. How will the transport decision affect this patient both short and long term?

DISCUSSION

Amputation is the severance, removal, or detachment, either partial or complete, of a body part. Although infrequently seen by paramedics, traumatic amputations are some of the most unnerving injuries they may encounter. Whereas the amputation site often draws a great deal of attention, the patient who suffers a traumatic amputation often will be a multisystem trauma patient and have other, possibly more severe injuries that may not be as obvious. Although care of the amputation site and the part that has been amputated are important considerations for the paramedic, the patient must be systematically evaluated and treated for all associated injuries and illnesses. For example, a person with an amputated foot and a pelvic fracture may be more at risk for hypovolemia from the pelvic injury than that of the extremity. EMS providers must not be distracted by the graphic nature of the injury to the point of neglecting the patient's other more immediate needs.

Effective trauma care requires the paramedic to perform a full trauma assessment to determine the patient's condition and to provide treatment for life-threatening injuries as they are discovered. The ABCs of patient care must always be performed to detect immediate threats to life and to begin the process of trauma resuscitation. Upon completion of the initial assessment a transport decision must be made whether to resuscitate on scene or en route to the medical facility. A transport decision tool such as the CUPS (for critical, unstable, potentially unstable, stable) classification system is useful for making these decisions. Some EMS systems also require that a trauma score be calculated to help make appropriate transport destination decisions. The paramedic must always be mindful of the time spent on scene and the goal of using no more than the "Platinum Ten" minutes before initiating transport.

Traumatic amputations are most commonly seen in patients between 20 and 40 years old. Males are four times more likely to experience a traumatic amputation than are females. The digits, lower leg, hand and forearm, and the distal portion of the foot are the parts of the body most frequently amputated. These injuries are commonly associated with occupational trauma, especially in workers who operate power tools and machinery, and with motor vehicle crashes. Farm workers are quite susceptible to traumatic amputation. The force required to cause a body part to be amputated is capable of causing multisystem trauma.

Although significant hemorrhage is a serious potential complication of traumatic amputation, the arteries of the injured body part usually retract and bleeding is not as great as one might expect. To control any bleeding that is present, direct pressure over the bleeding stump is generally sufficient. A tourniquet is rarely necessary and can cause additional trauma to the limb. The stump should be covered with a sterile trauma dressing and monitored carefully for resumption of bleeding.

Recovery and care of the amputated part is an important component of the paramedic's overall treatment of the amputation patient. This task, however, should be accomplished coincidentally with care for the patient and should not detract from resuscitative efforts. As soon as possible, the amputated part should be rinsed with sterile saline solution to remove any gross contamination, wrapped in sterile dressings, and placed in a plastic bag. The wetting of the dressing is controversial; therefore, local protocol should be followed. The plastic bag should be placed on crushed ice and transported with the patient. This two-layer method avoids direct contact between the part and the ice. The purpose of cooling the part is to preserve the tissue and prevent decomposition. One hour of warm ischemia is equal to about 6 hours of cool ischemia. Do not place the severed part directly on the ice or use dry ice or other chemical additives. Freezing of the part may cause powerful enzymes to escape from ruptured lysosome sacs and damage the healthy tissue that will be necessary for a replantation attempt.

If the severed part cannot be located or prepared for transport when the patient is ready for transport, the part should be packaged and sent to the same hospital as the patient by other emergency workers. If the amputated part is not located prior to transport to the hospital, law enforcement and rescue personnel should institute a search for the part. Regardless of the condition of the amputated part, it is imperative that it be retrieved and brought to the patient. Even if replantation is not possible, the tissue of the amputated part may be useful for grafting of skin, bone, or blood vessels.

The replantation of severed body parts has improved greatly with the development of the operating microscope in the early 1960s. Microsurgical techniques now offer traumatic amputation victims the opportunity of having a severed body part or limb successfully replanted. Therefore, it is important to these patients that the paramedic make the most appropriate transport decision. Although the survival of the patient takes precedence over the replantation of a severed body part, the microsurgical capabilities of the receiving facility should be considered before the paramedic makes a transport decision. When in doubt, the patient should always be transported to the closest, most appropriate hospital to ensure his survival, preferably a level I trauma center. If replantation is possible after the critically injured patient is successfully resuscitated, the patient may be transferred or a specially trained surgical team brought in.

Psychological care of the traumatic amputation patient is also a concern of the paramedic. The patient may or may not know that the amputation has occurred because a phenomenon known as "phantom pain" may give the patient a false sensation that the limb is still intact. In most cases the paramedic should avoid telling the patient that a body part has been amputated. It is often best left to the emergency physician and hospital staff who are better able to deal with the psychological trauma that almost certainly will follow. In all cases, however, the paramedic should reassure the patient that he is receiving the best care possible and that he is being transported to a medical facility that is capable of providing a high level of continuing care. Informing a patient not to worry because the amputated part will be replanted is never appropriate. Determining the viability of a replant attempt is far beyond the scope of the ALS provider and may only raise false hopes for the patient.

RETURN TO THE CASE

The paramedic calculates the patient's revised trauma score to be 12. Because this patient is considered to be unstable (U on the CUPS scale) the decision is made to begin transport and continue the trauma resuscitation en route. When notified by the fire-rescue personnel that the severed limb has been found, the paramedic directs one of the EMTs to prepare the severed limb for transport. The leg had been badly crushed and was lying in the dirt beside the roadway so the EMT rinses it with saline solution and wraps it in a dry, sterile multitrauma dressing before placing it in a large plastic bag.

The patient is placed in the ambulance for transport to the trauma center. In this case, the helicopter ETA is too great for the condition of the patient and medical dispatch is notified to cancel the request for its response. Because there are two trauma centers with relatively the same transport time, it is decided to transport the patient to the level I trauma center approximately 5 minutes farther from the scene than the level II center. ETA to the level I trauma center is 15 minutes or less.

The on-scene fire-rescue unit makes a call to its station with a request for crushed ice and a large container in which the severed leg can be placed during transport to the trauma center. When the ambulance passes the station en route to the trauma center, the ice will be obtained and the severed leg will be placed in the container to cool and preserve it.

As the patient is placed in the ambulance, a second large-bore IV is established, and a focused assessment is performed en route to the trauma center. The patient is still conscious and complaining of pain to the right side of his body. The focused assessment reveals contusions around several ribs and a swollen deformity of the right forearm. The paramedic splints the forearm and encourages the patient to take full breaths. The pulse oximetry reading for this patient is 96% on a nonrebreather mask, so assisted ventilation is not performed. The patient is closely monitored during transport to the trauma center. Upon admission to the emergency department, the patient receives further trauma resuscitation, starts on antibiotics, and is evaluated for replantation of the amputated leg. After surgical consultation, it is decided that the stump of the tibia is too short and too badly damaged to permit replantation of the leg. The patient is stabilized and then brought to the operating suite where the leg is surgically amputated above the knee. He is released from the hospital a week later and begins rehabilitation. Eventually, the patient is fitted with a prosthesis and otherwise completely recovers from the incident.

REFERENCES

Bledsoe, Bryan E., Robert S. Porter, and Richard A. Cherry. *Trauma Emergencies*. Vol. 4 of *Paramedic Care: Principles & Practice*. Chapter 5, "Soft-Tissue Trauma." Upper Saddle River, NJ: Brady/Prentice Hall Health, Pearson Education, 2001.

Langdorf, M. "Replantation." *eMedicine Journal* 2, no. 5 (2001): 2–5. Available at http://www.emedicine.com.

Owen M. Lander, MD
Carlo L. Rosen, MD

27

BLUNT CHEST TRAUMA

CASE PRESENTATION

You are called to a construction site for a worker who has fallen 15 feet onto firmly packed soil. Assessing the scene for safety, you and your partner notice no clear hazards in the area or overhead. You find the patient supine on the ground 10 feet from the base of the building, surrounded by several coworkers. Your initial survey reveals a man in his late 20s, with no obvious extremity deformity or open wounds. He is responsive to voice only. Your primary survey reveals sonorous spontaneous respirations at a rate of 6 per minute. A jaw thrust with in-line stabilization corrects the sonorous respirations and reveals an oropharynx with secretions but no blood in the airway. The patient has decreased breath sounds on the left and tenderness over the left lateral chest wall (evidenced by groaning to palpation) with deformity at the level of ribs six through nine. Radial pulses are strong bilaterally at a rate of 76. Your partner begins BVM ventilations with 100% oxygen and cricoid pressure. You immobilize the patient and obtain IV access. A brief neurological assessment reveals that the patient opens eyes to command, has equal and reactive pupils, and is spontaneously moving all extremities. The patient has a respiratory rate of 12 (by BVM), a heart rate of 80, a blood pressure of 138/64, and an oxygen saturation of 95%.

Because of the continued compromise of the patient's airway due to secretions, you elect to intubate the patient for definitive airway control prior to transport. Orotracheal intubation with in-line stabilization is performed using facilitated intubation with midazolam (see Case 15 on facilitated intubation). Endotracheal tube placement is confirmed with end-tidal capnography. Breath sounds are present on the right, but absent on the left. Now there is subcutaneous air palpable in the left chest wall and increased airway resistance with bagging. The oxygen saturation has dropped to 88% despite intubation and ventilation with 100% oxygen. Reassessment shows the endotracheal tube to be at 22 cm, a heart rate of 110, and blood pressure of 80 by palpation.

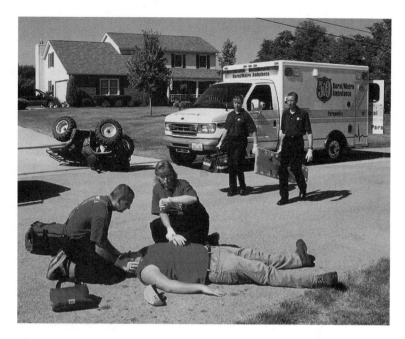

Chest injuries are common to blunt trauma mechanisms such as ATV and motor vehicle crashes and falls from heights.

QUESTIONS

1. What are the potential causes of your patient's clinical deterioration?
2. What procedure is indicated at this point?
3. What is the pathophysiological mechanism of tension pneumothorax, and what treatments are available?

DISCUSSION

In trauma patients the ABCs of patient care must be continuously reassessed. After securing the airway, the next step is to assess for life-threatening chest injuries, especially those that may require treatment in the field. This should include an assessment for massive hemothorax, pneumothorax (PTX), and flail chest. Other significant blunt chest trauma injuries include pulmonary contusions and shearing injuries to the aorta, but these injuries are hard to diagnose in the field and their prehospital treatment is limited to supportive care only.

Pneumothorax is defined as air within the potential space between the parietal and visceral pleura of the lung that are normally in continuous contact. Air can be introduced into the pleural space either through an external wound that violates the chest wall or by internal injuries to the lung that allow air to escape from the lung into the pleural space. A simple pneumothorax occurs when air leaks into the pleural space but does not communicate with the atmosphere or distort the mediastinum. This can be well tolerated in the short term. However, a tension pneumothorax is not well tolerated and is a life-threatening emergency that will result in respiratory and cardiovascular collapse if not corrected immediately. Tension pneumothorax occurs when a "one-way" valve mechanism exists, resulting in an increasing amount of air entering the pleural space with each inspiration that is not expelled during expiration. Progressive increase in the size of the pneumothorax results in collapse of the lung on the effected side and shift of the mediastinum to the opposite side. The net result is compromise of venous return to the heart and a drop in cardiac output and blood pressure, culminating in cardiovascular collapse and death. Positive-pressure ventilation (PPV) that occurs after endotracheal intubation can convert a simple pneumothorax into a tension PTX, as ventilations under pressure continue to expand the pneumothorax.

The diagnosis of this life-threatening complication must be made based on the clinical presentation, and must be treated quickly. Any trauma patient with an open chest wall injury or multiple rib fractures, as well as any chest trauma patient undergoing PPV, should be carefully monitored for the development of a tension pneumothorax. The clinical presentation is hypotension, tachycardia, and respiratory distress. There is unilateral loss of breath sounds with ipsilateral hyperresonance. Subcutaneous air in the chest wall or neck may result from air tracking out of the pleural space into the subcutaneous tissues. Decreasing oxygen saturation is frequently one of the earliest signs. The intubated patient will become difficult to ventilate due to increasing airway pressures. Eventually, patients will develop increased jugular-venous distention (JVD) due to impeded venous return to the heart. Tracheal deviation and cyanosis are late and ominous signs. Needle chest decompression is indicated in unstable chest trauma patients with any of these clinical findings suggestive of tension PTX.

The prognosis of an untreated tension PTX is poor due to compromise of both breathing and circulation. Volume resuscitation will not correct the hypotension or alter the ultimate outcome. The definitive therapy is the placement of a chest tube. In the prehospital setting, however, needle decompression is a life-saving, temporizing measure. This is performed with a large-bore angiocatheter (14- or 16-gauge), which is introduced into the pleural space. A rush of air and clinical improvement indicate successful decompression of the tension pneumothorax. The needle is then withdrawn, and the catheter is secured and left in place. Multiple one-way-valve devices exist to allow the continued expulsion of air from the pleural space while preventing reaccumulation. A simple device for a one-way valve may be fashioned from the finger of a rubber glove that has been cut off to form a tube. This is taped over the hub of the angiocatheter, allowing the free end to act as a flutter valve.

Two different approaches to needle decompression of the pleural space are recognized. The first approach is over the superior edge of the third rib (to avoid the subcostal vessels and nerves, which run along the inferior border of the ribs) in the second intercostal space in the midclavicular line. The advantage to this approach is ease of access in the boarded, supine patient. This has been the traditional approach on the assumption that the trapped air will rise preferentially to this area in the supine patient. Disadvantages to this technique include difficulty in assessing landmarks and the need to traverse significant soft tissue to access the pleural space. There is also a risk of bleeding from internal mammary or subcostal vessels due to improper technique. The alternative approach is lateral and posterior to the pectoralis major muscle and anterior to the latissimus dorsis in the midaxillary line just superior to the fourth or fifth rib. The concern that the trapped air may lie more anteriorly and be "missed" on this approach does not apply in the setting of a hemodynamically significant tension PTX, when most of the lung tissue will be collapsed away from the chest wall, both laterally and anteriorly. The advantage of this approach is that landmarks are easily appreciated even in the muscular individual. Because there is a minimal amount of soft tissue interposed between the skin and the target pleural space, the risk of bleeding is minimized both by the lack of major blood vessels and the reduced likelihood of inappropriate subcostal placement. Due to these technical considerations, the lateral approach is recommended when feasible.

The possible complications of needle decompression are similar to those of any invasive procedure and include bleeding and infection. Because of the risk of introducing infection within the chest cavity, needle chest decompression should never be attempted through an existing chest wall wound.

Another possible cause of decreased unilateral breath sounds and tachycardia is hemothorax due to bleeding from a vascular injury. The small diameter of an angiocatheter is unlikely to relieve hemothorax fully. However, needle decompression will not worsen a hemothorax, and it may lead to clinical improvement if there is a hemopneumothorax (both blood and air in the pleural space).

Another potential cause of unilateral right-sided breath sounds in a setting of trauma is right main stem intubation. Right main stem intubation with subsequent collapse of the left lung may result in hypoxia with decreased breath sounds on the left. Confirming proper tube placement should be the first step to remedy this.

Another controversy that exists concerning emergent chest decompression is whether definitive placement of a chest tube in the field is a preferred method. In certain settings such as the rural EMS system with long transport times or in helicopter transport systems, chest tube placement is an alternative to needle chest decompression. A 6-year review of both methods in the prehospital setting found that scene time was significantly increased with the placement of a chest tube (25.7 vs. 20.3 minutes), yet fewer patients were pronounced dead-on-arrival in the ED (7% vs. 19%) if they had chest tube placement versus needle chest decompression. A limitation of this study was that it included only patients transported by air, which theoretically has the potential to complicate pneumothorax because of the lower air pressure in the environment. The report also included a significant number of patients with either hemothorax or hemopneumothorax. Chest tube placement is a significantly more involved procedure with an increased potential for complications and an increase in scene time. At present, needle decompression remains the rapid intervention of choice in the hemodynamically unstable patient with suspected tension pneumothorax in the prehospital setting.

Any victim of blunt or penetrating chest trauma with decreased breath sounds, respiratory compromise, hypotension, and tachycardia should be presumed to have a tension PTX once simple causes such as improper endotracheal tube placement have been excluded. Because tension PTX can rapidly progress to hemodynamic collapse, chest decompression should be performed in the field as soon as the diagnosis is suspected.

RETURN TO THE CASE

A 14-gauge angiocatheter is placed using the left lateral approach, which results in an audible rush of air. Ventilation becomes markedly easier, the patient's blood pressure increases to 126/72, and his oxygen saturation returns to 95%. You deliver the patient to the emergency department without further complications. In the emergency department a left chest tube is placed and a chest radiograph is performed revealing the chest tube in good position and the left lung reexpanded. The work-up reveals multiple rib fractures on the left with pulmonary contusion, three thoracic spine fractures, and a subarachnoid hemorrhage. The patient is extubated on hospital day 2 and is discharged to a rehabilitation center on hospital day 4.

REFERENCES

Barton, E. D., M. Epperson, D. B. Hoyt, D. Fortlage, and P. Rosen. "Prehospital Needle Aspiration and Tube Thoracostomy in Trauma Victims: A Six-Year Experience with Aeromedical Crews." *Journal of Emergency Medicine* 13, no. 2 (1995): 155–163.

Bledsoe, Bryan E., Robert S. Porter, and Richard A. Cherry. *Trauma Emergencies*. Vol. 4 of *Paramedic Care: Principles & Practice*. Chapter 2, "Blunt Trauma." Upper Saddle River, NJ: Brady/Prentice Hall Health, Pearson Education, 2001.

Dan S. Mosely, MD

28

BURNS

CASE PRESENTATION

You are preparing to eat your lunch at the station when a call comes over the dispatch to respond to a possible burn victim at a location not far from the station. Within 5 minutes you arrive at a house and are directed to the backyard by a number of frantic individuals. When you get there it is obvious that there was preparation for a cookout, but your attention is immediately drawn to a small crowd surrounding a man lying supine next to a charcoal grill who is screaming in agony. You learn that the man was trying to light the charcoal with gasoline when the fire jumped up to the can he was still holding and, as the man was trying to throw the can, he was covered with gas over his shirt, which then started to burn.

As you approach the patient, you clear the bystanders from the immediate area and move the patient away from the still-burning grill. You simultaneously have the fire department dispatched to take care of the potential hazard. Your initial impression is that the man is in his mid-30s, in obvious pain, and with charred skin and clothes over his groin, torso, and upper extremities. His clothes are not actively burning, but most of his shirt and the upper part of his pants are still smoldering. You extinguish the smoldering areas with a nearby garden hose.

You remove the remaining clothing and perform an initial assessment. This reveals that his airway is patent and there are no singed hairs on his face or in his nares. He is breathing rapidly, there is no stridor, and breath sounds are clear bilaterally. His heart rate is elevated at 132, but his blood pressure is slightly elevated at 142/85. Pulses are palpated and strong in all four extremities, including the injured left upper extremity. He is in obvious pain but he is otherwise oriented.

QUESTIONS

1. How do you rapidly assess for life-threatening airway obstructions from burns?

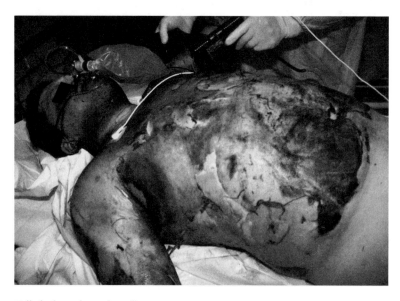

Full-thickness burns from flame injury.

2. How do you rapidly determine the percentage of body surface area (BSA) covered by the burn for adults, children, and infants?

3. How do you treat the exposed burn?

DISCUSSION

Burn injuries are a major source of morbidity and mortality, with approximately 1.25 million presentations to emergency departments each year in the United States. Understanding the basic principles of burn care and wound management is critical in minimizing the complications associated with any burn.

Many factors influence the prognosis of burn patients, including the presence of inhalation injury, the depth of the burn, other injuries, the patient's age, and the presence of comorbid diseases. Shock can result from direct metabolic derangements of the damaged tissue as well as significant volume loss through burned tissue that can no longer control its fluid loss or evaporation rate. The patient must be continually monitored for any change in the vital signs that might indicate a worsening clinical status.

Of primary importance in the assessment and management of any burn patient is a rapid and continual appraisal of the patient's airway. Thermal damage to the glottic and subglottic region can lead to edema and closure of the airway that can occur minutes to hours from the time of initial exposure. The paramedic must be aware of the following signs of a potential inhalation injury:

- Facial burns or singed facial hairs
- Carbonaceous material in the mouth or nose

- Explosion injury with burns to the head and torso
- Acute inflammatory changes in the oropharynx presenting as stridor, drooling, hoarseness, etc.

If a potential airway obstruction is considered likely given any of the findings above, the paramedic should have a low threshold for endotracheal intubation as further swelling will make this increasingly difficult. Even when the possibility of an airway burn is unlikely, all patients should be placed on 100% oxygen via nonrebreather face mask.

Estimating burn size is important because it will dictate the management of the patient. The size of the burn may be quantified based on the percentage of body surface area (BSA) involved. An easy method of determining burn size in adults is the "Rule of Nines." This method divides the body into segments that correlate with a BSA that is either 9% or multiples of 9% of the whole body, with the perineum forming the remaining 1%. Note that this method must be modified for infants or children as they have relatively larger heads and smaller legs. Another quick method for smaller burned areas is to use the back of the patient's hand (not including the fingers) as a reference; this area roughly equals approximately 1% of the BSA for that patient.

The depth of burn is also important because it gives an idea of the extent of injury and a fairly accurate prognosis for healing and return of function. The depth of burn has historically been described in degrees: first through fourth. Recently, however, the accepted standard is to describe the burn based on the need for surgical intervention. In this system, burns are described as superficial partial-thickness, deep partial-thickness, and full-thickness.

Once the size and depth of the burn is determined, the classification is further broken down into one of three categories: major, moderate, and minor burns. This classification is important because it determines the type of treatment facility (burn center vs. hospital) that the patient will need. For transportation purposes, however, patients should be taken to the closest appropriate emergency department based on their clinical status unless local EMS protocols dictate otherwise. Further evaluation and stabilization will then determine the patient's ultimate disposition. The American Burn Association has established criteria for when it is appropriate to transfer a patient to a specialty burn center. These criteria include

- Partial-thickness burns greater than 15% BSA
- Full-thickness burns greater than 5% BSA
- Significant burns to the face or head, feet, hands, or perineal areas
- High-voltage electrical injuries
- Inhalation injuries
- Chemical burns causing progressive tissue destruction
- Associated significant injuries
- Associated significant comorbidities such as diabetes or peripheral vascular disease

Prehospital assessment is divided into initial and detailed assessments. During the initial assessment, any immediately life-threatening emergencies should be identified and treated. This process is the same as for any trauma victim with the exception noted above that delayed airway closure may be seen. The secondary survey is a complete head-to-toe assessment during which burn size and depth is calculated and other related injuries can be identified.

Treatment of the burn patient involves removal of any burning clothing and jewelry, particularly bracelets and rings because these may become constricting bands as extremities continue to swell. Oxygen should be delivered via face mask at 100% FiO_2 (fractional concentration of inspired oxygen). Intravenous lines should be started, preferably in non-burned extremities. If access cannot be otherwise obtained, peripheral access through burned skin is acceptable. Crystalloid solution can be started at 200 cc/hr. Precise formulas (such as the Parkland formula) are not generally necessary in the prehospital setting as these calculations will be adjusted once the patient reaches definitive care. Once the patient is completely exposed, cover him with clean or sterile sheets, particularly over burned areas. Because burned skin loses many of its thermoregulatory mechanisms, the patient should also be covered with a blanket to ensure that hypothermia does not occur. Initially, many full-thickness burns are not painful because the nerves have been destroyed, but partial-thickness burns may be intensely painful and will likely require prehospital parenteral analgesia. Use existing pain control protocols or online medical authority to give narcotic or other effective analgesics to burn patients as needed to control their pain.

RETURN TO THE CASE

During your initial assessment, you recognize that the patient has a patent airway and has no apparent risk factors for an airway burn, but your index of suspicion remains high. You remove the charred clothing from the patient and all jewelry from the extremities. He does not have a medical alert bracelet. He is given 100% O_2 by face mask. You calculate the burns as 30% full-thickness (torso and portions of the upper extremities) as well as areas of deep partial-thickness burns. A peripheral intravenous line is started in the right antecubital fossa and an infusion of crystalloid solution is initiated at 200 cc/hr. He is then covered with clean sheets and a blanket. The patient is transported to the nearest trauma center with burn facility support. While en route, you obtain permission from medical control to give 5 mg of morphine for pain control.

After initial treatment in the emergency department, the patient is admitted to the burn center for continued treatment with topical antibiotics and skin grafting. He is discharged 1 month later and returns home. He will undergo four additional skin graft surgeries over the next year.

REFERENCES

Bledsoe, Bryan E., Robert S. Porter, and Richard A. Cherry. *Trauma Emergencies*. Vol. 4 of *Paramedic Care: Principles & Practice*. Chapter 6, "Burns." Upper Saddle River, NJ: Brady/Prentice Hall Health, Pearson Education, 2001.

Limmer, Daniel, Michael F. O'Keefe, Harvey D. Grant, Robert H. Murray, J. David Bergeron, and Edward T. Dickinson, ed. *Emergency Care*. 10th ed. Upper Saddle River, NJ: Prentice Hall, 2005.

Dan Gabbey, MD

29

CERVICAL SPINE INJURY

CASE PRESENTATION

It is the Friday afternoon before a holiday weekend and there is a mass exodus from the city. Traffic is heavy. You receive a call for a serious motor vehicle crash (MVC) on the interstate. By the time you reach the incident, Highway Patrol has secured the scene but you are the first medical personnel to reach the injured.

You find that a small compact car has struck a retaining wall. The driver has extricated himself, is ambulatory, and is without complaint. However, the passenger remains entrapped, seated in the front. There is significant front-end damage and both airbags have deployed. As you approach the entrapped patient you quickly ascertain that she is awake but appears to be confused. There is no obvious respiratory distress and she is stating that both of her arms seem "weak."

As you start the primary survey, your partner has slipped into the backseat of the vehicle and is maintaining cervical spine immobilization. The patient's airway is secure and you briefly interrupt your primary survey to assist your partner in applying the cervical spine collar. The remainder of your survey reveals a stable blood pressure and no visible sign of injury. The patient is able to move all of her extremities, but you notice that although she grasps your hands symmetrically, both grasps are weak.

You are most concerned about a possible spinal cord injury and radio for a Medevac helicopter. While the fire department deploys the Hurst tool for extrication, you place the patient on a nonrebreather mask, and maintain manual cervical stabilization.

QUESTIONS

1. What are the indications for cervical spine immobilization?
2. What physical exam findings might tip you off as to a possible spinal cord injury in the unconscious patient?

DISCUSSION

The human spine consists of 33 bony vertebrae: 7 cervical, 12 thoracic, 5 lumbar, 5 sacral (fused into one), and 4 coccygeal (usually fused into one). The vertebrae are separated by flexible intervertebral disks and are uniformly connected by a complex network of ligaments. This vertebral column provides the basic structural support for the upright torso of humans and also protectively encases the spinal cord. Although evolution has afforded us the ability to walk upright, it has also resulted in a spinal cord that is easily subject to injury. The cervical spine injury in particular, by virtue of the head having a tremendous range of motion, can be easily injured in a trauma setting. It is for this reason that paramedics must be vigilant in their search for this type of injury because prehospital stabilization and intervention can sometimes limit the devastating consequences of a spinal cord injury.

Annually, there are nearly 6,000 fatalities, 5,000 new paraplegics, and 500 quadriplegics as a result of spinal cord injury. Approximately 50% of these injuries are caused by motor vehicle crashes. Since 1973 there has been a proportional decrease in vehicular accidents as acts of violence grow. The average age of injury is 31 and males are more commonly injured. Additionally, the approximate lifetime cost of caring for a quadriplegic is in excess of $2 million. More important, the emotional costs for both the patient and the family, especially because this is largely a medical problem of the young, far surpass any financial burden that may incur.

The modern EMS systems and the principles of in-the-field resuscitation and stabilization of the patient with a spinal cord injury owe their development to the National Highway Safety Act of 1966 and the Emergency Medical Services Act of 1973. Prior to

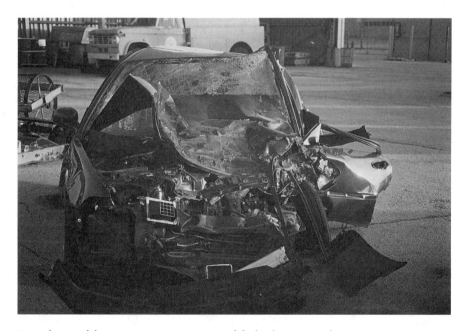

Heavy front-end damage, requiring extrication with hydraulic rescue tools.

these policy decisions, there was no organized means for prehospital care for multitrauma victims in the United States.

The ultimate management of a patient with a spinal cord injury is very involved and numerous complications may ensue. Fortunately, the role of the prehospital provider, although vitally important, is fairly straightforward. It involves maintaining vital organ function, preventing further neurological injury during transport, and rapidly transporting the patient to a well-qualified hospital center that has the capacity to care for the spinally injured patient.

Any trauma patient should be considered spinally injured until proven otherwise. The initial approach is the same for all patients and ABCs must be strictly followed. Severe head injury and even diaphragmatic paralysis may be encountered in this setting, and securing the airway is of paramount importance. As part of the primary survey, it is incumbent upon the paramedic to quickly and accurately assess the "D" or *disability* of the patient. Asking the patient to move her fingers and toes and ensuring that she has symmetric feeling and strength in her extremities is adequate initially. A more thorough secondary survey must also be performed because it may become apparent after the patient is exposed that other injuries are present.

It is fairly common in the prehospital setting to fully immobilize a patient with a cervical collar and a long board in the trauma setting. Recently, the National Association of EMS Physicians (NAEMSP) Board of Directors issued a position paper on the indications for spinal immobilization. Specifically, application of a cervical collar and long board should take place when any of the following are present: altered mental status, evidence of intoxication, a distracting painful injury, gross neurological deficit, or spinal pain or tenderness. Usual distracting injuries include long bone fractures. Although not mentioned in the NAEMSP position paper, if there are signs of significant head injury or a profound mechanism of injury, spinal injury precautions should be taken. In one well-known neurosurgical study, 71% of patients who were ejected from their vehicle sustained a cervical spine injury. If none of these clinical criteria are present and there is *no* mechanism with a potential for causing injury, the patient may possibly be transported without c-spine immobilization in a position of comfort if allowed by local EMS protocols.

As was stated earlier, the prehospital provider must have a healthy respect for the potential sequelae of a spinal cord injury. Nearly 40% of cervical spine injuries produce neurological deficit and fully one quarter of these injuries are thought to be caused by improper handling. Cadaver studies have confirmed that the best way to stabilize the cervical spine is to use a collar with adjoining head blocks and to secure the head and collar to the long board with tape. Should intubation become necessary, maintenance of in-line cervical spine stabilization by a second person is the safest method. Furthermore, the use of a Miller blade for intubation has been shown to cause the least amount of movement of the cervical spine in all three planes.

The pathoanatomy of spinal cord injury is complex. There are numerous primary injury mechanisms including burst fractures, fracture dislocations, missile injuries, and ruptured disks. These injuries invariably result in an ischemic insult to the spinal cord, followed by an inflammatory response, causing damage that may be irreversible. One of the initial interventions in the emergency department for select patients (those who sustained blunt trauma) is the administration of high-dose steroids. Methylprednisolone helps to quiet this inflammatory response, but has been shown effective only when given within 6 hours of injury.

The initial neurological evaluation of the patient with a suspected spinal cord injury begins with simple observation. For instance, obvious bruising about the head or neck or an abnormal breathing pattern ("C4 and 5 keep the diaphragm alive") may provide important clues to a cervical injury. Palpation of the spine may also reveal areas of tenderness or deformity. Of equal importance is a good motor and sensory assessment. Be certain to ask the patient to move all of her extremities against resistance and be certain to document any impairment of sensation (asking the patient if she feels you touching her in a symmetric fashion is more than adequate in the prehospital setting).

A thorough physical examination can provide a great deal of information and may help the provider to pinpoint the possible location of injury. A *complete* spinal cord lesion is defined as total loss of motor power and sensation distal to the site of a spinal cord injury. There are many *incomplete* spinal cord lesions, but one of the more important ones is called a *central cord syndrome*, seen most commonly in elderly people (because of degenerative arthritis of the cervical vertebrae) or in those patients subject to significant hyperextension of their cervical spine. These patients have a greater neurological deficit in the upper extremities than in the lower extremities. Last, neurogenic shock may result from spinal injury. Hypotension and bradycardia (one would normally expect to see a compensatory tachycardia in the setting of hypotension) are pathognomonic in neurogenic shock. Prehospital interventions should consist of administering atropine for profound bradycardia, fluid resuscitation for hypotension, and placing the patient in the Trendelenburg position if tolerated.

RETURN TO THE CASE

Another EMS crew arrives to assist you with the extrication after the door and roof are removed by the fire department. You continue to maintain C-spine immobilization manually (in addition to the collar) and the patient, as a unit, is placed onto a long board. A large-bore intravenous line is started, she is fully exposed, and you start your secondary survey. Her vital signs remain stable. The patient states that she experienced a whiplash effect when the car suddenly decelerated. There are no visible injuries and she is not complaining of neck tenderness on examination. However, she still has diminished motor strength in her upper extremities with symmetrical sensation. Correctly, you maintain full spinal precautions. Just as you finish your survey, the Medevac helicopter lands and the patient is taken to the regional trauma center. She is emergently evaluated by neurosurgery and an MRI reveals that she indeed suffered a central cord syndrome. She is given high-dose steroids and, 2 months later, has regained only partial restoration of motor function in her upper extremities.

REFERENCES

Bledsoe, Bryan E., Robert S. Porter, and Richard A. Cherry. *Trauma Emergencies*. Vol. 4 of *Paramedic Care: Principles & Practice*. Chapter 9, "Spinal Trauma." Upper Saddle River, NJ: Brady/Prentice Hall Health, Pearson Education, 2001.

Bracken, M. B., M. J. Shepard, W. F. Collins, T. R. Holford, W. Young, D. S. Baskin, H. M. Eisenberg, E. Flamm, L. Leo-Summers, J. Maroon, et al. "A Randomized, Controlled Trial of Methylprednisolone or Naloxone in the Treatment of Acute Spinal-Cord Injury." *New England Journal of Medicine* 322, no. 20 (1990): 1405–1411.

Domeier, R. "Indications for Spinal Immobilization." *Prehospital Emergency Care* 3, no. 3 (1999): 251–252.

Andrew W. Stern, NREMT-P, MPA, MA

30

HEAD INJURY

CASE PRESENTATION

Just after going into service on the night shift, the dispatcher transmits a third-party call for a fight, with injuries, at a local bar. The scene is not yet secure and your unit is instructed to stage in the area until the police confirm the area is safe to enter. A few minutes later you receive a transmission that the police are on the scene and it is now secure, with the police reporting one patient who has been assaulted with a baseball bat. Along with a fire department first response unit, you proceed onto the scene. As you enter the bar you see a male with blood covering his face lying supine and moaning. A police officer informs you that according to witnesses, the patient was hit a number of times—a few times to the stomach and at least one blow to the side of the head.

Your partner checks the level of consciousness and determines that the patient is responding only to painful stimuli. The ABC assessment identifies snoring respirations of 16 and a pulse that is thready and rapid. You observe external bleeding on the side of the head, but it is not profuse. Your partner performs a jaw-thrust maneuver while in-line stabilization is applied. The snoring ceases with this maneuver. With the help of the first responder unit, the following vital signs are obtained:

Respirations	16 bpm
Pulse	110
Blood pressure	100/70
Glasgow Coma Scale (GCS)	12 (eyes—3/open to voice) (verbal—4/confused) (motor—5/localizes pain)
Oxygen saturation (SpO$_2$)	92% (room air)

You make the decision to rapidly transport to the trauma center. The patient has already been placed on oxygen by nonrebreather. After inspecting and palpating the neck,

155

Prevention of hypoxia and hypotension are essential in the management of patients with significant head injuries.

Courtesy of Edward T. Dickinson, MD.

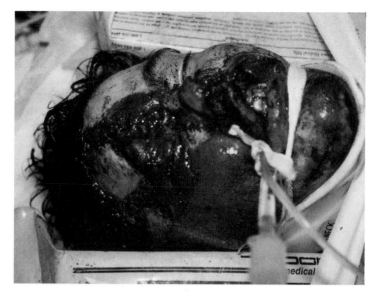

you apply a cervical collar. In preparation for transport, you and your partner secure the patient to a long backboard. While you are doing this, you observe that the patient's breathing has become more labored, and you determine that the rate is now 10. You reassess the eye opening, motor, and verbal responses and calculate a GCS score of 8. You decide to immediately start assisting ventilations with a bag-valve mask with 100% oxygen at a normoventilation rate of approximately 12 per minute. You load the patient into the ambulance and while en route you initiate an IV of normal saline with a 16-gauge needle. After 250 cc are infused, you obtain a new set of vital signs. The transport time to the trauma center is 17 minutes. Your clinical impression is that the patient may have a severe traumatic brain injury as well as internal bleeding in the abdomen.

QUESTIONS

1. Should this patient be intubated and, if yes, what is the most appropriate way of accomplishing the intubation?

2. When assisting ventilations with a bag-valve-mask (BVM) on a patient with a traumatic brain injury, what assessment criteria should be used to determine when a hyperventilation rate is clinically appropriate?

3. Why are hypotension and hypoxia significant issues with traumatic brain injury?

DISCUSSION

Until recently, prehospital assessment of traumatic brain injuries focused on Cushing response (also known as Cushing's Reflex), a group of vital signs changes that include decreasing pulse rate, increasing blood pressure, and erratic respirations (usually described as Cheyne-Stokes respirations) caused by increasing intracranial pressure (ICP) that compresses the upper brainstem.

In the last few years, research has identified additional patterns of response to brain trauma. While the Cushing response may indeed be observed, other responses that are even more likely to be observed involve hypotension (a decreased blood pressure) and hypoxemia (decreased arterial oxygen saturation) or hypoxia (decreased tissue oxygenation). In a review of the literature by a team of experts under a grant from the National Highway Traffic Safety Administration (NHTSA), the following was reported:

> One central concept is now known: All neurological damage does not occur at the moment of impact [primary injury], but rather evolves over ensuing minutes, hours, and days [secondary injury]. The secondary brain injury can result in increasing mortality and more disabling injuries.

> [t]he precise definition of hypotension and hypoxemia are unclear in these patients [with traumatic brain injury]. However ample evidence exists regarding hypotension, defined in these studies as a single observation for a systolic blood pressure (SBP) <90 mmHg, or hypoxia, defined as apnea or cyanosis in the field or an arterial oxygen saturation (SpO_2) <90%. The evidence indicates that these values must be avoided, if possible, or rapidly corrected in severe head injury patients.

In other words, the primary injury—the injury sustained at the moment of impact (e.g., when the patient was struck by the bat)—can produce significant secondary injury resulting in brain tissue death from lack of oxygen and decreased blood flow to the brain (ischemia). Therefore, although some head injury patients may manifest with Cushing response (decreased pulse, increased blood pressure, erratic breathing), others may present with hypoxia and hypotension associated with secondary brain injury.

As noted in the research results above, hypoxia in the context of traumatic brain injury is defined as an oxygen saturation of below 90% and hypotension as a systolic blood pressure below 90 mmHg. One study found that when a patient with a traumatic brain injury had just one episode of hypoxia or a single occurrence of hypotension, it resulted in a poor outcome (severely disabled, vegetative, or dead) of 55% and 74% respectively. When patients were found to have *both* hypoxemia *and* hypotension, a poor outcome was observed 94% of the time.

This study points up the need for frequent assessment of head injury patients with rapid interventions to reduce hypoxia and prevent hypotension in the prehospital setting. The study reported that patients whose hypotension was not corrected in the field had a worse outcome than those corrected prior to arrival at the emergency department. Therefore, it is essential to gain immediate control of the airway and ensure effective oxygenation and an SpO_2 of greater than 90%. Hypotension must be rapidly treated with fluid replacement to maintain a systolic blood pressure greater than 90 mmHg.

Additional patterns of response have been identified as associated with brain trauma that is severe enough to cause herniation. These include pupil abnormalities and posturing. Head trauma results in brain herniation when increased pressure forces structures such as the medulla oblongata to shift or be pushed downward through the foramen magnum. As a consequence, pressure may be exerted on cranial nerve III, resulting in pupils that are dilated and unresponsive to light either unilaterally or bilaterally. Other findings that may be observed, depending on the amount of herniation and the part of the brain affected, are extensor (decerebrate) posturing to painful stimuli or the patient being completely flaccid as a result of the pressure progressing down the brainstem. Many patients with cerebral herniation will also be found to be either unconscious or unresponsive even to painful stimuli.

The Glasgow Coma Scale (GCS) is an assessment tool that helps quantify the severity of a head injury. Three subscores are determined: eye opening, verbal response, and motor response. The numeric values assigned to each of these categories are added together to obtain a total GCS score ranging from 3 to 15 points. (See Figure 30-1.) Comparing sequential GCS scores against the baseline is an indicator of possible outcome. One study of head-injured patients found that an increase of 2 or more points over the emergency department GCS score was a predictor of discharge with little or no neurological deficit. In this same study, those patients who had little or no GCS score increase ultimately had a major deficit or died. Scores of 3 to 5 have been shown to have a predictive value of poor outcome (severely disabled, vegetative, or dead) as high as 84%.

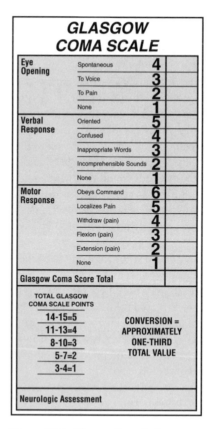

Figure 30-1 Glasgow Coma Scale.

The assessment process is the key to determining what type of treatment needs to be provided to the brain-injured patient. Level of consciousness, best determined in the field by using the Glasgow Coma Scale (GCS), along with blood pressure, pupillary response, and oxygen saturation are the four findings that will provide most of the information needed to make decisions about treatment.

Treatment of the head-injured patient always starts with the standard resuscitation ABCs. Remember that many head injuries are not isolated, so it is important to consider the mechanism of injury and perform as complete an assessment as time and resources permit. The goal for all brain-injured patients is to minimize hypoxia to maintain an oxygen saturation above 90% and to maintain a blood pressure greater than 90 mmHg.

There is a critical determination to make before deciding what sort of ventilation to provide, and that is whether herniation is or is not present. The signs of herniation are dilated unreactive pupil(s), unresponsive to painful stimuli, and extensor posturing or flaccid. If there is no sign of herniation, normoventilation with high concentration oxygen at a rate of 12 ventilations per minute should be provided in an adult. *Note that in this situation, when herniation is not suspected, hyperventilation is not recommended because hyperventilation may result in vasoconstriction in the brain which, if excessive, is potentially harmful.* When providing an IV, crystalloid, dextrose-containing IV solutions should be avoided unless hypoglycemia has been specifically determined. Monitor the patient closely to avoid fluid overload or providing inadequate amounts that could result in sudden hypotension.

A patient found with signs of brain herniation should be hyperventilated in an attempt to slow the rise of intracranial pressure. (Again, the signs of herniation are dilated unreactive pupil(s), unresponsive to painful stimuli, extensor posturing or flaccid.) Hyperventilation is an increase of approximately 10 breaths per minute over the normal ventilation rate adjusted for the age group (adult, child, infant). If the patient has a GCS score of less than 9, the airway will probably need to be protected. Endotracheal intubation is the most effective way to accomplish this. Depending on local protocol and the level of consciousness, the use of sedation or rapid sequence intubation (RSI) may help facilitate the intubation. The use of sedatives and paralytics will also help control the agitation and combativeness that can increase intracranial pressure (ICP). Lidocaine is thought to prevent an increase in ICP that occurs with endotracheal intubation. Although no human studies have demonstrated that a transient increase of ICP occurs during airway manipulation, many prehospital protocols recommend the use of lidocaine. Before giving a sedative or paralytic agent, it is important to obtain a baseline GCS score as the effect of these medications will make the GCS score invalid.

In the case of significant traumatic brain injury, repeat GCS scoring and vital signs at least every 5 minutes. The importance of assessment and reassessment to establish trends in the patient's condition cannot be overemphasized—particularly with patients who have ingested either alcohol or drugs, which make assessment more difficult.

RETURN TO THE CASE

While the patient continues to have assisted ventilations, you obtain a new set of vital signs, including a check of the pupils, and calculate a GCS score.

Respirations	BVM assisted with 100% O_2 at 12 bpm
Pulse	120 (thready)
Blood pressure	90/60
Skin	pale and diaphoretic
Glasgow Coma Scale (GCS)	7 (eyes—2/open to painful stimuli) (verbal—2/incomprehensible sounds) (motor—3/flexion to painful stimuli)
Pupils	left pupil dilated and unresponsive right pupil responds to light
Oxygen saturation (SpO_2)	95 (100% O_2)

You decide to intubate the patient and administer lidocaine and midazolam. With good visualization of the cords, the endotracheal tube is easily inserted. After verification of placement you secure the tube to minimize movement and possible displacement and ventilate the patient at 12 breaths per minute. Your partner performs a rapid physical assessment and notes a 6 cm contusion in the right parietal region as well as rebound tenderness in the upper right abdominal quadrant. An additional 250 cc of normal saline is rapidly infused. Shortly thereafter, you notice that the patient exhibits extensor (decerebrate) posturing and no longer responds to painful stimuli. You initiate hyperventilation at approximately 20 ventilations per minute.

Soon after arrival at the hospital, the patient has a CT scan of the brain and abdomen that shows an epidural hematoma and a liver laceration. He is taken to the operating room to evacuate the epidural hematoma. The decision is made to treat the abdominal injury nonoperatively. The patient remains hospitalized for two weeks and is discharged to a rehabilitation facility. He remains in rehab 1 month and then is able to return to work with some diminished capacity.

REFERENCES

Baxt, W. G., and P. Moody. "The Impact of Prehospital Emergency Care on the Mortality of Severely Brain-Injured Patients." *Journal of Trauma* 27 (1987): 365–369.

Bledsoe, Bryan E., Robert S. Porter, and Richard A. Cherry. *Trauma Emergencies.* Vol. 4 of *Paramedic Care: Principles & Practice.* Chapter 8, "Head, Facial, and Neck Trauma." Upper Saddle River, NJ: Brady/Prentice Hall Health, Pearson Education, 2001.

Brain Trauma Foundation. *Guidelines for Prehospital Management of Traumatic Brain Injury.* New York: Brain Trauma Foundation, 2000. Also available at http://www.braintrauma.org.

Chestnut, R. M., L. F. Marshall, M. R. Klauber, B. A. Blunt, N. Baldwin, H. M. Eisenberg, J. A. Jane, A. Marmarou, and M. A. Foulkes. "The Role of Secondary Brain Injury in Determining Outcome from Severe Head Injury." *Journal of Trauma* 34 (1993): 216–222.

Winkler, J. V., P. Rosen, and E. J. Alfrey. "Prehospital Use of the Glasgow Coma Scale in Severe Head Injury." *Journal of Emergency Medicine* 2 (1984): 1–6.

31

Lawrence Mottley, MD, MHSA

BLUNT MULTIPLE TRAUMA

CASE PRESENTATION

A telephone lineworker is working in an elevated power "bucket" when the bucket truck is struck by another vehicle. Although the worker remains in the bucket because of the restraining safety belt, the bucket arm collapses under the strain and falls to the ground. The nearby police officer radios in the call and you arrive in less than 2 minutes. You survey the scene carefully, and ensure that the electrical wires are in place and the telephone poles intact before entering the scene. Bystanders are placing a tourniquet on the left leg of the patient, where there is a gaping wound with bone protruding.

You ignore the extremity injury and focus your attention on the patient's overall appearance. She is a woman in her 30s with obvious severe facial and head trauma manifested by bilateral periorbital swelling and blood from her left external ear canal. You perform a primary survey and find rapid, deep, and snoring respirations at a rate of 32. There are unequal breath sounds, right better than left, with crepitus to palpation of the left lateral chest. You place an oropharyngeal airway and oxygen on the patient and perform the secondary survey. The secondary survey reveals a firm abdomen, an unstable pelvis and open fracture of the left tibia or fibula with a tourniquet in place, as well as worsening periorbital ecchymoses. The Glasgow Coma Scale is 5 (verbal = 1; eye = 1; motor = 3).

You are 2 minutes from the community hospital and 15 minutes from a trauma center by ground. The ETA of the medical helicopter is 12 minutes.

QUESTIONS

1. What are the treatment priorities in patients with multiple serious injuries?
2. What factors enter into the decision as to whether to utilize the medevac helicopter?

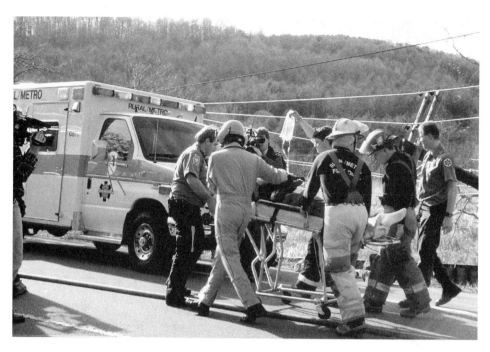

Multiple trauma patients should be managed with rapid assessment, immediate life-saving interventions, and timely transport to an appropriate hospital.

DISCUSSION

Definitive care of the trauma patient can take place only in the hospital setting. The role of EMS in trauma care is threefold: to correct immediately life threatening conditions; to prevent further injury; and to provide rapid transport to the most appropriate hospital. These three goals are in a dynamic tension, as satisfying one impedes the other two. The paramedic must use good judgment to optimally balance these needs. The exam of the multiply injured patient follows the A-B-C-D-E (**A**irway-**B**reathing-**C**irculation-**D**isability-**E**xposure) approach.

AIRWAY

The search for life-threatening injuries begins with the primary survey. The primary survey is designed to quickly identify life-threatening injuries in priority order.

The airway is always the first priority, and in the trauma patient is combined with protection of the cervical spine. Although we concentrate on ALS maneuvers, the initial step is always to simply open the airway through basic life support (BLS) maneuvers. In the case of trauma, this means the jaw-thrust method since the C-spine cannot be extended. The most common source of airway obstruction is still simply the tongue falling posteriorly.

Patients with a GCS of 8 or less are optimally treated by intubation for airway protection, usually in the prehospital phase (see Case 15 on facilitated intubation), but patients with GCS greater than 8 may require intubation for diverse reasons such as facial fractures, chest trauma, or coexisting drug use. If intubation is required in a patient with a GCS of 3, medication may not be needed. Many patients with a GCS of 3 and the majority of patients with a GCS greater than 3 who require intubation will require medication-facilitated intubation.

Nasotracheal intubation is an alternative, but is used with great caution in the patient with head or neck trauma and is relatively contraindicated in facial trauma ("trauma above the clavicles"). Surgical airways should be reserved for patients in extremis who are not intubatable. As part of the airway assessment, the cervical spine must be immobilized. As the cervical collar is placed, look for the jugular-venous distention (JVD) or a deviated trachea—telltale signs of cardiac tamponade or tension pneumothorax. A tension pneumothorax identified in the field can and should be treated with needle thoracostomy with the same priority as any other airway compromise.

BREATHING

The second part of the primary survey is the determination of the adequacy of breathing or respiration.

One way of assessing both the airway and breathing is to speak loudly to the patient as you approach. If the patient answers, she both has an airway and is breathing (and has a pulse as well), although the adequacy of the breathing will need further assessment. Adequacy of breathing is determined by assessing both the rate and quality of respirations as well as the presence of bilateral breath sounds and stability of the chest wall.

Identification during the breathing assessment of tension pneumothorax or flail chest permits prehospital treatment by the paramedic. Identification of cardiac tamponade or suspected hemothorax may permit the ED team to prepare for immediate intervention on arrival in the ED.

All multiple trauma patients are given high-concentration oxygen.

CIRCULATION

The third definitive care priority is to stop gross bleeding, usually arterial. These maneuvers are within the realm of basic life support, and when sufficient help is on-scene, the paramedic may delegate this task to concentrate on needed ALS interventions. Direct pressure is almost always sufficient to control hemorrhage. Blood-soaked dressing should not be removed but additional layers applied. In the extremely rare instance when tourniquet control is required for uncontrolled bleeding of an extremity, make careful notation of the time of its application.

Once your exam has reached this stage it is time to begin transportation. You must consider the appropriate destination hospital. If the patient is in cardiac arrest—and your protocol requires treatment and transportation—you should proceed to the nearest emergency department regardless of its trauma designation or diversion status. The vast majority of these patients will not survive; those who do survive need intensive hospital-level care within minutes of the onset of arrest. Patients who have a palpable pulse do have a blood pressure and should be transported to a trauma center, if one is available. Local protocols will determine the time or distance paramedics may travel to reach a trauma center instead of a community hospital, but protocols commonly use either transport time or total prehospital time to make that determination (e.g., "May transport 20 minutes past the nearest hospital" or "If total prehospital time does not exceed 1 hour").

Helicopter medical evacuation (Medevac) is a useful adjunct, especially in the rural setting. The benefit of aeromedical helicopter use in the suburban setting is less clear, and Medevac in the urban areas should be extremely rare. Although speed from point to point is much faster in a helicopter, there are inherent delays that often make the actual time from scene to emergency department longer than if ground transport had taken place. Sources of delay include awaiting helicopter arrival, reassessment of the patient by the Medevac team, landing sites distant from the emergency department, and the like. Helicopter evacuation should be performed for two reasons: first, if it brings a needed higher level of medical care to the scene and second, if the ETA to the destination hospital is clearly faster than that of the ground ambulance.

DISABILITY

While en route to the hospital, a brief assessment of the patient's neurological status should be performed. The EMS crew may be the only health care providers to see the patient before coma occurs. The patient should be assessed for ability to move her extremities, respond to questions, and perceive touch or pain. In the patient with altered mental status, pupil status and eye deviation should be noted.

EXPOSURE

During transport, the patient should undergo a visual inspection of the head, neck, and trunk for occult injuries, and, if time and treatment permit, a head-to-toe exam—the secondary survey—for less serious injuries.

RETURN TO THE CASE

Your patient has a number of serious injuries, but you direct your attention to the airway. The presence of rapid deep respirations in this setting strongly suggests central neurogenic hyperventilation, indicative of severe brain trauma. Because she has facial trauma as well, you elect to attempt intubation. The combination of the patient's low GCS plus topical spray of Cetacaine in the oropharynx allows you to orotracheally intubate the patient while a first responder manually immobilizes the neck. You verify endotracheal tube placement with a colorimetric $ETCO_2$ detection device and begin BVM ventilations. Her tidal volume is sufficient, so you add supplemental oxygen. Manual palpation and visual inspection show crepitus and subcutaneous emphysema of the left chest. When your partner reports decreased breath sounds on the left, you note the trachea starting to shift to the right. This, combined with the fact that she is increasingly difficult to ventilate by BVM, makes you suspect that a tension pneumothorax has developed. You perform a needle thoracostomy with a 14 gauge angiocatheter on the left side of the chest, with an audible release of air and improvement in both tidal volume and breath sounds. A cervical collar is placed and the patient is carefully logrolled onto a backboard.

At this point, having effectively treated the immediately life threatening conditions, you begin transport to the trauma center. Vital signs are blood pressure 90/40, pulse 120, and oxygen saturation 94%. You note that the patient has a flexion response to pain in her upper extremities, but no response of her lower extremities. A large-bore IV of normal saline has been initiated in each arm, and because you know that even a single episode of hypotension in severe head injury more than doubles the mortality rate, you run the solution in rapidly.

You place a saline-moistened battle dressing over the open fracture and release the tourniquet, carefully noting how long it had been in place. Your secondary survey also reveals a grossly unstable pelvic fracture. You call your medical control physician to see if medical antishock trousers (MAST) use is indicated. The medical control physician, who finished his ED residency in 1995, has never heard of MAST trousers, and instead tells you to tie a sheet firmly around the sides of the pelvis to stabilize the fractured pelvis.

You arrive at the trauma center after a 17-minute transport time. The emergency department team immediately verifies the endotracheal tube placement and begins their trauma assessment. The patient is taken to the CT scanner for imaging of the head, abdomen, and pelvis. The head CT shows several small areas of contusion but no injuries that will require neurosurgery. The abdominal CT shows a high-grade splenic injury that will require immediate surgery. The patient is taken to the operating room (OR) and the trauma surgeon performs a splenectomy. With the splenectomy completed, the orthopedic team comes to the OR and provides fixation of the leg fracture and applies an external fixator to the pelvis for stabilization. The patient is extubated 4 days later and discharged to a rehabilitation hospital on the eleventh hospital day.

REFERENCES

Bledsoe, Bryan E., Robert S. Porter, and Richard A. Cherry. *Trauma Emergencies*. Vol. 4 of *Paramedic Care: Principles & Practice*. Chapter 2, "Blunt Trauma." Upper Saddle River, NJ: Brady/Prentice Hall Health, Pearson Education, 2001.

Campbell, John Emory. *Basic Trauma Life Support*. 5th ed. Upper Saddle River, NJ: Brady/Prentice Hall Health, Pearson Education, 2004.

Steven J. Busuttil, MD

32

RUPTURED ABDOMINAL AORTIC ANEURYSM

CASE PRESENTATION

Your squad is working a typically slow Friday afternoon. You are called to an ophthalmologist's office to see a 73-year-old white male patient. He and his wife were waiting to see the doctor when he relatively suddenly developed abdominal and back pain. He was having trouble sitting still, and started pacing the waiting area where he collapsed.

Upon your squad's arrival, the patient is in an exam room with the exam chair fully reclined. You note he is awake and conversant, but lethargic. You also note he is pale and diaphoretic. Vital signs taken by the office staff immediately after the collapse were a heart rate of 120 bpm, systolic blood pressure 60 mmHg, and respirations at 20 bpm. The vital signs you obtain are similar except the blood pressure has risen to 85/55 mmHg and the heart rate is now 100 bpm. The patient complains of constant tearing or burning pain going through his abdomen to his back. He is very uncomfortable. From interviewing the patient and his wife, you find he has a long history of hypertension, and moderate to severe COPD (chronic obstructive pulmonary disease). He has cut back, but still smokes approximately one pack per day of tobacco. He has an active senior life and has not had any cardiac complaints or history. The patient tells you that his father died in his 60s of a "burst blood vessel" and he has an older brother who had an aneurysm repaired several years ago. Your exam reveals that carotid and femoral pulses are palpable and equal. His abdomen is moderately distended and moderately tender; in addition, he has a pulsatile mass that can be palpated above his umbilicus.

You are currently located 2 to 3 minutes from a small 50-bed hospital and approximately 15 minutes from a tertiary hospital with a full complement of triage, anesthesia, and surgical staff.

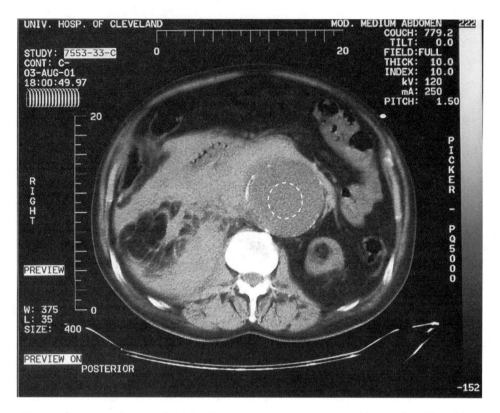

CT scan of patient with ruptured AAA. Notice aortic aneurysm surrounded by calcific wall, and large retroperitoneal hematoma. Dotted circle in center of aneurysm indicates normal aortic diameter.
Courtesy of Steven J. Busuttil, MD.

QUESTIONS

1. What treatment for shock should be instituted in the field and during transport (e.g., IV fluid resuscitation, etc.)?
2. Is there a role for medical antishock trousers (MAST) and pneumatic antishock garment (PASG) protocols?

DISCUSSION

An aneurysm is a pathologic dilation of an artery. Abdominal aortic aneurysms (AAAs) are a fairly common disorder of elderly people with an incidence of 2% to 5% in the population greater than 60 years of age. Ruptured AAA accounts for approximately 15,000 deaths and is currently the 13th leading cause of death in the United States.

Approximately 85% of AAAs are undiagnosed. The vast majority of patients have no symptoms until the aneurysm expands rapidly or ruptures. In-hospital mortality of ruptured AAA is still between 40% and 70%. If cardiac arrest occurs prior to arrival at the hospital, even if the patient is initially resuscitated, the mortality from ruptured aortic aneurysm is close to 90%.

Abdominal aneurysms usually occur in patients in the sixth to eighth decades of life and is seven times more common in males. A history of smoking, atherosclerosis, hypertension, and COPD are common. The section of the aorta from the renal arteries to the iliac bifurcation is the area involved in 95% of AAAs ("infrarenal aneurysms").

The risk of rupture is directly related to the size of the aneurysm. Small aneurysms of less than 5 cm have a low risk of rupture (less than 5% per year) and the risk of rupture increases to greater than 30% per year for an aneurysm greater than 7.5 cm in diameter.

The abdominal aorta is separated from the free abdominal cavity by the retroperitoneum. This allows blood to be contained in the retroperitoneal space early during rupture. Aneurysms that leak into the free abdominal cavity usually result in rapid uncontrolled hemorrhage, exsanguination, and death. These patients rarely make it to the hospital alive. The majority of aneurysms rupture on the left posterior-lateral side, thus the early hemorrhage from rupture is tamponaded in the retroperitoneum. These are the patients who maintain a measurable blood pressure, and arrive alive at the hospital, to be able to undergo emergency AAA repair.

Of patients whose aneurysms rupture, the classic symptoms include hypotension, abdominal and/or back pain, and a pulsatile abdominal mass. Presence of all three symptoms in the triad is highly suggestive and should be considered a ruptured AAA until proven otherwise. Unfortunately, less than 50% of patients exhibit all three symptoms at the same time, making the diagnosis more difficult. Other symptoms associated with rupture include tachycardia, anorexia or vomiting, abdominal distention, urinary or groin pain, and ischemic symptoms or mottling of lower extremities. The physical exam usually reveals a pulsatile abdominal mass.

Once at the hospital, the diagnosis is confirmed by one of several methods. Patients who are unstable hemodynamically and have the appropriate symptomology are brought directly to the operating room usually following ECG and blood work. In the OR an exploratory laparotomy confirms the diagnosis and allows for repair. Patients in whom the diagnosis is unsure and are hemodynamically stable should undergo a CT scan of the abdomen and pelvis. The diagnosis can be confirmed or other pathology identified in a short time with the fast CT scans today.

Prehospital care of patients with ruptured AAA is supportive and not unlike that for any other patient with significant hemorrhage. Following the basic ABCs, an airway assessment should be made. This usually is a concern only if the patient is unconscious due to hypovolemic shock. Breathing and oxygenation should be supported with 100% oxygen therapy. Aggressive support of circulation is the only area where there is controversy. Clearly, all patients should have vital signs and ECG monitoring en route; large-bore IV should be started en route as well, if possible. Because surgical repair is necessary for survival, expedient transport to an institution with the surgical resources immediately available to perform emergent repair is key for survival.

Circulatory support with large volumes of IV fluids to replace the hypovolemia due to hemorrhage is controversial in the management of AAAs. Most vascular surgeons agree with Dr. Crawford's suggestion in 1990 that patients with ruptured aneurysms should not be aggressively fluid resuscitated and even be allowed to maintain a systolic blood pressure as low as 50 or 70 mmHg. Blood pressures that are greater, or closer to normal, are felt to interfere with the tamponade of hemorrhage in the retroperitoneum, resulting in increased blood loss. Although there are no prospective randomized studies that confirm controlled hypotension as the optimal strategy, several retrospective studies have shown equal, or improved, survival utilizing this strategy.

Also controversial is the use of the pneumatic antishock garment (PASG). One small study with 18 AAA patients suggested increased survival and decreased blood loss with the use of the PASG. This is contrasted with the results from a number of studies in hypovolemic trauma patients in which no benefit was shown. Due to the increased time involved for placement and removal, and the difficulty in performing an adequate physical exam by the receiving surgeon, the use of PASG should be limited to situations where there will be a substantial delay in definitive therapy.

RETURN TO THE CASE

As you are preparing the patient for transport, you contact the medical command physician who requests you transport the patient to the larger tertiary hospital that can render definitive care. She also advises you she will contact the receiving ED to have a surgical team ready for this presumed ruptured AAA patient. You administer oxygen via a mask and place a large-bore IV during transport. The patient remains with a systolic blood pressure of between 80 and 100 mmHg; therefore, only a small amount of fluids are given. The patient remains awake, alert, and continues to complain of pain.

Upon arrival at the hospital, the vascular surgeon and the anesthesiologist are in the ED awaiting the patient. The patient receives an ECG and Foley catheter, and bloods are drawn for type and cross match. In addition, the anesthesiologist places a second large-bore IV for interoperative IV fluid and blood replacement. Within several minutes of arrival the patient is brought to the operating room and undergoes repair of his ruptured abdominal aortic aneurysm.

Postoperatively, he spends several days in the intensive care unit and several more days recovering and receiving physical therapy. He is home recovering within 10 days and feels back to normal after 2 months. He and his family are reassured to know that as a survivor of a ruptured AAA, his long-term life expectancy returns to normal and he lives with his wife and family for years afterward.

REFERENCES

Bledsoe, Bryan E., Robert S. Porter, and Richard A. Cherry. *Trauma Emergencies*. Vol. 4 of *Paramedic Care: Principles & Practice*. Chapter 10, "Thoracic Trauma." Upper Saddle River, NJ: Brady/Prentice Hall Health, Pearson Education, 2001.

Halpern, V. J., R. G. Kline, A. J. D'Angelo, and J. R. Cohen. "Factors That Affect the Survival Rate of Patients with Ruptured Abdominal Aneurysms." *Journal of Vascular Surgery* 26 (1997): 939–948.

O'Connor, R. E., and R. M. Domeier, "An Evaluation of the Pneumatic Anti-Shock Garment (PASG) in Various Clinical Settings." *Prehospital Emergency Care* 1, no. 1 (1997): 36–44.

Claudia E. Goetter, MD
Rajan Gupta, MD
Vicente H. Gracias, MD

33

SHOCK IN PENETRATING INJURY TO THE CHEST

CASE PRESENTATION

You respond to a reported shooting. You are initially told to stage two blocks from the scene, but while en route you are told that the scene is secured by the police and there is a single patient with a gunshot wound to the chest. As you arrive at the scene, you note a young male lying on the ground with a small amount of blood next to the right side of his chest. His eyes are open and his breathing is spontaneous, although it is somewhat labored. Auscultation reveals decreased breath sounds on the right side. He has weakly palpable femoral and radial pulses. He is moaning and unable to answer any questions. As you expose him, you identify a single gunshot wound (GSW) on the right side of his anterior chest. A small amount of blood is exuding from the wound.

You apply a face mask for supplemental oxygen, and establish intravenous access in his right arm. The initial systolic blood pressure is 80 mmHg and the heart rate is 70 bpm. You begin crystalloid infusion and load the patient for transport to the trauma center. Your scene time is 7 minutes.

QUESTIONS

1. Is this patient in shock? What are the potential etiologies of this patient's hypotension?
2. What interventions does this patient require to start treatment for the hypotension? Was the location and timing of the IV access appropriate?
3. What other precautions must you consider as you prepare to transport this patient?

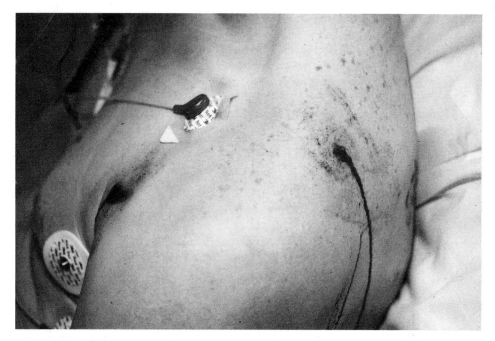

Gunshot wound to the chest.
Courtesy of Edward T. Dickinson, MD.

DISCUSSION

Shock is defined as a lack of perfusion to vital organs. Clinical signs of shock include decreased level of consciousness, cool and/or pale skin, slow capillary refill time, tachycardia, weak or absent pulses, and hypotension. The trauma patient in shock may manifest any or all of these signs. Hypotension is typically thought to be due to hypovolemia, specifically hemorrhage. However, there are many other potential causes of acute shock in this population:

- Restrictive (cardiac tamponade or tension pneumothorax)
- Neurogenic (spinal cord injury)
- Cardiogenic (blunt myocardial injury or concurrent cardiac disease)

RESTRICTIVE

Patients with penetrating injury may cause even more confusion because it is quite rare that hypotension is due to causes other than hemorrhage. Therefore, establishing IV access, starting volume resuscitation, and rapid transport remain the most important interventions for the trauma patient in shock after airway and breathing have been addressed. Recently, some have questioned whether hypotensive patients who have sustained penetrating injury to the torso should be aggressively volume resuscitated. The basic principle underlying the argument not to aggressively resuscitate these patients is that until definitive surgical control of the bleeding sites can be obtained, restoring "normal" blood pressures will lead to further hemorrhage. Conversely, prolonged hypotension leads to decreased perfusion and worsens the shock state. In large urban areas with high volumes of truncal penetrating injury and short transport times to trauma centers, adopting a policy of less aggressive volume resuscitation may be feasible. However, this concept is not applicable to the majority of the prehospital EMS systems where there is not immediate access to a trauma center available.

The location of IV access can also be very important. If a patient has sustained most of the traumatic injury to one side of the torso, he is at risk for injury to the large veins draining that side. This is especially true in penetrating injury. Thus, attempts should be directed toward placing the IV on the relatively less injured side whenever possible.

Additional interventions to treat shock are also important. Simple maneuvers such as direct pressure to bleeding sites and immobilization of fractures can help reduce the volume of blood loss. However, these may not be necessarily applicable in penetrating injury to the torso. Use of the pneumatic antishock garment (PASG) is contraindicated in torso injury as the increased afterload (higher pressure) in the lower extremities results in increased bleeding from injuries not within the garment. After exposing and examining the patient, it is also very important to keep the patient warm. Hypothermia exacerbates the physiologic derangements of the shock state such as acidosis and can induce a loss of normal blood clotting (coagulopathy). Warm fluids and blankets are important adjuncts in the care of patients such as the one presented in this case study.

Knowledge of the possible etiologies of shock is vital to carry out further possible interventions. If the knife or bullet injured the lung or tracheobronchial tree, it could result in a tension pneumothorax. Thus, one must always consider the potential utility of a decompressive needle thoracostomy. Another injury pattern that would lead to a restrictive type of physiology resulting in hypotension is cardiac tamponade. A direct injury to the heart or coronary vessels can easily result in pericardial tamponade. The best treatment for this entity in the prehospital setting is volume resuscitation to maximize the heart's preload and attempt to optimize cardiac output while buying time until arrival at a trauma center where definitive care is available.

NEUROGENIC

Neurogenic shock secondary to spinal cord injury (SCI) may be present even in the patient sustaining penetrating injury to the chest. Bullets and knives can injure the vertebral bodies as well as the spinal cord itself. An injury to the spinal cord at the cervical or high thoracic level results in a loss of sympathetic innervation and subsequent vasodilation. Clinically, this is usually manifested by hypotension *without* an associated tachycardia. In fact, some patients may even be relatively bradycardic. This type of injury pattern highlights some important concepts in the prehospital management of these patients. It emphasizes the importance of assessing disability. This part of the evaluation is part of the primary survey, immediately following circulation. In these particular patients, it may become a part of assessing circulation. Simply noting whether the patient moved all extremities or just the upper ones would potentially raise one's suspicion for SCI. This remains an important adjunct in penetrating injury to the chest. This type of injury pattern also emphasizes the importance of immobilization during transport of these patients. One must recognize that this type of injury can occur in penetrating injury to the torso, and may be the primary etiology of hypotension and shock. Proper immobilization principles should always be consistently followed when spinal injury is suspected.

CARDIOGENIC

Cardiogenic shock secondary to underlying cardiac disease is not commonly seen in patients sustaining penetrating injury to the chest. This is due to the epidemiological factor that most patients sustaining this injury pattern are young and live in urban environments. Therefore, restricting volume resuscitation because the patient may be suffering from congestive heart failure is not appropriate in penetrating injury to the chest until hemorrhage can be definitively excluded. Similarly, septic shock is also rarely encountered in the prehospital care of the trauma patient. This type of shock usually develops later during the course of the patient's hospitalization, most commonly due to infection.

RETURN TO THE CASE

On arrival to the trauma center, the patient's airway is intact, his breath sounds are decreased on the right, and he has palpable femoral pulses. He opens his eyes spontaneously and intermittently follows commands with his upper extremities. He is moaning and does not answer questions. His initial vital signs are significant for a heart rate of 90 and a blood pressure of 60/30 mm Hg. The patient is examined and is found to have a single gunshot wound in the right anterior axillary fold. Intravenous access in the left arm is obtained, and the crystalloid resuscitation is redirected toward a blood products resuscitation. A chest radiograph (Figure 33-1) demonstrates an opacity in the right side of the chest, and a foreign body consistent with a bullet on the left side. A chest tube is placed on the right side, initially draining approximately 400 cc of blood. The potential transmediastinal trajectory of the bullet raises concerns for injury to the heart and/or great vessels. However, an ultrasound of the pericardium does not demonstrate fluid, although this diagnostic technique is less reliable in the presence of a hemothorax. At this point, a reevaluation of the data already obtained changes the focus of the possible etiology of this patient's instability. The patient's heart rate is relatively slow for the degree of hypotension, and the patient is not moving his lower extremities. Thus, neurogenic shock becomes the leading concern, and vasopressors are started. Subsequently, a CT scan of the chest (Figure 33-2) is obtained to determine the potential trajectory of the bullet. This demonstrates a fracture of the second thoracic vertebral body with probable spinal cord transection. Thus, the resulting loss of sympathetic tone as demonstrated by hypotension with relative badycardia is the cause of his shock.

This patient is clearly in shock at the prehospital setting. Volume resuscitation is appropriate, and placement of the IV in the left arm was appropriate. IV access is appropriately obtained at the scene as it does not result in a delay in transport. One might consider

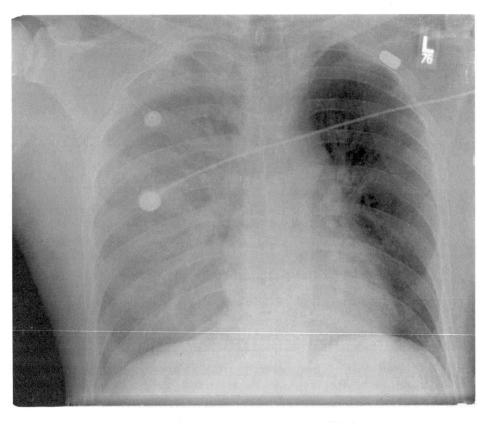

Figure 33-1 Chest x-ray shows right hemothorax and a bullet in apex of left chest.
Courtesy of Vicente H. Gracias, MD.

a needle decompression of the right side if the patient demonstrated signs of tension physiology. However, the patient is not immobilized for spinal precautions during transport, and shortly after arrival to the trauma center SCI is found to be the primary etiology of his instability. A simple gross assessment to check for motor ability in all extremities would have identified the injury. Although diagnosing this in the prehospital setting is not always possible, it must be considered and every patient should be appropriately immobilized prior to transport when signs and symptoms consistent with a spinal cord injury are found in penetrating trauma. This patient's acute injuries are managed in the trauma center, and approximately 1 week later he is transferred to a spinal cord injury rehabilitation center.

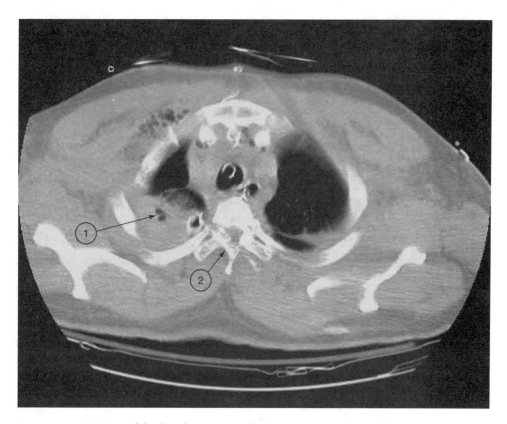

Figure 33-2 CAT Scan of the chest demonstrates right lung injury (1) and a spinal fracture (2).
Courtesy of Vicente H. Gracias, MD

REFERENCES

American College of Surgeons. *ATLS—Advanced Trauma Life Support for Doctors*. 6th ed. Student Course Manual. Chicago: American College of Surgeons, 1997.

Bickell, W. H., M. J. Wall Jr., P. E. Pepe, R. R. Martin, V. F. Ginger, M. K. Allen, and K. L. Mattox. "Immediate versus Delayed Fluid Resuscitation for Hypotensive Patients with Penetrating Torso Injuries." *New England Journal of Medicine* 331, no. 17 (1994): 1105–1109.

Bledsoe, Bryan E., Robert S. Porter, and Richard A. Cherry. *Trauma Emergencies*. Vol. 4 of *Paramedic Care: Principles & Practice*. Chapter 10, "Thoracic Trauma." Upper Saddle River, NJ: Brady/Prentice Hall Health, Pearson Education, 2001.

Vicente H. Gracias, MD

34

STAB WOUND

CASE PRESENTATION

You are called to respond to a patient who is reportedly the victim of stabbing. The dispatcher reports that police are already on the scene and you may proceed directly without staging. When you arrive at the scene, despite the police presence, a crowd has gathered around the victim and it is difficult to approach. As you push your way through, identifying yourself, you first notice that the patient is a male approximately 20 years old and there is a small amount of blood on the front of his shirt.

He is sitting up and is complaining of shortness of breath. As you attempt to lay him back down, he sits up and complains that he can't breathe when he is lying down. You remove his shirt and notice a small 2 cm puncture wound in the anterior portion of his left chest wall midclavicular line 3 cm below the clavicle. Auscultation reveals decreased breath sounds on the left. Your partner obtains IV access in an antecubital vein and you administer oxygen by mask. Vitals signs at this point are normal.

You place the patient on a stretcher and transport him to your unit. Your scene time was 11 minutes. En route to the hospital the patient begins complaining of worsening shortness of breath (SOB), coughs up blood, and drops his systolic pressure to 90 for the first time.

QUESTIONS

1. With penetrating trauma in this location, what is the appropriate site for IV access?
2. If the patient complains of SOB with penetrating trauma to the chest, how does hypotension change your emergent management of him?
3. If the patient experiences hemoptysis (coughing up blood) from his penetrating chest injury, what is the appropriate position for the patient while transporting him to a care facility?

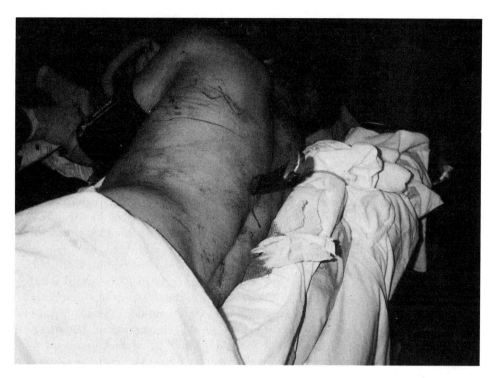

A stabbing with impalement of the knife.
Courtesy of Edward T. Dickinson, MD.

DISCUSSION

Upon your arrival to a scene where a crowd has gathered, caution must always be maintained for your safety as well as the patient's, even when law enforcement is already on the scene. Always identify yourself and move as quickly as possible to the patient's side. Clear a work area for yourself and concentrate on the needs of the patient.

When confronted with any patient suffering from penetrating injury you must always remember the ABCs of trauma care. This patient's airway is intact and he appears to be maintaining a stable airway. With complaints of shortness of breath, oxygen should be administered as soon as possible. Assess the patient's comfort level with the use of face-mask oxygenation. Some patients may resist placement of a face mask in this situation and a nasal cannula may need to be used, since some oxygen is better than none. Although complaints of SOB may be related to anxiety, in this patient with worsening SOB secondary to supine positioning you must consider the possibility of a pneumothorax. If decreased breath sounds are also present on the side of the penetrating injury, the diagnosis is almost certain. If the patient has a pneumothorax but does not have associated hypotension—the hallmark of tension pneumothorax—he does not need any immediate intervention other than supplemental oxygen and continued monitoring for signs of hypotension. If hypotension develops with a clinical picture of pneumothorax, then immediate needle decompression of the affected side of the chest is indicated.

In a patient who has suffered penetrating injury, it is often prudent to achieve IV access on the unaffected side, if you are able to assess a unilateral injury to a specific limb or side of the torso. Therefore, this patient with a stab wound near his clavicle on the left has risk for injury to his subclavian vessels; thus, the IV should be placed in the right antecubital vein if possible.

IV access can be obtained either rapidly while on the scene prior to transport or while in transport mode to the hospital. Traditional trauma and EMS teaching limits the on-scene time in major trauma cases to 10 minutes or less. Attempts at establishing an IV should never delay transport to the definitive care of the emergency department or operating room.

During transport the patient's vital signs should be continuously monitored as well as his SOB and response to therapy (e.g., oxygen). Once the patient has documented hypotension the possibility of tension pneumothorax must be considered and needle decompression is warranted. Needle decompression of the chest should be performed in standard fashion as per local EMS protocol. A large-bore angiocatheter is inserted in the second intercostal space just below the rib in the midclavicular line on the side with the decreased or absent breath sounds. The angiocath should be pushed all the way in as there should be minimal risk to someone with collapsed lung and tension physiology. Appropriate decompression of the thorax in patients with tension pneumothorax is a life-saving intervention that cannot be delayed until ED arrival. Following decompression, the patient's respiratory status and vital signs should be monitored to assess the response to therapy.

The occurrence of hemoptysis in this patient with penetrating trauma presents a unique clinical problem that may occur with patients who suffer penetrating injury to the chest and lung. If the penetrating injury involves not only lung parenchyma but a larger bronchial tributary, the patient can bleed from the stab wound in the lung into his own airway and subsequently suffocate in his own blood unless appropriate measures are taken by the EMS providers. The patient with penetrating thoracic trauma and associated hemoptysis should preferably be placed with the effected side of thorax down to prevent bronchial bleeding from crossing into the unaffected lung. If the patient cannot tolerate this, then the patient should be maintained in a sitting position, with as much of the effected side in a dependent position as possible. Should the hemoptysis worsen, the patient should be immediately intubated and positive-pressure ventilation applied in an attempt to insufflate the affected portion of lung and tamponade the bleeding.

The change in the patient's status should be reported immediately to the receiving emergency department so that appropriate surgical response can be waiting for the patient upon arrival to the hospital.

RETURN TO THE CASE

With the patient's clinical deterioration, the paramedic immediately performs a needle decompression of the patient's left side in the appropriate location and notes a hissing sound from the angiocath. The patient's shortness of breath improves remarkably and the paramedic is able to lay the patient supine. Upon the first signs of hemoptysis the paramedic places the patient's affected side in the dependent position. Supplemental oxygen is administered using mask and the patient tolerates this well until he presents to the trauma resuscitation bay of the hospital.

The regional trauma center and waiting trauma team receive the patient. The patient is quickly assessed. Left-tube thoracostomy is performed and the patient is noted to be saturating well on 50% FIO_2 mask with no further hemoptysis. The patient is taken immediately for a CT scan of the chest which shows a large parenchymal bleed within the left upper lobe of the lung. A subsequent pulmonary angiogram performed due to the patient's history of hemoptysis reveals no extravasation of contrast and therefore no further bleeding into the airway or lung. The patient does well, the chest tube is removed on day 3 of admission, and he is discharged to home.

REFERENCES

Bledsoe, Bryan E., Robert S. Porter, and Richard A. Cherry. *Trauma Emergencies*. Vol. 4 of *Paramedic Care: Principles & Practice*. Chapter 2, "Penetrating Trauma." Upper Saddle River, NJ: Brady/Prentice Hall Health, Pearson Education, 2001.

Jonathan Halpert, MD

35

TRAUMA ARREST

CASE PRESENTATION

You respond to the scene of an individual who has fallen from scaffolding. On arrival you find an adult male who has been partially buried by a large amount of scaffolding and roofing material. Assessment of the scene verifies no danger of secondary collapse.

The initial call for help was placed via cell phone by a coworker of the victim, who observed the collapse. The patient was partially buried by the construction debris, with aspects of the face, head, torso, and arms involved. The coworker began manual disentanglement of the victim, and was joined shortly thereafter by the first arriving police unit. Working quickly, the two achieve complete extrication of the patient as your unit arrives on scene, 12 minutes after the original call to the regional 911 center was made. A second ALS provider joins you, simultaneous to your arrival on the scene. The BLS ambulance arrives 10 minutes after your arrival.

Initial observation reveals the patient sustained a two-story fall. He landed on a grassy surface, and was struck and partially buried by the wood and pipe scaffold structure he had been working on, along with pallets of roofing slate that the scaffold had been bearing. The total weight of materials involving the patient is grossly estimated at 1,000 pounds.

The primary survey is initiated, and you note that the patient is unresponsive. His airway appears compromised, as debris in the mouth is obvious. There is also profuse bleeding involving the midface, nose, and mouth, with multiple avulsed teeth and a gaping, jagged laceration of the lower jaw evident. The patient is apneic; the chest wall is marked by multiple contusions; and there is no open wound, bony crepitus, or palpable subcutaneous air. His skin is remarkably pale, and you detect thready, very tachycardic carotid pulses; radial pulses are not palpable. Other than the obvious facial and head injuries, there is no readily evident source of gross exsanguination. The Glasgow Coma Scale is 3, and his pupils are estimated to be 4 mm bilaterally and are nonreactive.

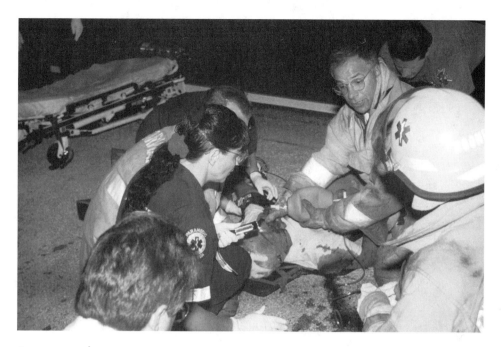

A traumatic cardiac arrest.

Your partner manually stabilizes the cervical spine, and opens the airway with a jaw thrust. You suction out the oral pharynx with difficulty because copious bleeding about the mouth is encountered. Ventilation is then begun using a bag-valve-mask with 100% oxygen supplement. Direct laryngoscopy is rapidly performed; the vocal cords are obscured by the large volume of blood that continues to occupy the airway, though the glottic opening is vaguely identified by the presence of bubbling in the hypopharynx. An endotracheal tube is passed into the glottis. The patient ventilates easily, with symmetric chest rise, diminished but clear bilateral breath sounds, absent borborygmi, and appropriate colorimetric findings on end-tidal CO_2 detector. Following intubation, carotid pulses are lost. CPR is initiated, and the ECG monitor is attached, revealing pulseless electrical activity, or PEA (sinus tachycardia). The patient is logrolled onto a long spine board. Two milligrams of epinephrine are instilled into the endotracheal tube, and the patient is placed into the now waiting ambulance. The patient continues to bleed from his facial injuries. Total on-scene time is 12 minutes.

QUESTIONS

1. What mechanisms can cause cardiac arrest following application of positive-pressure ventilation in a hemodynamically unstable trauma patient?

2. What is the significance of ongoing exsanguinating hemorrhage from the face and head in the trauma patient?

DISCUSSION

Establishing and securing the airway of a critically injured patient is one of the fundamental principles regarding management of a victim of multiple trauma. Regardless of the mechanism of injury and extent of other modalities utilized to manage the trauma patient, failure to open and maintain the airway of such a patient will result in significantly increased morbidity and mortality.

The introduction of direct laryngoscopy and endotracheal intubation to the prehospital setting revolutionized emergency medical practice. Placement of an invasive airway dramatically reduces the risk of pulmonary aspiration related to blood and clot, as well as the passive regurgitation of gastric contents. Additionally, bag-to-tube ventilation markedly reduces dead space considerations. This technique also facilitates rescuer manipulation of the upper airway anatomy, the failure of which results in complications related to gastric insufflation and aspiration, with resultant poor oxygenation and ventilation, and worsening acidosis. Endotracheal intubation markedly improves alveolar oxygenation and ventilation and limits rescuer fatigue, which allows for the application of longer-duration and more effective resuscitation techniques.

It has been documented that, although the benefits of endotracheal intubation are many, there are certain well-known potential hazards to the utilization of such devices. It can be anticipated that in certain circumstances, patients may experience a measure of decline in their physiologic status, even after proper placement of an endotracheal tube.

In the case of this patient, though direct visualization of the vocal cords was not possible, he was promptly and correctly intubated. However, he became pulseless almost immediately after the intubation event. Cardiac arrest immediately following endotracheal intubation can be the result of several factors, which must be immediately addressed to reverse the situation. Chief among the factors requiring correction would be that the administration of positive pressure ventilation has converted a simple pneumothorax to a tension pneumothorax—a pneumothorax involving air under tension.

In pneumothorax, the inciting event is a pulmonary parenchymal defect, which allows air to leak from the alveolar airspace into the pleural space by way of defects in the lung parenchyma and visceral pleura. Although several mechanisms exist that explain how patients develop these defects, in the case of a blunt trauma victim it is typically related to barotrauma. The classic example is the rapid application of an unusually large compressive force to the exterior chest, suddenly compressing the intrathoracic volume. This can occur simultaneous to the patient holding the glottis closed after having taken a deep breath, in anticipation of impending impact (the "paper-bag" effect). The application of these abnormal forces against an area of predisposed weakness in the lung parenchyma results in rupture and subsequent development of an air leak.

In and of itself, a small defect in the pleural-parenchymal boundary may not necessarily produce a cataclysmic event. If the defect is small, or the defect occurs in a subsequently apneic individual, the result often is a simple pneumothorax, not necessarily involving intrathoracic air under tension.

Application of positive pressure ventilation via the endotracheal tube can, however, cause the pleural leak to manifest itself in a particularly malignant fashion. As air is pumped into the lung at high pressures via the ventilator and endotracheal tube, it leaks through the pulmonary defect and rapidly accumulates in the pleural space, causing intrapleural pressures to elevate. Significantly increased pressure can result in a shift of mediastinal structures away from the site of the air leak. Should mediastinal shift occur, right heart filling pressures markedly decrease, as this shift can cause relative vena caval occlusion due to rotation away from its normal axis. Loss of normal right heart preload results in subsequently decreased left heart filling. Lacking adequate preload to the left heart, cardiac output falls; this event is typically associated with a dramatic drop in systemic blood pressure.

During the development of a pneumothorax, the function of the affected lung becomes increasingly more compromised. Thus, the body's physiologic requirement pertaining to oxygenation and ventilation shifts to the unaffected lung. In the case of tension pneumothorax, an additional effect of mediastinal shift is encountered. The unaffected lung parenchyma can easily become compromised due to the collapsing, shifting lung moving away from the site of accumulating intrapleural air, resulting in compression of the contralateral lung.

As compression of the originally unaffected lung progresses, pulmonary functions become dramatically altered. Decreased pulmonary blood flow secondary to diminishing preload results in loss of carbon dioxide offloading, whereas parenchymal compression results in decreased alveolar membrane surface area available for oxygenation and gas exchange. This precipitates profound hypoxia and hypercarbia, with resultant worsening acidosis.

Given this patient's acute need for a definitive airway and positive-pressure ventilation (PPV), there is no choice but to manage the patient with the most definitive device available. Securing the airway early in the management of the multiple trauma patient with an endotracheal tube is requisite. This patient rapidly deteriorated into a state of cardiac arrest following this required intervention, which necessitated rapidly addressing the possibility that there was causality between the two events. As it is well documented that PPV can transform a simple pneumothorax into a tension pneumothorax, and that a tension pneumothorax occurring in the physiologically frail state of a multiple trauma patient can have catastrophic implications, there is little choice but to address this possibility as soon as possible with needle thoracostomy emergently performed to relieve a possible tension pneumothorax. The most common airway-related reasons for abrupt decompensation of the intubated patient are described by the mnemonic D-O-P-E (tube Displaced/Obstructed, Pneumothorax, Equipment failure). In this case pneumothorax—the P in D-O-P-E—seemed to be the most likely cause.

Another problem with positive pressure ventilation is that it has the potential to produce significant negative hemodynamic side effects, even in the absence of an underlying pneumothorax. It is common to encounter some degree of hypotension following the introduction of an endotracheal tube and subsequent PPV. In the case of a rapid sequence intubation protocol utilizing induction agents such as midazolam or propofol, hypotension is expected. Because of this side effect, these agents should be used with great care or not at all in the hemodynamically unstable patient. Even in the absence of these particular medications, a measure of hypotension is often encountered following initiation of PPV. This phenomenon is especially apparent in those individuals with baseline physiologic alterations, such as dehydration, hypovolemia, anemia, or acidosis.

This effect may be a function of arrhythmia, as airway manipulation with the laryngoscope can mediate significant increases in vagal tone, which can provoke bradycardic and even asystolic cardiac rhythm responses.

Postintubation hypotension is believed to be most often a function of increased intrathoracic pressure. It is not the intubation that incites this phenomenon so much as the increase in intrathoracic pressure that endotracheal tube mediated PPV facilitates. This occurs secondary to the change from normal, physiologic negative-pressure ventilation to that of externally driven, positive-pressure ventilation. In a normal situation, an individual takes a breath due to contraction and flattening of the diaphragm. This motion increases the volume of the lung, creating lower internal pressure relative to external atmospheric pressure. Air subsequently rushes in to fill the low-pressure void, and a breath is taken. A subject undergoing PPV has air (or oxygen) introduced by a device, utilizing pressures considerably above that of atmospheric. This consequently causes the lungs to fill, but at significantly higher pressures than usual.

Increased intrapulmonary pressure is transmitted throughout the chest as intrathoracic pressure. Drastically increased intrathoracic pressures can adversely impact other intrathoracic structures (e.g., the mediastinum). In a physiologically challenged individual, the effects of this phenomenon can be measurable, and potentially have a profound negative impact on the patient.

For example, increased intrathoracic pressures can result in decreased cardiac output. There are several reasons for this. The hyperventilated, hyperoxygenated state of the initially intubated patient results in significantly increased pulmonary capillary blood flow. This effectively allows blood to pool in the pulmonary capillary beds between the right and left hearts, functionally precluding normal preloading of the left atria and ventricle, producing decreased cardiac output. Additionally, increased intrathoracic pressures tend to impede venous return to the right heart, further decreasing preload. Also, a component of both right- and left-sided ventricular dysfunction has been described with this condition. Decreased ventricular muscle relaxation results in incomplete ventricular filling. The ventricle is unable to completely stretch to accommodate the load it is given. This results in further compromising the ability of the ventricle to satisfactorily eject blood, and decreases cardiac output. All of these factors have been described to occur most significantly in the volume-depleted patient, and are responsive to aggressive isotonic crystalloid volume loading either prior to or following institution of endotracheal intubation and positive-pressure ventilation.

Exsanguinating hemorrhage is, of course, a significant challenge to the stability of the multiple trauma patient. Bleeding control remains a fundamental tenet of managing the patient during the primary survey. However, it is often overlooked by even the most knowledgeable providers. This is most likely due to a failure on the part of caregivers to accurately perceive the quantity or significance of ongoing external blood loss. Oftentimes it is difficult to appreciate bleeding that occurs on the posterior aspect of a patient lying on a spine board or stretcher. Occasionally, a patient is not fully exposed during the course of initial evaluation, and vigorously bleeding wounds are simply not recognized, given all else that may be going on with treating a critically injured patient.

Head wounds can present several kinds of challenges. Scalp hair can disguise wounds. A patient immobilized to a long board, with cervical collar and head immobilizer in place, presents little exposed surface area for visual evaluation. Failure to recognize and treat potentially serious head wounds prior to placing these external devices can be devastating. The skin of the scalp and face are incredibly well vascularized structures. A small wound often presents with fairly dramatic associated bleeding. A large defect can bleed catastrophically. The need to control bleeding from head wounds may seem to fly in the face of the conventional pre-hospital dogma that head injuries are incapable of producing shock (except in the very young). This is true of closed head injuries, because there is so little room inside the skull that internal bleeding is suppressed. It is not true of open, externally bleeding head wounds, which must be controlled.

Treating the bleeding scalp of the multiply traumatized patient while en route to the hospital can be challenging. Concern over appropriate spinal precautions typically results in difficulty accessing the occipital scalp for the placement of direct pressure. Equally challenging is the application of elevation techniques for bleeding control. In the well-perfused patient, it is possible to elevate the head of the spine board somewhat, to keep the patient supine but with head to some extent above the heart. In the hypotensive, unstable, or arrested patient, elevation of the head is contraindicated because this maneuver would result in further decreased cerebral perfusion. Utilization of pressure dressings is required. Although bulky dressings will contain a good deal of blood, in and of themselves they may not achieve hemostasis in a vigorously bleeding wound. That, however, may be all that can be utilized over the occipit of a supine, boarded patient. Digital, fingertip pressure in conjunction with a discreet amount of dressing material applied directly to a wound may be what is required to get temporary control over a rapidly or persistently exsanguinating site. Exsanguinating facial or airway wounds must be similarly addressed. Suction equipment must be used liberally to keep the airway clear of blood and clot. Dressing materials in the form of either sponges or packs should be placed into the oral pharynx, around the nose and face to minimize blood loss. Failure to do so will result in a catastrophic chain of events, including anemia, volume depletion, hypothermia, coagulopathy, shock, and death.

Patients who suffer traumatic cardiac arrest have a very poor prognosis. This is true for both blunt and penetrating trauma. In most studies, patients found to be in traumatic arrest upon arrival of the EMS units die despite maximal ALS interventions. Trauma patients who arrest in the presence of EMS may have a very narrow window of possible resuscitation if they are rapidly transported to an appropriate medical facility and "reversible" causes of the arrest such as tension pneumothorax, hypovolemia, or pericardial tamponade are immediately identified and treated either by ALS or immediately upon emergency department arrival.

Management of the traumatic cardiac arrest patient relies on strict adherence to emergency patient care fundamentals. Specifically, exquisite attention to airway, breathing, and circulatory assessment, intervention, and reassessment cannot be overstressed.

RETURN TO THE CASE

A priority 1 transport is initiated, with an additional 2 mg of epinephrine instilled into the endotracheal tube. A brief secondary survey reveals clear ears, no Battles or raccoon signs, severe contusions to the lower face, flat neck veins, midline trachea, a soft, nondistended abdomen, and a stable pelvis. Peripheral IV access is gained en route to the hospital, with 14- and 16-gauge catheters placed. Aggressive fluid resuscitation is started with normal saline. A total of 5 L of IV fluids are pressure infused prior to transfer to the trauma center.

The case is discussed with online medical control while en route to the trauma center. You are directed to perform a bilateral needle thoracostomy. No air rush or change in status is noted immediately following the decompressions. ACLS resuscitation protocol is followed, with the patient receiving additional epinephrine and CPR during the 20-minute transport time. Five minutes prior to arriving at the trauma center, a return of spontaneous circulation is observed, with carotid and radial pulses detected. A palpable systolic blood pressure of 100 is measured. The patient remains flaccid with a GCS of 3. Oozing bleeding from the face continues.

Once in the hospital, the patient receives maximal resuscitation effort per ATLS guidelines. Bilateral tube thoracostomies, pericardiocentesis, blood transfusion, and ongoing pharmacological therapy are furnished. The nasal and oral pharynx is packed, and the facial wounds are whip stitched for reapproximation, in an effort to obtain hemostasis. The patient experiences recurrent episodes of PEA (pulseless electrical activity) and VF (ventricular fibrillation) during his stay in the emergency department. Ultimately, he experiences disseminated intravascular coagulation, has uncontrollable hemorrhage from all wound and puncture sites, and suffers cardiac arrest refractory to further pharmacotherapy. He is pronounced dead 3 hours after the inciting trauma has occurred.

REFERENCES

American College of Surgeons. *ATLS—Advanced Trauma Life Support for Doctors*. 6th ed. Student Course Manual. Chicago: American College of Surgeons, 1997.

Bledsoe, Bryan E., Robert S. Porter, and Richard A. Cherry. *Trauma Emergencies*. Vol. 4 of *Paramedic Care: Principles & Practice*. Chapter 4, "Hemorrhage and Shock." Upper Saddle River, NJ: Brady/Prentice Hall Health, Pearson Education, 2001.

Deakin, C. D. "Prehospital Management of the Traumatized Airway." *European Journal of Emergency Medicine* 3, no. 4 (December 1996): 233–243.

Dickinson, E. T. "Prehospital Trauma Triage." In R. Sing and P. M. Reilly, eds., *Trauma Decision Making—Initial Management of Injuries*. London: BMJ Publishing, 2001.

Stock, M. C., and A. Perel. *Handbook of Mechanical Ventilatory Support*. Baltimore: Williams & Wilkins, 1997.

Tobin, M. J. "Mechanical Ventilation." *New England Journal of Medicine* 330, no. 15 (April 14, 1994): 1056–1061.

Raquel Schears, MD, MPH, FACEP

36

ADVANCE DIRECTIVES

CASE PRESENTATION

Your unit is dispatched to the local nursing home for an 82-year-old woman in cardiopulmonary arrest. Staffers tell you she has widely metastatic lung cancer and advanced dementia. She was warm, unresponsive, and pulseless when found on morning rounds. She had lived in the nursing home for 6 months but neither her daughter (designated as power of attorney for health care on an intake form) nor her primary doctor could be reached. Someone recalled that on her last hospital discharge summary there was mention of a living will, but it was not copied nor transferred back with her to the nursing home. Her facility medical records contained no affirmation of her determination not to have her life prolonged by artificial means.

As you approach her bedside, your initial impression is that she is extremely cachectic, without obvious signs of life, and centrally cyanotic. You determine this patient's unwitnessed arrest has been going on for a minimum of 10 minutes prior to EMS arrival. The nurses have CPR in progress without a backboard in place or BVM oxygen, and the providers are tiring. You observe no airway adjuncts or IV access, and on your portable monitor the patient is in asystole. The nurses are very focused on expediting the care and transfer of this resident to the ambulance for transport to the ED, although privately they concede their belief that death is a foregone conclusion. Nervously, they tell you they want to be able to inform the daughter that "everything was done."

QUESTIONS

1. Are there options available to the paramedics in treating patients without advance directives (ADs) when death is expected and 911 is called?

2. Should the trained preoccupation with preservation of life be applied to *all* patients regardless of their wish for a natural death at the end of life?

3. Is there an ethical or medicolegal difference between withholding and withdrawing life-sustaining treatment?

DISCUSSION

Without a valid EMS-DNR (do not resuscitate) order, proceeding with an adequate trial of resuscitation per ACLS protocol is the standard of care in the nonhospital setting. This practice occurs even in cases such as this case where the patient has an extremely poor prognosis and death is the most likely outcome. Ethically, nonhospital resuscitation cannot be denied to any group of patients without their express permission because doing so would endanger the good that could be achieved by such ADs for those patients who do not want CPR. As well, "Hollywood" or pseudo-CPR is unethical, medically unsound, and violates the tenet of therapeutic trust—it cannot be condoned.

Once initiation of resuscitation has begun, maximal effort is required for *any* accrual of benefit. The probability of surviving sudden cardiopulmonary arrest is extremely poor, and the chances of surviving with normal neurological status are even more remote. It is well known that prognosis deteriorates quickly as time in arrest lengthens, even if good CPR is performed. As the sole treatment for cardiac arrest, CPR confers a survival benefit of less than 5%. Survival declines 10% for each minute defibrillation is delayed in the first 5 minutes of arrest. By the time asystole occurs, successful resuscitation is very unlikely. Nonetheless, the ACLS *Guidelines 2000* indicate ALS efforts should be continued for at least 20 minutes in patients with unwitnessed arrest. As in this case, even if the bystanders are not prepared to treat fully, at least they must provide chest-compression-only CPR, shown superior to no CPR in early arrest. Coronary perfusion pressure cannot be generated without some form of chest compression.

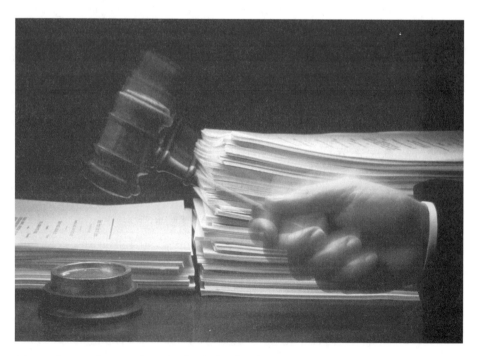

Advance directives have significant legal and ethical implications.

This case illustrates a common scenario in the United States. Medical technology and the moment of death are usually knit together, orchestrated by well-intentioned professionals paid, and often constrained, to act as if death is avoidable. This sentiment is a side effect of the media misrepresenting actual medical achievements in extending life expectancy, and it's fueled by the mutual self-deception found in patient–medical provider communication. Truth is, most Americans fear death yet few plan for its inevitability. Discussing death makes doctors uncomfortable. Paramedics usually called by 911 networks come fully prepared to deny it, protocol ready to fight it. We have been taught that death is equivalent to failure. We have believed that however limited life is, it is still better than death. Last, as this case suggests, we don't want to take the blame for the moment death happens because we fear family reprisal through litigation.

The public recognizes the existence of fates worse than death. Over the last 20 years patients have increasingly been occupying the driver's seat in making their own medical decisions. It is socially, ethically, and medicolegally acceptable for *competent* patients to refuse treatment, including life-sustaining interventions. Advance directives (ADs) are the vehicles commonly used by patients to portray their wishes if and when incapacity occurs. (There is no consensus on handling *incompetent* patients with no AD, proxy, or surrogate decision maker.) Living wills and health care power-of-attorney designations are examples of AD devices available to consumers to limit unwanted care especially at the end of life.

Paradoxically, having an AD is no guarantee against CPR, and the last decade has revealed the difficulties in applying AD theory to practice in nonhospital settings. Once activated, the EMS system is heavily weighted toward saving lives and treating illness. To expect such a system to function as well in reverse may be as unrealistic as the expectations dying patients have that all their wishes will meet with instant compliance. EMS personnel have little time to make determinations of patient identity and nonuniform document validity while trying to resuscitate. Thus, the human error remains to err on the side of life, or full resuscitative care for the patient with most ADs. Providers treat fully and perhaps transport to the hospital. When the pace of the arrest settles, and if the patient lives, the issues of identity, currency, and AD validity can be scrutinized. At that point, if necessary, it remains possible to undo the temporary trespass, and realign with the patient's AD wishes. In this way, much of the patient's (and EMS providers') control over end-of-life decisions is overwhelmed by situational urgency, overruled by physicians, and undermined by organizational complexity. Many EMS systems have tried to remedy this situation by instructing families on the frontiers of dying, *not to dial 911*. This may be the only way to provide choice, certainty, and control over death.

So far, the legal community has concurred with the resuscitation instincts of the medical profession where document ambiguity exists, and has upheld an interest in the preservation of life. Families of plaintiffs with ADs to forego life-sustaining interventions who have sued for "wrongful life" following resuscitation, have also not been successful. Additionally, the Federal Patient Self-Determination Act passed in 1991 was aimed at encouraging hospitals and nursing homes that participated in Medicare and Medicaid programs to honor patients' requests regarding end-of-life decisions. The mandate directs institutions to provide patients with information about ADs (but not forms), and place completed ADs in the patient medical record. Unfortunately, there is no requirement that patients document their ADs, or discuss DNR status with their physician.

DNR orders accomplish the same goals as the ADs previously described, but are slightly different because they incorporate the considered judgment of a licensed physician, as evidenced by his or her signature. In nonhospital settings, these directives are referred to as EMS-DNR orders. The vital distinction is that these orders represent physician buy-in with respect to patient wishes. (Exceptions exist in Kentucky, Louisiana, and Oklahoma where an EMS-DNR can be created by a patient *without* a physician signature.) Overall, the legal protection afforded the EMS community acting as agents of the EMS-DNR is clearer, with physician orders subject to higher professional practice standards and public accountability. Forty-two states now have statewide EMS-DNR protocols in place as of September 1999; however, little has been published on these nonhospital protocols.

In most states EMS providers acting in good faith are protected from criminal prosecution, civil liability, or administrative action when withholding or withdrawing resuscitation in accordance with EMS-DNR statute. All states require that comfort care be provided to patients. Most states also detail instances in which EMS personnel would not have to comply with a DNR order. These exceptions vary from state to state, but the categories include (a) when the DNR is revoked, canceled, or of questionable validity; (b) when EMS is unaware of the DNR order; (c) when someone objects to the DNR order, or if administering CPR is necessary for safety, or to relieve pain or suffering; and (d) when the EMS providers' conscience renders them unable to comply with a DNR order.

Despite the preceding list of excuses aimed at overlooking EMS nonadherence with EMS-DNR orders, emergency providers have a higher moral imperative to comply with patients' wishes at the end of life. This is argued for several reasons. First, if few nursing home patients have ADs to limit care as they near death, the solution is not to find new ways to ignore them all, but to accept them all—even the expired or imperfectly executed ones. After all, the reason EMS-DNR orders were invented in a climate rife with other forms of advance direction, was not to make it procedurally harder for patients to refuse unwanted treatment, but to make it easier. Morally, to say we want to err "on the side of life" is foolish when the cost of cheating death temporarily is the patient's involuntary suffering and indignity. Second, the idea that caution should be exercised in following through on an EMS-DNR order in patients at the end of life because the patient may have changed her or his mind is seriously flawed. Incompetent patients have lost the ability to think and therefore have no minds to change. Nonetheless, these same patients have not surrendered their constitutional rights—which include the right to refuse treatment. Third, to provide resuscitation over an EMS-DNR order to halt treatment does not obviate the need to medically care for that patient and surrogates present. To do "everything" indicated under the circumstances, being mindful of the human context within which we practice, is a better goal than doing everything possible to avoid the truth.

Last, there is no moral difference between withdrawing a treatment that is felt to offer no benefit and withholding one that is not indicated. However, the ease with which nonbeneficial treatments are withheld or withdrawn, once instituted, may be relative to the practice setting. This latter distinction leads practitioners to feel more exposed to certain medicolegal risks. For example, frontline emergency providers feel it is harder to withhold life-sustaining treatment than to start it and eventually stop it, whereas downstream ICU providers find it harder to withdraw a nonbeneficial treatment already started than to withhold starting additionally pointless procedures. The two actions feel different because both sets of providers have a training bias toward providing cures and not end-of-life care to ensure the comfort of dying patients and their families.

Prior research has established the medical pointlessness of continued ED resuscitation efforts for patients in cardiac arrest who fail to respond to nonhospital ACLS. Yet even into the late 1990s there is continued transport of many patients to hospitals fitting this description. There has been little research into this phenomenon and no development of protocols that focus on nonmedical factors, which influence transport decisions in this situation. One study did look at family acceptance of terminating unsuccessful prehospital arrests in the field. The findings indicated families did not expect that EMS treatment always include transport to a hospital, and were satisfied with ending unsuccessful arrests at the scene. Although these results are encouraging, they have not been replicated in nursing homes or for arrests outside the home.

Guidelines 2000 states it is permissible for EMS to suspend ACLS after an adequate trial if unsuccessful (no return of spontaneous pulse during 20 minutes) and terminate the resuscitation effort, regardless of the location. Jurisdictions differ in whether physician radio backup or even on-site medical doctors are employed to terminate unsuccessful arrests in the field. State law defines who can legally determine that extraordinary procedures not be used to continue a human life, and who can implement such an order. Without exception, only a licensed physician can direct such an order and the order cannot be delegated to a layperson. Interestingly, in a recent small study of field experience with nonhospital ADs 28% of EMS providers admitted to implementing prehospital AD *without* medical control.

RETURN TO THE CASE

Paramedics immediately move the patient to the floor and begin full resuscitation per ACLS algorithm for asystole. After two rounds of IV medications, and a successful intubation, the rhythm remains unchanged. The arrest is terminated in the nursing home, after discussion with the local ED medical command physician. The nurses are finally able to contact the daughter to inform her of her mother's arrest and unsuccessful resuscitation. The daughter is very upset at the heroic measures employed at the end of life for her mother who never would have wished for such interventions. When asked why she had neglected to make her mother's wishes part of the nursing home medical record, the daughter stated she feared her mother's care would be abandoned once labeled a DNR patient. She thought she'd have more time to personally make clear her mother's desire for a peaceful death.

Because advance directive laws are different in each state, it is important to familiarize yourself with your state's law. Partnership for Caring: America's Voices for the Dying, a national not-for-profit organization, is an invaluable resource for health care professionals and their clients. Partnership for Caring developed the first living will over 25 years ago and today remains the nation's largest distributor of free state-specific advance directives. State laws regarding nonhospital EMS-DNR are also tracked. Its expert staff of educators, lawyers, social workers, and nurses will answer questions about the complex issues of patients' rights and end-of-life medical treatment.

Many of the questions Partnership for Caring fields come from health care professionals who are unsure of their legal rights and duties when honoring a patient's medical treatment wishes. To speak to someone at Partnership for Caring about end-of-life decision making, place bulk orders for educational materials or advance directives for your facility, or to order a free advance directive packet, you can call toll-free at 1-800-989-WILL, or write to Partnership for Caring, 1620 Eye Street NW, Suite 202, Washington, DC 20006, or visit the Web site at http://www.partnershipforcaring.org.

REFERENCES

American Heart Association and International Liaison Committee on Resuscitation. "Guidelines 2000 for Cardiopulmonary Resuscitation and Emergency Cardiovascular Care." *Circulation* 102 (August 2000 Suppl.): I-1–384.

Berg, R. A., K. B. Kern, R. W. Hilwig, and G. A. Ewy. "Assisted Ventilation during 'Bystander' CPR in a Swine Acute Myocardial Infarction Model Does Not Improve Outcome." *Circulation* 96, no. 12 (December 1997): 4364–4371.

Bledsoe, Bryan E., Robert S. Porter, and Richard A. Cherry. *Introduction to Advanced Prehospital Care*. Vol. 1 of *Paramedic Care: Principles & Practice*. Chapter 6, "Legal Aspects of Advanced Prehospital Care." Upper Saddle River, NJ: Brady/Prentice Hall Health, Pearson Education, 2000.

Diem, S. J., J. D. Lantos, and J. A. Tulsky. "Cardiopulmonary Resuscitation on Television: Miracles and Misinformation." *New England Journal of Medicine* 334 (1996): 1578–1582.

Lombardi, G., E. Gallagher, and P. Gennis. "Outcome of Out-of-Hospital Cardiac Arrest in New York City." *Journal of the American Medical Association* 271 (1994): 678–683.

"No Liability for Unwanted Resuscitation. *Wright v. The Johns Hopkins Health Systems Corp.*" *Hospital Law Newsletter* 17, no. 5 (March 2000): 1–5.

O'Brien, L. A., and J. A. Grisso. "Cardiopulmonary Resuscitation in Nursing Homes." *American Journal of Medicine* 98, no. 3 (1995): 316.

Partridge, R. A., A. Virk, A. Sayah, and R. Antosia. "Field Experience with Prehospital Advance Directives." *Annals of Emergency Medicine* 32 (1998): 589–593.

Sabatino, C. P. "Survey of State EMS-DNR Laws and Protocols." *Journal of Law, Medicine and Ethics* 27 (1999): 297–315.

37

Dan Limmer, AS, EMT-P

ATTEMPTED SUICIDE

CASE PRESENTATION

You are dispatched to a call for an "attempted suicide" at 1426 Maxwell Road. Dispatch advises you to stage at Maxwell and Creekside until police secure the scene.

After you are advised to respond in, you do so carefully, observing as you approach. You see two police cars outside with an officer standing at the front door waving you in. As you approach the officer tells you that parents came home and found their son with a gun in his room. He is not injured, but is intoxicated and seemingly depressed. The police officer requests transport to the local psychiatric facility. You are assured that the scene is safe and that the patient is weapon-free. You approach the patient.

The patient is sitting on his bed. You observe a 23-year-old male patient who is alert and oriented with a clear airway and apparently normal respirations. He does not have external injury. You introduce yourself as a paramedic and assure the patient that you are there to help. The patient does not make eye contact but verbally acknowledges your presence. He eventually states that he had planned on killing himself with a rifle but his parents interrupted him. He acknowledges ingesting about a pint of bourbon over the past 3–4 hours. The patient denies medical or traumatic problems. A brief physical exam with full vital signs are all within normal limits.

A brief scan of the scene reveals packing material for the weapon which appears to have been recently opened. You do not observe any medications, illegal substances, or other possible mechanisms of injury present. The police report that a suicide note was found indicating issues with a recent divorce.

The parents further acknowledge that they have been concerned about their son's alcohol use which has increased after the patient's separation and divorce. He attempted suicide one other time over a year ago with nonprescription medications. They recently opened mail and found new credit cards. The parents suspect that the son opened a credit card solely to purchase the rifle he was to use to kill himself. The parents were a

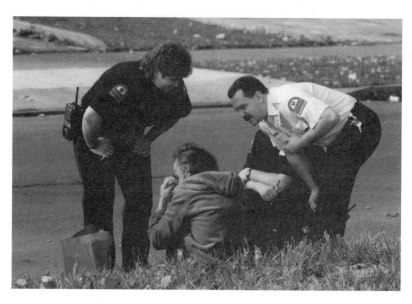
Depression is the most common trigger for attempted suicide.

bit surprised at today's events because they thought that their son had been doing dramatically better (less depression) recently.

QUESTIONS

1. What risk factors has this patient shown for suicide?
2. Is there significance to the previous suicide attempt more than a year ago?
3. What is a suicide plan? Are there elements of a plan? How does a suicide plan relate to the success of a person committing suicide?
4. Why did the patient appear "better" recently?

DISCUSSION

Suicide is the eighth leading cause of death overall and is third in the 15–24-year age group. In this specific group suicide is third after accidental trauma and nonaccidental trauma (homicide) as the leading causes of death.

Attempted suicide and other psychological issues are harder to deal with than most of the medical and traumatic cases handled by paramedics because there are no physical signs or symptoms. The paramedic's attitude toward suicide as a personal and social issue can also affect perception of the patient, the patient's condition, and whether the attempt was "real" or not.

When a patient has previous suicide attempts, it is a common attitude among EMS providers that the patient is "looking for attention" and that this, as with previous suicide attempts, is "not real." Patients with prior suicide attempts are in fact at a higher risk of successful suicide. Experiences transporting patients with multiple attempts can cause paramedics to overlook critical facts leading toward a significant suicide attempt.

One mechanism that is not thought of as a common method may be surprisingly common. As many as 10% to 15% of single-occupant motor vehicle accidents may be suicide attempts. This should be differentiated from single-vehicle accidents because a person could cross over the center line and strike another car head-on as a means of suicide. Finding a patient who has survived a significant crash but remains depressed or speaks of suicide may be an indicator of this phenomenon. Suicide notes may be found in the car or in another location (e.g., home or mailed to relatives) in times around the incident.

When any patient experiencing a psychiatric emergency is taken to the hospital, valuable clues are left behind at the scene. The mental health professionals who examine the patient will perform a mental status exam. This exam is comprised of many components including history, observations of the patient and scene, social factors, thought processes, and living arrangements. In cases of attempted suicide, additional specific information such as the suicide note, observations of family or witnesses, and evidence of a detailed suicide plan (discussed below) is important. Some of these items are available only at the scene. Your documentation of the patient and his surroundings—and communicating these to the hospital or psychiatric facility staff—is crucial.

There are many commonly accepted risk factors for suicide such as depression, alcoholism, and significant relationship issues, including estrangement and divorce. Suicide has been linked with a profound sense of hopelessness. There is a higher risk of suicide for those who have had a family member commit suicide and an even higher risk if the family member was a same-sex parent.

Noted specifically in the scenario was the formation of a suicide plan. A detailed suicide plan significantly increases the risk of successful suicide. In this case the patient had obtained a credit card, waited for the card to arrive, and then purchased the weapon to be used in the suicide attempt. He left a note that related marital problems, a risk factor for suicide.

One other cause of concern is that the parents felt that their son had been doing better and had been less depressed recently. This may indicate that the patient has decided to commit suicide and put a plan into motion. The improvement gives family and friends false hope. It also promotes guilt because loved ones let their guard down and feel that the patient has improved. The subsequent death of the patient would be felt with compounded guilt by the surviving family.

Suicidal patients will require both medical and psychological care. Medical care comes first, although psychological care may be performed concurrently. Medical care includes evaluating the patient for medical and traumatic conditions as a result of suicide attempts and looking for potential hidden causes (e.g., overdose presenting as altered mental status). Patients who have depression and other psychological conditions may be taking prescribed medications with life-threatening complications in the event of overdose.

There are many types of such medications. The tricyclic antidepressant is still widely available, although many new classes of drugs are available for depression such as the selective serotonin reuptake inhibitor (SSRI). The tricyclic class of drugs is known for a profound and deadly course in the event of overdose including cardiac dysrhythmias, hypotension, seizures, and coma. Although potentially dangerous, SSRIs are not reported as having such a severe impact. Of course many overdoses are performed with multiple drugs and alcohol, making effects and outcome unpredictable.

Whereas the assessment and treatment of the wide range of traumatic and medical conditions possible in attempted suicide are not in the scope of this chapter, it is worthy to note the potential dangers and clinical issues inherent with many of these sources. Safety from dangerous mechanisms (e.g., firearms) is critical as well as a need to carefully take body substance isolation (BSI) precautions. Dangerous environments such as carbon monoxide are also possible.

Patient safety and BSI remain a concern as well. The need for airway and breathing support and control are critical. Cardiac dysrhythmias, hypotension, seizures, and coma require careful cardiac and hemodynamic monitoring and interventions. Naloxone may be appropriate in narcotic, mixed, or unknown overdoses. The availability of narcotic substances for analgesia make suicide by these medications possible.

The psychological care is not governed by a definite set of clinical guidelines (e.g., an algorithm) but rather by interpersonal interaction and compassion. Many EMS providers are hesitant to discuss the actual suicide attempt with the patient because the provider feels awkward. If the patient senses this awkwardness, he is much less likely to relate any details or information on his problems of the suicide attempt. Although it may not be necessary or in the scope of the paramedic to obtain detailed psychological information, some discussion of the events are necessary and inevitable.

In general, show interest and compassion when dealing with the patient. Do not express either disdain or pity—even casually—as this will be observed by the patient. Use positive body language and take some time (don't rush) when talking to the patient. Using the word *suicide* may make some patients uncomfortable, so use the terms spoken by the patient when you ask about what happened. For example, if the patient says "I wanted to end it all," you may ask: "Can you tell me why you wanted to end it all?" This terminology for the suicidal act is now acceptable to both the patient and the rescuer.

There are many schools of thought on whether the police should ride along (or in some cases at least follow) when an ambulance is transporting a psychiatric patient of any type. The presence of police is more likely in an involuntary transportation; however, a request for an officer to accompany you in the back of the ambulance should be made whenever you feel it is necessary. This may prevent harm to EMS personnel or prevent the escape of the patient who has consented to transport with the intention of escaping on the way to the hospital.

The incidence of injury to providers in this area has not been unusually high but safety during assessment, care, and transportation is always the primary concern.

RETURN TO THE CASE

The patient consents to transport and is brought by ambulance to the regional psychiatric facility. Because of its link with an adjoining hospital, the patient is able to obtain medical clearance as well as a psychiatric evaluation. The patient is nonviolent and due to the close proximity to the hospital, the police do not ride with the patient. Transport is uneventful, with some discussion of the patient's feelings and attempted suicide. Vital signs remain stable and unchanged. As per the regional protocol, the patient is transported to the emergency department to be "medically cleared" prior to his transfer to a psychiatric facility. Medical clearance includes a detailed physical examination as well as blood tests, including serum ethanol and aspirin and Tylenol levels, to ensure that no unreported overdose occurs. Following his medical clearance, the patient is turned over to the staff at the psychiatric facility for psychiatric evaluation.

Due to the potentially deadly mechanism of injury and the likelihood of completion of the attempt had his parents not returned home, the patient remains at the psychiatric facility for 72 hours and is then turned over to the care of his parents with a strong outpatient therapy regimen and antidepressant medications. The patient is also introduced to a twelve-step recovery program for alcohol addiction.

REFERENCES

American Psychological Association. *Diagnostic and Statistical Manual of Mental Disorders IV-TR*. Washington, DC: American Psychological Association, 2002.

Bledsoe, Bryan E., Robert S. Porter, and Richard A. Cherry. *Medical Emergencies*. Vol. 3 of *Paramedic Care: Principles & Practice*. Chapter 12, "Psychiatric and Behavioral Disorders." Upper Saddle River, NJ: Brady/Prentice Hall Health, Pearson Education, 2001.

Dernocoeur, Kate Boyd. *Streetsense: Communication, Safety, and Control*. 3rd ed. Redmond, WA: Creative Options 1996.

National Center for Injury Prevention and Control, Centers for Disease Control and Prevention. *Suicide Surveillance Summary, 1980–1992. Violence Surveillance Summary Series No. 1*. Atlanta: National Center for Injury Prevention and Control, Centers for Disease Control and Prevention, 1995.

Joseph Heck, DO, FACOEP/FACEP

38

CARE UNDER FIRE

CASE PRESENTATION

Your agency has an agreement with the local police department to provide medical support for their special operations. You are the senior paramedic on duty and you and your partner are assigned by your agency to cover any incidents that might occur during your shift. After running a few routine calls, you get a page telling you to report to a staging location where the tactical team is preparing to deploy on a hostage/barricade situation. Upon arrival you make contact with the team leader and are informed that patrol officers responded to a "public disturbance" call at the local high school and upon approaching the building, shots were fired from an upper floor window, followed by shouts that if anyone came near the school "people will die." The tactical team leader also tells you that the crisis negotiation team has made contact with a suspect and is attempting to bring the standoff to a peaceful resolution, but he wants you to be prepared to support an entry team if negotiations fail. You return to your unit, give your partner the details, and gear up.

After several hours of negotiations, the suspect becomes increasingly agitated and is firing shots randomly from several windows. The decision is made to make entry. Your agency's standard operating procedure is for one medic to stay with the tactical van, where additional supplies are stored, and for the senior paramedic to approach with the team and to hold at the last point of cover. The team enters through a rear door and you remain at the threshold. Within minutes, shots are heard followed by shouts of "medic up!" A tactical officer returns to your location and escorts you inside the school to a hallway where you find an officer with gunshot wound to the midthigh and another to the distal forearm. You are told the suspect fired down the hallway and then ran. Your escort remains with you as the remainder of the team continues to clear the building.

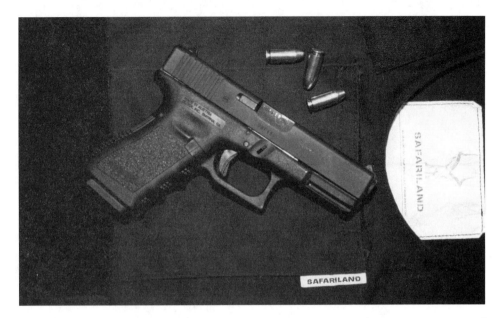

Rendering emergency medical care in a tactical environment requires specialized training to assure personal safety and optimized patient care.
Courtesy of Edward T. Dickinson, MD.

QUESTIONS

1. How does your approach to this patient differ from the routine assessment of a trauma patient?
2. What are your immediate concerns and actions in caring for this patient?

DISCUSSION

When rendering aid in a hostile environment it is imperative that a risk–benefit determination be made prior to instituting any treatment. Will the benefit of the treatment outweigh the risk of prolonged or increased exposure to a threat? To answer this question it is helpful to determine in what *zone* the care will be provided. Most law enforcement operations are divided into perimeters, which can be thought of as a series of concentric circles (Figure 38-1). The center circle is the target, which is surrounded by the inner perimeter. The tactical team usually controls the inner perimeter, and entry into or exit from this area is extremely limited. The outer perimeter is that area furthest from the target, marking the outermost boundary of police operations, and is usually secured by patrol officers. Although perimeters are useful for police operations, they are static determinations and do not take into account the dynamic nature of an evolving incident where areas of safe refuge can rapidly change with the movement of a suspect to different locations within the inner perimeter.

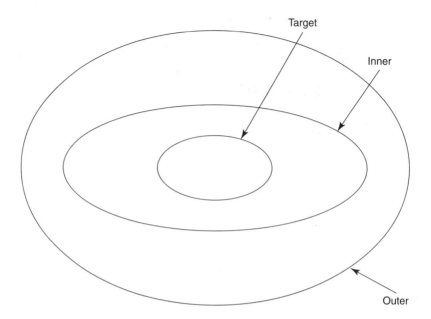

Figure 38-1 Zone systems such as this are used in tactical medical operations.

To better assess the intervention risk–benefit ratio, it is helpful to divide the medical area of operations into three zones (Figure 38-2). The *cold zone* is a secured area, either by cover or distance, where there is no threat. Here, medical care should follow routine prehospital procedures. The *hot zone* is that area where a threat is imminent, such as a suspect aiming a weapon in that direction. In this zone the only acceptable care is self-aid or immediate extraction. Risking additional personnel will only hinder the operation. The area that most affects the decision-making process is the *warm zone*. This is the area where a threat is present, but not immediate. An example would be an armed suspect known to be somewhere in the target location.

Care in the warm zone should follow a modified primary survey, sometimes referred to as the "tactical primary survey," based on the special circumstances of providing care under fire. The tactical primary survey follows the acronym SABCDE.

Securing the patient takes priority because this will render the immediate area safer and decrease the risk to the caregiver. Injured law enforcement officers should have their weapons secured, preferably by another officer, and perpetrators as well as unknown persons should be handcuffed and quickly searched for weapons.

Airway maintenance remains the cornerstone of prehospital care in the tactical setting, but may require changes in technique. Obtunded patients should have a nasal airway placed as the primary method for securing a patent airway. If this is unsuccessful, then more definitive airway control will be required. Techniques that require minimal equipment and positioning are preferred and digital intubation has become a popular method of endotracheal intubation in the tactical environment. Alterna-

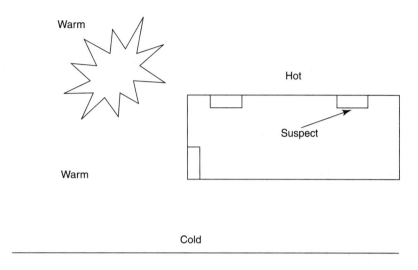

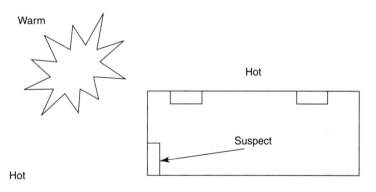

Figure 38-2 Modification of zones of medical operations based on the location of the suspect.

tive airways include dual lumen tubes and the laryngeal mask airway. In the event endotracheal intubation is not possible, a surgical airway should be performed. Conventional orotracheal intubation by direct laryngoscopy is more time consuming and requires additional equipment. Pharmacologically facilitated intubation is usually not indicated due to the requirements of intravenous access and additional medications, which will result in potentially prolonged exposures.

Bleeding and breathing are the next assessments in the tactical primary survey. Ten percent of those who die from penetrating trauma do so from peripheral exsanguinating hemorrhage, therefore controlling bleeding with the early and liberal use of tourniquets warrants consideration. Once the patient is evacuated to a cold zone, the tourniquets can be removed and bleeding controlled by other methods. After hemorrhage control, the patient's ability to adequately ventilate should be examined.

Another 9% of those who die from penetrating trauma will succumb to a tension pneumothorax. Hence, any patient with penetrating trauma to the thorax and respiratory distress, after a patent airway is secured, should be considered as having a tension pneumothorax and undergo immediate needle thoracentesis on the affected side. The warm zone is not the place to check for the absence of breath sounds and waiting for the late occurring signs of jugular-venous distention and tracheal deviation may result in an increased morbidity and mortality. If there is no relief after needle decompression of the effected side, the opposite side should undergo needle thoracentesis: remember, once the projectile enters the thorax its exact path is unknown.

The use of occlusive dressings in the treatment of penetrating chest trauma should be reserved for those patients who continue to have respiratory distress after needle decompression. A sucking chest wound requires the defect in the chest wall to be approximately two-thirds the diameter of the trachea for air to preferentially travel through the hole and not down the trachea. This is seldom the case with gunshot wounds. Additionally, the paramedic supporting law enforcement special operations may not have the ability to closely monitor the patient after application of an occlusive dressing and could potentially miss the development of an iatrogenic tension pneumothorax.

Circulation involves the assessment of two distinct entities: the need for intravenous fluid resuscitation and cardiopulmonary resuscitation. The role of fluid resuscitation in trauma patients has recently been called into question, with some studies advocating withholding fluids during the prehospital treatment and others suggesting that limited fluids result in better outcomes. In the warm zone the ability to start and maintain an IV will be severely impeded. General guidelines dictate that a patient who is normotensive—that is, a patient with a clear sensorium demonstrating adequate cerebral perfusion—does not require immediate fluid resuscitation. A hypotensive patient, demonstrated by an altered level of consciousness and controlled peripheral hemorrhage, may benefit from a fluid bolus to increase cerebral perfusion. Last, a hypotensive patient with uncontrolled intraabdominal or intrathoracic hemorrhage should receive intermittent fluid boluses to maintain cerebral perfusion.

CPR should generally not be performed in the warm zone because traumatic cardiac arrest has a universally poor outcome. Possible exceptions would be in cases of cardiac arrest due to toxic exposures, where antidotes may reverse the arrest, electrocution, an arrest as a result of a suspected myocardial infarction, or in the case of drowning. In each circumstance, the risk to the medical provider of increased exposure to hostile threats and the risk to the other team members due to the use of scarce resources must be carefully evaluated.

Disability is assessed by quickly checking pupillary size and response and documenting the patient's mental status using the AVPU mnemonic. The Glasgow Coma Scale is a cumbersome tool that was initially developed to assess the mental status of patients suffering closed head injuries and has never been validated in other types of trauma or medical presentations. Using the parameters of *awake*, responds to *verbal* stimuli, responds to *painful* stimuli, or *unresponsive* allows the paramedic to make a quick initial, and subsequent, determination of the patient's level of consciousness.

Exposure is to remind the paramedic to look for additional wounds and injuries and then to protect the patient from further exposure to the environment and hostile threats.

RETURN TO THE CASE

Because the exact location of the suspect is still unknown, your security officer tells you extraction is not advisable. You conclude that you are in a warm zone and must render the appropriate care. Your escort secures the injured officer's weapon. The patient is able to talk to you and responds appropriately to your questions, indicating that he has a patent airway and no further intervention is required. A tourniquet is applied to the upper thigh to treat a suspected arterial injury and a dressing is placed over the forearm wound. The patient is slightly tachypneic, but you find no evidence of thoracic trauma and assess this is secondary to anxiety and pain. Since the peripheral hemorrhage is controlled and the patient's sensorium is clear, an IV is not initiated. The patient's pupils are round and reactive and he is awake. No other injuries are identified and your security officer maintains a vigilant watch over you and your patient.

Approximately 45 minutes later the suspect is found hiding under a classroom desk and subdued. You now safely evacuate your patient to your unit and transport him to the local trauma center. Plain x-rays of the injured extremities fail to reveal any evidence of bony trauma. An emergent angiogram reveals a lacerated femoral artery. The trauma surgeon tells you that without the tourniquet, the officer would have bled out within approximately 30 minutes. He is taken to the operating room where a graft is placed and he completes an uneventful recovery.

REFERENCES

Bellamy, R. F. "The Causes of Death in Conventional Land Warfare: Implications for Combat Casualty Care Research." *Military Medical* 149 (1984): 55–62.

Bledsoe, Bryan E., Robert S. Porter, and Richard A. Cherry. *Special Considerations/Operations*. Vol. 5 of *Paramedic Care: Principles & Practice*. Chapter 12, "Crime Scene Awareness." Upper Saddle River, NJ: Brady/Prentice Hall Health, Pearson Education, 2001.

Butler, F. K., J. Hagmann, and E. G. Butler. "Tactical Combat Casualty Care in Special Operations."

Pope, A., G. French, and D. E. Longnecker, eds. *Fluid Resuscitation: State of the Science for Treating Combat Casualties and Civilian Injuries*. Washington, DC: National Academy Press, 1999.

Arthur Cooper, MD

39

CHILD ABUSE

CASE PRESENTATION

You and your partner are called to the home of an 8-month-old boy who has become increasingly sleepy in association with numerous episodes of vomiting over a 12-hour period. The emesis was initially clear, but has since become greenish in color. When you enter the apartment, you notice that it is poorly kept, although there appears to be no immediate danger to yourself, your partner, or your patient. The mother quickly relates the above history.

As you approach your patient, who is lying quietly on his mother's bed, you note that he appears slightly lethargic, with poor muscle tone. Work of breathing is slightly increased, whereas circulation to the skin seems diminished because central color is pale.

QUESTION

1. What is your first impression, according to the Pediatric Assessment Triangle? What does this mean regarding further assessment and treatment?

DISCUSSION

The Pediatric Assessment Triangle (Figure 39-1) is the optimal method for characterizing your general impression in the pediatric patient. It consists of three components—appearance, work of breathing, and circulation to skin—which are assessed visually, "from the doorway," without physically examining the patient. It generates, in effect, a mental snapshot of the child's condition when first encountered. Abnormalities in any one of the three components categorize a child as seriously ill or injured, and in need of urgent care in an emergency facility. Abnormalities in the Pediatric Assessment Triangle also indicate the

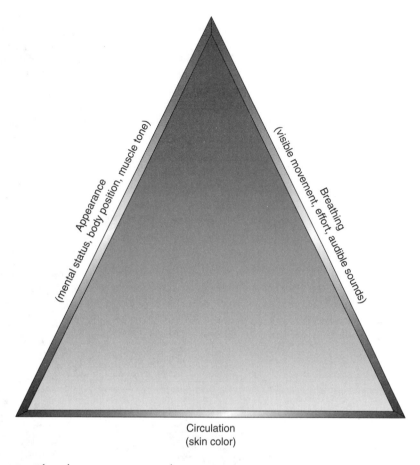

Figure 39-1 The pediatric assessment triangle.
Reproduced with permission of the American Academy of Pediatrics.

need to proceed immediately to a hands-on initial assessment of the ABCDEs, and to complete the focused history and detailed physical examination only if the child is found to be clinically stable on initial assessment.

In applying the Pediatric Assessment Triangle, prehospital professionals will look for abnormalities of appearance, which include altered mental status, unusual body position, or poor muscle tone; work of breathing—respiratory effort that is increased, labored, or decreased, or respiratory rate that is increased, decreased, or absent; and circulation to skin—pale, mottled, cyanotic, or ashen skin or mucous membrane color. In this case, the Pediatric Assessment Triangle demonstrates abnormal appearance—altered mental status and poor muscle tone; abnormal work of breathing—increased work of breathing; and abnormal circulation to skin—pale central color. Singly or together, they indicate that the child's condition is urgent; therefore, you should proceed with the ABCDEs without obtaining additional information.

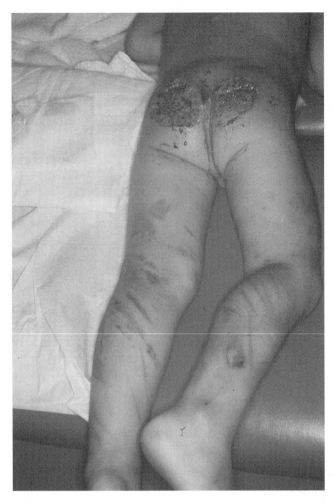

Injuries typical of child abuse. Note the linear markings on the child's legs.

RETURN TO THE CASE

You proceed with initial assessment of the ABCDEs. Your partner places the head and neck in a sniffing position. The airway is clear, without gurgling, stridor, hoarseness, or snoring. You evaluate the breathing, confirming adequate chest rise and bilateral air entry, although both the respiratory effort and the respiratory rate appear slightly increased. The respiratory rate is 40 breaths per minute, and the pulse oximeter indicates that the oxygen saturation is 98% on room air. You next assess the circulation, measuring a pulse rate of 140 at the brachial artery, with weakly palpable brachial and femoral pulses, extremely thready, barely perceptible radial and pedal pulses, and a capillary refill time of 4 to 5 seconds. No active external bleeding is detected. You then determine the degree of disability. The pupils are equal and reactive, whereas the neurological check reveals an alternately alert and anxious, then sleepy but arousable infant responsive to verbal stimuli. You then expose the infant fully, taking care to keep him warm. Moderate abdominal distention is noted on inspection, and marked abdominal tenderness on palpation.

QUESTIONS

1. Do your findings indicate partial or complete upper airway obstruction? respiratory distress or failure? compensated or decompensated shock? altered mental status or altered level of consciousness?
2. What treatments are needed, if any? What is your overall assessment at this point?

DISCUSSION

The airway is open and requires no intervention beyond positioning. The breathing is increased, consistent with respiratory distress (not failure) for which 100% oxygen via a non-rebreather mask or blowby is indicated. The circulation is decreased, but peripheral pulses, though very weak, are still barely palpable, consistent with compensated shock, for which no treatment other than supplemental oxygen is indicated. The disabilities you elicit are indicative of altered mental status, for which low tissue oxygen content, or hypoxia, is the most important cause, as is likely in this case. The exposure phase reveals a distended, tender abdomen. The infant likely has serious intraabdominal illness or injury. Based upon the above findings, keeping the child warm and rapid transport to the hospital are warranted.

RETURN TO THE CASE

The child is transported to the hospital. While in the ambulance, your partner obtains a SAMPLE history from the mother, who reiterates that the child began to vomit earlier in the day, but became sleepier as the emesis turned from clear to yellow to green. The child has no known allergies, takes no regular medications, has no significant past medical history, last retained formula about 12 hours previously, and had been entirely well until earlier in the day. Your partner also performs a detailed physical examination, finding small, oval, mixed reddish, bluish, and greenish patches on both upper arms in a symmetrical pattern, and slight reddish discoloration of the abdominal wall above and to the left of the navel. On arrival in the emergency department, you relate the findings of your scene survey, general impression, initial assessment, focused history, and detailed physical examination to the nurse in charge. He, in turn, relates them to the physician on duty. She confirms your findings, and admits the child to the hospital for evaluation.

QUESTIONS

1. What is the underlying cause of the child's medical condition?
2. What are the additional responsibilities of prehospital professionals in cases such as these?

DISCUSSION

Although this infant presents with a "classic" history of acute gastrointestinal illness, (which could be caused by infectious organisms such as bacteria or viruses, or by less common conditions such as intussusception—a condition in which a proximal segment of intestine telescopes into a distal segment, causing intestinal obstruction—or even appendicitis which is rare in infancy), the patient described in this case presentation is a victim of major blunt abdominal trauma due to child abuse. Circumstances and findings that may lead you to suspect child abuse can be very subtle. In this case, the parents' apartment was not well kept, but this should not, in and of itself, lead you to suspect the possibility of child abuse. In addition, the history offered by the child's mother is not atypical for a child with an acute gastrointestinal illness—vomiting followed by lethargy, as the dehydration caused by the vomiting becomes more severe. What leads the experienced clinician to suspect the possibility of child abuse in this case are the discolored spots on the child's upper arms. Their small, oval, symmetrical appearance and reddish, bluish, and greenish discoloration suggest the possibility of finger marks, as the child is forcibly grasped and possibly shaken. The fact that the small oval "fingerprints" are in different stages of healing indicates that the marks resulted from more than one episode of grabbing. The child's altered mental status thus could be the result either of dehydration due to repetitive vomiting, or a head injury. Other telltale signs of possible abuse include the slight reddish discoloration of the abdominal wall, indicating bruising, although such markings will be present in no more than about 50% of all cases of major blunt abdominal trauma due to child abuse. Fortunately, major blunt abdominal trauma due to child abuse is relatively rare, comprising fewer than 5% of all cases of major physical child abuse. However, the presentations in such cases can be sufficiently misleading, resembling the presentations of infants and children with natural diseases such as acute gastroenteritis. Thus, the possibility of child abuse warrants special attention, chiefly because delay in diagnosis is the major contributor to poor outcome in these patients—as many as 50% of whom may die if the underlying cause is not recognized in a timely manner.

In the case described, findings are due to a ruptured duodenum—the first part of the small intestine—which resulted from a severe blow to the upper abdomen. Spillage of intestinal contents from the duodenum causes marked inflammation of the abdominal lining, or peritonitis, as well as increasingly severe dehydration. Although there is no evidence of traumatic brain injury in this case, such injuries are fairly common among physically abused children. Because of the high frequency of trauma to the head and neck in such patients, complete spinal immobilization, including application of a cervical extrication collar, and fixation on a long spine board or similar device is indicated, in addition to the treatment already provided.

Whereas symptoms and signs of child abuse can be nonspecific and subtle, prehospital professionals should suspect child abuse whenever there are any of the following: unexplained delays in seeking treatment for children's illnesses or injuries; the history offered does not match the physical findings observed; the story they are given just doesn't seem to make sense; there has been hospital or doctor shopping; the parent blames the child, a sibling, or a third party; or the parent protects the spouse rather than the child. Specific signs of child abuse include bruises in various stages of healing; bruises in unusual locations or patterns; whip, restraint, gag, or strangulation marks; scald burns in a glove, stocking, or buttock distribution; scald or contact burns in unusual locations or patterns; and thigh fractures in children too young to walk. Prehospital professionals have a legal responsibility in all states and territories of the United States to report instances of suspected child abuse to appropriate authorities, although the details of who must make and receive the report differ slightly from state to state. Prehospital professionals also have an obligation to report suspected cases of child maltreatment to the physician or nurse on duty in the hospital emergency department, and to record their findings on the prehospital care report in a straightforward, factual, nonjudgmental, and nonaccusatory way. It is good advice to recall that confrontation and accusation typically delay treatment and transportation, and have no place in the prehospital management of suspected child abuse in the field.

Dealing with suspected child abuse can take a heavy emotional toll in prehospital professionals, particularly if they were themselves abused as children. Often it seems as though the systems in place for handling serious child abuse are ineffective because so few cases are ultimately found to be substantiated, or proven, whereas many more cases are deemed to be "unfounded," or unproven. The social welfare systems established to prevent and manage cases of child maltreatment clearly are not perfect; however, they represent our only hope of ensuring that potentially abused children receive the help that they need. Prehospital professionals must therefore resist the urge "not to get involved," since failure to report a case of suspected child abuse not only carries stiff penalties in most jurisdictions if failure to report is willful but also runs the far more serious risk that an opportunity will be missed to get the abused child and family into appropriate treatment, before more severe injury or death occurs.

REFERENCES

Bledsoe, Bryan E., Robert S. Porter, and Richard A. Cherry. *Special Considerations/Operations*. Vol. 5 of *Paramedic Care: Principles & Practice*. Chapter 2, "Pediatrics," Chapter 4, "Abuse and Assault." Upper Saddle River, NJ: Brady/Prentice Hall Health, Pearson Education, 2001.

Cooper, A., T. Floyd, B. Barlow, M. Niemirska, S. Ludwig, T. Seidl, J. O'Neill, J. Templeton, M. Ziegler, A. Ross, R. Ghandhi, and R. Catherman. "Major Blunt Trauma Due to Child Abuse." *Journal of Trauma* 28 (1988): 1483–1487.

Foltin, G., M. Tunik, A. Cooper, D. Markenson, M. Treiber, A. Skomorowsky, V. Ferrante, and S. Gilbert, eds. *Paramedic Teaching Resource for Instructors in Prehospital Pediatrics (TRIPP)*. New York: Center for Pediatric Emergency Medicine, 2002.

Foltin, G., M. Tunik, A. Cooper, D. Markenson, M. Treiber, A. Skomorowsky, V. Ferrante, and S. Gilbert, eds. *Teaching Resource for Instructors in Prehospital Pediatrics (TRIPP)*. New York: Center for Pediatric Emergency Medicine, 1998.

Kornberg, A., and S. Ludwig, eds. *Child Abuse: A Medical Reference*. 2nd ed. New York: Churchill Livingstone, 1992.

Markenson, David, George Foltin, Michael Tunik, Arthur Cooper, Hedda Matza-Haughton, Lenora Olson, and Marsha Treiber. "Knowledge and Attitude Assessment and Education of Prehospital Personnel in Child Abuse and Neglect: Report of a National Blue Ribbon Panel." *Annals of Emergency Medicine* 40 (2002): 89.

40

Elizabeth M. Datner, MD
Iris Reyes, MD

DOMESTIC VIOLENCE

CASE PRESENTATION

You are called to the scene of a domestic disturbance for an injured person. The police are on scene and they report the scene is secure prior to your arrival. You arrive at the scene to find neighbors standing outside of an apartment building talking about the constant police calls to this apartment. You proceed into the apartment. The police are talking in the hallway to a man who appears to be angry and intoxicated. You are directed to a woman in a back bedroom who is sitting on the bed holding her upper arm.

As you approach the patient your initial impression is that she is not ill or severely injured. She appears disheveled and is intermittently crying and arguing with the accompanying police officer. You notice two small children in the next room watching the activity through the doorway, and hear a baby crying in the next room.

Upon questioning the patient, she tells you that she tripped and fell down the stairs. She notes that her left upper arm hurts. She denies hitting her head, passing out, or having neck pain. She has no prior medical or surgical history and denies allergies to medications. She mentions that she just found out she is pregnant. The primary survey reveals that the patient's airway is intact. She has equal bilateral breath sounds. Her blood pressure is normal and she is mildly tachycardic. You note an ecchymotic right eye, an abrasion over the deltoid area of her left arm, and an ecchymosis on her upper back (see photo). You place a sling on the patient's left arm and prepare to position her on a long spine board with a cervical collar in place. As your partner turns to leave the room to retrieve the board you notice the man from the hallway watching you.

When your partner arrives with the board and collar the patient states, "I'm not getting on that thing, I'm not going anywhere."

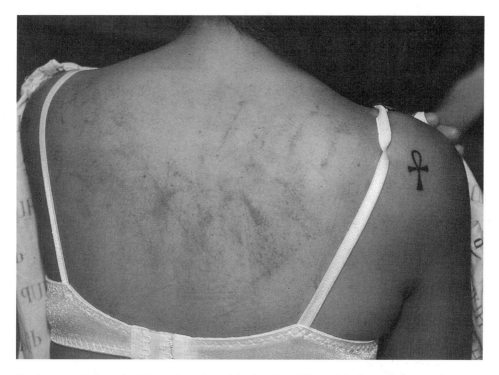

Hand print on the upper back. Note the outline of the thumb medially, and the finger marks extending superiorly toward the right shoulder.

Courtesy of Edward T. Dickinson, MD.

QUESTIONS

    1. Should you leave the scene because the patient is refusing transportation?

    2. Should you involve the husband in the medical and transportation decisions?

    3. What are the risk factors for high-risk domestic violence situations?

DISCUSSION

It is estimated that one in four women will be abused by an intimate partner during her lifetime. Domestic violence (intimate partner abuse, domestic abuse) is understood to be a set of assaultive and controlling behaviors that one partner employs as a means to exert power and control over the other. The behaviors may encompass or be a combination of physical violence, emotional abuse, and social or economic isolation. They may vary in severity from controlling access to financial support or medical services to severe physical trauma or rape. Threats of violence toward the partner, other family members, pets, or children are another means of maintaining control.

Perpetrators of domestic abuse tend to be male, although perpetrators and victims may be of either gender and involved in either heterosexual or homosexual relationships. The majority of incidents of domestic violence, however, tend to be perpetrated by males on female victims. Abusers tend to be more likely to use or abuse tobacco, alcohol, and or illicit drugs than nonabusers.

Abuse during pregnancy is reflective of domestic violence (DV) in general; however, it may be more frequent and more severe. Estimates of abuse during pregnancy range from 4% to 17% of pregnant women being current victims of domestic violence. Additionally, women who are abused during pregnancy report more severe and frequent assaults during pregnancy than other non-pregnant domestic violence patients. A study by Campbell, Oliver, and Bullock of women abused during pregnancy reports several general themes to which the violence was attributed: (1) jealousy toward the fetus (i.e., more attention directed at the fetus than to the adult partner); (2) pregnancy-specific violence not directed toward the fetus (i.e., increased stress in the relationship); (3) anger toward the fetus (i.e., unwanted pregnancy); and (4) "business as usual" or anger directed at the partner (i.e., beaten prior to the pregnancy with continuance). Regardless of the stimulus for the violence, the consequences are severe. A recent review of maternal mortality by Horon and Cheng found that homicide was the number one cause of maternal death.

Identifying victims of DV serves a dual purpose. It not only provides a clue to a potentially dangerous situation for the patient but may also provide a window of opportunity to avert significant injury or psychological trauma to children. There is a known high correlation between DV and child abuse, with a study by Strauss and Gelles showing that 50% of men who abuse their partners frequently also abuse their children. Partner abuse tends to precede child abuse, allowing for a window of opportunity to protect children if DV victims are identified early. Additionally, having witnessed abuse in your family as a child is the greatest risk factor for becoming either a victim or a perpetrator of violence as an adult.

Victims of DV may immediately disclose the DV or, paradoxically, attempt to hide the cause of their injuries. They may not have injuries at all or have nonspecific complaints but called 911 in an attempt to avert a potentially violent situation and get help quickly. A study performed by the author and colleagues suggests that DV victims are more likely to access the 911 system than non-DV victims but only for situations related to DV, not for other medical complaints. When presented with a patient who does not have a clear medical indication for having called for medical assistance, questions should be asked to glean the possibility of safety at home. In the case of an injury, the medical team should be attentive to all suspicious lesions and be alert to the possibility of the injury being caused by another person regardless of the history given by the patient. For example, a black eye is an unlikely injury from a fall down a flight of stairs; it is most commonly caused by a direct blow to the orbit. Other clues to potential DV victims include frequent calls, refusal of care once medics are on the scene, and presence of a partner who is controlling or may seem overly concerned and will not leave the victim alone in the care of the medics.

Patients should be asked about DV in a direct, nonjudgmental way. Phrasing questions to mention the specific acts are more likely to yield positive results than asking if the patient is "abused" as this is a matter of perception. It is also helpful to begin with a brief introductory statement to assure the patient that he or she is not alone and that you are comfortable dealing with DV—a statement such as "We see so many women who have been injured by their partners that we now ask about it routinely." This statement may be followed by "Did another person cause this injury in some way?" "Have you been hit, punched, or kicked by someone? Did someone injure you with an object?" "Do you feel afraid of someone?" "Did someone threaten to hurt you or your children?" "Did someone threaten to use a weapon against you or your children?"

Clearly, these questions should be asked in a safe environment, out of range of visual contact or the hearing of other people including children. It is paramount for the victim to feel that she and her children are safe prior to the interviewing. Part of feeling safe requires that the victim be assured that the perpetrator, who may still be present, does not learn of her disclosure. Assurance of confidentiality is essential. However, there are certain circumstances that require reporting to authorities. Most states require reporting of injuries that result from knives or guns. Injuries to noncompetent patients, including mentally incompetent adults, elderly patients, or children, must be reported to appropriate authorities. Some states require reporting of suspected or known DV to police. You should be aware of the mandatory reporting requirements of your state. If there is no mandatory-reporting requirement in your state for DV, the decision about leaving the home is solely at the discretion of the patient.

If a patient admits DV and refuses transportation to a medical facility, safety assessment and counseling are essential. The patient can be asked, "Do you feel safe staying here?" If the patient does not feel safe, he or she should be encouraged to accept transportation to a medical facility, shelter, DV advocacy facility, or the home of a friend or family member. *Children should never be left behind.* Other indicators of highly dangerous situations include pregnancy, presence of weapons in the home, increasing frequency or severity of abuse, injuries to children or pets, threats of homicide or suicide, use of alcohol and drugs, disclosure of the abuse, and recent attempts by the victim to leave the relationship.

RETURN TO THE CASE

The patient continues to adamantly refuse transportation to the hospital. You ask the police to distract the husband so that you can speak to the patient. The husband leaves the house and heads down the street swearing. You question the patient about DV. She discloses to you that her husband did in fact cause her injuries. He punched her in the eye and threw her down the stairs. She managed to call 911, which she has done on multiple occasions. The patient admits that she had disclosed her pregnancy to the husband. She admits that he owns a gun, which he carries with him and has threatened her with it in the past. She denies that he has injured the children. She maintains that she does not want to go to the hospital and that she does not want to make a detailed report to the police or file for a protection from abuse order. You determine that the patient is not clinically intoxicated and appears to be mentally competent. You have the patient complete the Refusal Against Medical Advice form.

You leave the house after giving the patient a DV resource card and the national DV hotline number (1-800-799-SAFE).

Prior to clearing the scene you advise the police sergeant that the patient informed you that the husband may be armed. The police inform you that they are aware of the husband's volatile nature and that DV is an ongoing issue at the address.

That evening after your shift, you are watching the 11 o'clock news and notice a report of a homicide-suicide in the neighborhood where you saw that patient. They report that the woman was trying to leave the apartment with her three children when her husband returned and shot her and then turned the gun on himself. The children will be placed in foster care.

REFERENCES

Bledsoe, Bryan E., Robert S. Porter, and Richard A. Cherry. *Special Considerations/Operations* Vol. 5 of *Paramedic Care: Principles & Practice*. Chapter 4, "Abuse and Assault." Upper Saddle River, NJ: Brady/Prentice Hall *Health*, Pearson Education, 2001.

Campbell, J. C., C. Oliver, and L. Bullock. "Why Battering during Pregnancy?" *AWHONN* 4 (1993): 343.

Datner, E. M., and A. A. Ferroggiaro. "Violence during Pregnancy." *Emergency Medical Clinics of North America* 17, no. 3 (1999): 645–656.

Datner, E. M., F. S. Shofer, K. Parmele et al. "Utilization of the Emergency Medical/911 System as an Identifier of Domestic Violence." *American Journal of Emergency Medicine* 17, no. 6 (1999): 560–564.

Horon, I. L., and D. Cheng. "Enhanced Surveillance for Pregnancy-Associated Mortality—Maryland, 1993–1998." *Journal of the American Medical Association* 285, no. 11 (2001): 1455–1459.

Strauss, M. A., and R. J. Gelles. *Physical Violence in American Families*. New Brunswick, NJ: Transaction, 1991.

James P. McCans, BS, NREMT-P, FP-C

41

EMS AND AIR MEDICAL SERVICE INTERACTION

CASE PRESENTATION

You are a paramedic assigned to an ALS and transport capable unit. You are dispatched to the scene of a truck versus truck MVC (motor vehicle crash) with a reported fire. Fire, rescue, and police units have all been dispatched as well. While approaching the general area you are requested to report to an intersection that is west, upwind, and uphill of the accident. You observe a large volume of smoke in the general area of the incident. You hear multiple radio transmissions on the fire department's channel regarding the presence of a suspected toxic substance and a burn victim. Upon hearing this message you contact your dispatch center and place a medical helicopter on standby. This request will give the medical helicopter additional time to prepare coordinates and confirm landing zone (LZ) information.

Moments later, an apparent victim approaches the ambulance with the assistance of a firefighter. The victim is in his mid-30s, approximately 6 feet tall and about 100 kilograms. The right side of his face appears to be red and facial hair is singed. Portions of his clothes are burned, particularly the front, right side and back of his shirt. The patient seems out of breath, anxious, in pain, and can provide only one-word answers between breaths. The firefighter informs you that the man has been burned in an explosion of a suspected hazardous material. The substance ignited after the victim's truck was struck broadside by another truck. As the victim ran from the cab, he turned to glance back when the vehicle erupted. His burns are the apparent result of his proximity to the fireball.

You have the patient lie down on a tarp and perform your ABCs. A quick exam shows the patient to be conscious, alert, and oriented, very anxious and in moderate pain. Some facial burns are noted and his mustache is singed. The patient, in a hoarse voice, complains of no throat or mouth pain. He states repeatedly that he ran for his life and is thankful to be alive. His respirations are 32 and shallow with bilateral wheezes. Your partner provides the patient with a nonrebreather mask at 15 L/min. Pulses are present in all extremities and capillary refill is greater than 2 seconds. His skin, in the unaffected areas, is pale, cool to the touch, and moist.

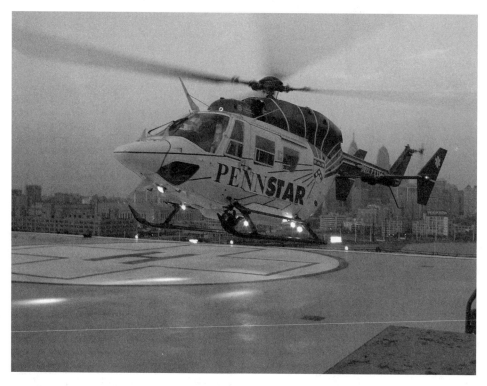

A medical helicopter landing on a hospital roof helipad.
Courtesy of James P. McCans.

As you remove the patient's clothing, your partner contacts the Incident Commander (IC) via radio and requests an LZ be designated for a possible medical evacuation and requests any information on the identity of the chemical(s) involved. The IC is also asked to provide a method of decontamination to the medical staging area.

Your assessment shows the patient to have a BSA (body surface area) of approximately 21% second-degree burns and approximately 5% first-degree burns. The patient is 90% saturated on supplemental oxygen, heart rate is sinus tachycardia at 128 bpm, and blood pressure is 108/56. You request, via the IC, that the helicopter be dispatched to the LZ.

Your treatment consists of two 16-gauge IVs placed in bilateral forearms. Lactated Ringer's (LR) is infusing at a rate consistent with the Parkland formula (3 cc to 4 cc per kilogram of body weight per percentage of BSA within 24 hours, with the first half of the solution in the first 8 hours). In this case, a rate of the LR infusion should be approximately 1 L/hr.

The IC advises you that the aircraft has a 12-minute ETA.

QUESTIONS

1. What do you foresee as a potential life-threatening situation for this patient?
2. How will this patient's exposure to a hazardous material affect his air medical evacuation?

3. By what means can you identify the hazardous materials involved in this case?
4. What role will communication between the ground providers and the aviation crew play in the care of this patient?

DISCUSSION

As in all aspects of EMS, the "preparation phase" is the first step in a rescue or resuscitation scenario. This phase should be dedicated to identifying needs, researching solutions, and seeking education to improve outcome. In cases involving an EMS helicopter this phase must include

- Identifying air medical services in order of potential use
- Developing protocol for air medical usage
- Training with these services to learn safety, aircraft specifications, and operational procedures
- Developing a review or critique system to improve on future interactions

An EMS unit's choice of air medical service support should not be limited to the geographically closest service. A factor in determining the order of helicopter utilization is the mission profile of the flight service, as some flight services are designated for hospital-to-hospital transport only or are outfitted solely for a specialty transport, such as pediatric transfers. Availability should also be taken into account because some services may utilize a 12-hour or part-time aircraft that may not be in service at the time of request. It stands to reason that geographic closeness is usually the dominant factor in determining choice of flight service.

A protocol for air medical transport should be created with the input of the EMS program's medical director, intended flight services, and representatives of the local tertiary facilities that will receive the patients. This protocol should take into consideration variables such as weather, changes in traffic patterns, and divert status of receiving facilities. Guidelines set forth by national organizations such as the American College of Surgeons, the Association of Air Medical Services (AAMS), and the National Association of EMS Physicians (NAEMSP) should be referenced for the creation of such a protocol to ensure that overusage as well as underusage does not occur. The NAEMSP guidelines for utilization of aeromedical services are outlined as follows:

A. Clinical Criteria
  1. General
     a. Trauma victims need to be delivered as soon as possible to a regional trauma center.
     b. Stable patients who are accessible by ground vehicles probably are best transported by ground.
  2. Specific
     Patients with critical injuries resulting in unstable vital signs require the fastest, most direct route of transport to a regional trauma center in a vehicle staffed

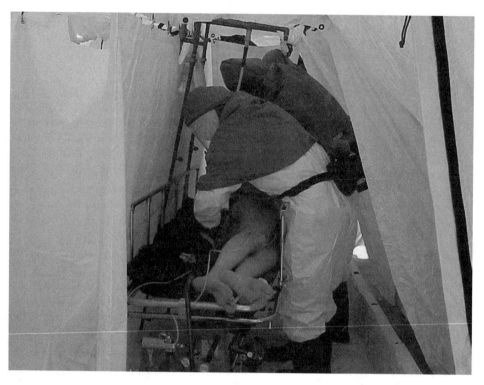

Field decontamination of a hazmat patient.

with a team capable of offering critical care en route. Often this is the case in the following situations:

a. Trauma score less than 12
b. Glasgow Coma Scale score less than 10
c. Penetrating trauma to the abdomen, pelvis, chest, neck, or head
d. Spinal cord or spinal column injury, or any injury producing paralysis of any extremity or any lateralizing signs
e. Partial or total amputation of an extremity (excluding digits)
f. Two or more long bone fractures or a major pelvic fracture
g. Crushing injuries to the abdomen, chest, or head
h. Major burns of the body surface area; burns involving the face, hands, feet, or perineum; burns with significant respiratory involvement; or major electrical or chemical burns
i. Patients involved in a serious traumatic event who are less than 12 or more than 55 years of age
j. Patients with near-drowning injuries, with or without existing hypothermia

    k. Adult patients with any of the following vital sign abnormalities:
        i. systolic blood pressure <90mm Hg
        ii. respiratory rate <10 or >35 per minute
        iii. heart rate <60 or >120 per minute
        iv. unresponsive to verbal stimuli

B. Operational situations in which helicopter use should be considered include the following:
    1. Mechanism of injury
        a. Vehicle rollover with unbelted passengers
        b. Vehicle striking pedestrian at greater than 10 miles per hour
        c. Falls from greater than 15 feet
        d. Motorcycle victim ejected at greater than 20 miles per hour
        e. Multiple victims
    2. Difficult access situations
        a. Wilderness rescue
        b. Ambulance egress or access impeded at the scene by road conditions, weather, or traffic
    3. Time or distance factors
        a. Transportation time to the trauma center greater than 15 minutes by ground ambulance
        b. Transport time to local hospital by ground greater than transport time to trauma center by helicopter
        c. Patient extrication time greater than 20 minutes
        d. Utilization of local ground ambulance leaves local community without ground ambulance coverage

Source: National Association of EMS Physicians.

Situations such as unavailable first-due aircraft or multiple patient scenarios require the EMS service to be familiar with the capabilities of all services that may be called upon to respond to the scene. This possibility requires the emergency service personnel to understand the capabilities of each supporting air medical service, including patient capacity, ETA, and communication ability. Regular drills, at least yearly, with primary and secondary flight services are recommended to update ground personnel with safety procedures, capabilities, and changes within the flight program's operational guidelines.

A safe landing zone is key to a successful helicopter operation. It is the responsibility of the LZ officer to designate an area that is large enough (100 ft × 100 ft) and level enough (less than 10 degree slope) to land the helicopter. This area should be void of major debris, such as trash, wood debris, or dusty soil (such as a baseball infield) that can cause damage when propelled by the aircraft's rotorwash. Safety considerations should include an approach path clear of obstructions including trees, wires, light standards, or any object that could damage the helicopter on its descent. White lights should not be used in the area of the LZ to avoid compromising the pilot's night vision; however, red and blue lights are acceptable and encouraged to assist the flight team in identifying the general LZ area. More information on proper LZ procedures can be found by contacting the National EMS Pilots Association at http://www.nemspa.org.

The importance of communication between the flight crew and the ground providers cannot be overemphasized. Both radio communication before landing and a concise and relevant verbal report to the flight crew at the time of the patient "hand-off" are essential components of patient care.

The final phase involves review and critique of trauma cases. Each of the groups involved in the selected case should present in an appropriate forum the challenges faced and the solutions that were employed. All involved should be open to honest constructive criticism. Proper steps should be taken to improve upon the areas identified as lacking. This last step will bring us full circle to the *preparation phase,* with both the ground and aviation agencies dedicated to identifying needs, researching solutions, and seeking education to improve patient outcome.

In the case presented, until the suspected hazardous substance involved is identified, you must assume that it is extremely hazardous, isolate the treatment area, and protect yourself. To identify the substance a number of methods can be used, and the best practice is to then verify the information by at least one other method. In this situation a direct interview with the driver may yield the fastest results. Visualization of a placard on the vehicle and cross-referencing with a current hazardous material book is also a quality means of identification. In many instances, the material safety data sheet (MSDS) and other documents pertaining to the product being transported are stored in the driver's side door of the truck's cab. In this case, the cab and material in it are destroyed by fire. Contact with the trucking company may lead to identification of a transported product if the truck's identification can be made through a license or serial number. Some of these chemical transport firms use an automated tracking system that may enable them to identify the vehicle and relay cargo information rapidly. Once identified, if applicable, it should be noted if the product is behaving in a manner consistent with the identification.

The substance and its current condition will dictate decontamination needs as well as the level of personal protection that is required for the responders. This information also needs to be passed on to the medical helicopter crew. A judgment will be made by the pilot in charge to accept the patient based on the properties of the contaminant. If the product could impair the pilot and cannot be fully removed from the patient, then air transport is not an option. In most cases a reliable identification with quality decontamination will result in a patient suitable for flight. All of the previously noted therapies must be performed with respect to decontamination procedures. Self-protecting equipment should be utilized until decontamination is complete or the chemical is identified as not requiring such measures.

This patient is showing signs of potential airway or respiratory compromise. This compromise may be due to thermal insult or chemical exposure to the respiratory tract. Although the patient is not in extremis yet, you must anticipate and prepare for the worst-case scenario. Care for his peripheral burns including pain management must be undertaken as well.

Your crew should discuss options with their medical command physician (MCP) for supporting the patient's respiratory status. A pulse oximetery reading of 90% with 100% supplemental oxygen in place is cause for concern. An albuterol treatment may be beneficial for this patient. The dilation of the bronchial airways may relieve some of this patient's distress, as chemical irritation of these structures may be a factor.

Morphine should be considered for pain relief, especially prior to a burn site being decontaminated. Great care must be used in the administration of this medication due to its possible depression of the patient's respiratory drive. The patient's anxiety may be relieved with the control of pain alone; however, the use of midazolam, also a possible respiratory depressant, may be indicated. Relief of anxiety will lead to a decreased oxygen demand. Vigilant monitoring will reveal any subtle changes due to the above therapies or the progression of this patient's respiratory collapse. If your ALS service has a protocol for an RSI (rapid sequence intubation), then this is a patient for whom it may be indicated. You should be prepared to perform a surgical or needle cricothyrotomy should this patient's airway constrict to the point of occlusion.

RETURN TO THE CASE

Decontamination includes complete removal of the patient's clothing and jewelry and thorough washing of all body areas including the burn sites. The patient states that the material he is hauling is Hexane (n-hexane CAS No. 110-54-3); the incident commander confirms this information with the trucking firm. You follow a gross decontamination protocol and clean the patient with a municipal fresh water source. As you clean the patient from head moving down the body, you establish an intravenous line of lactated Ringer's in the left wrist via a 16-gauge catheter once the site is cleaned. You administer 3 mg of morphine and begin an Albuterol treatment. When the patient is declared clean, he is moved to the waiting ambulance for transport to the LZ.

Despite these therapies, the patient remains anxious with a pulse oximetery reading of 92%. Medical command advises you to push another 2 mg of morphine and a 2 mg dose of midazolam. The patient relaxes somewhat but is still tachypneic with an unchanged pulse oximetery.

Upon arrival at the LZ, you give your report including the following information:

- A description of the incident and mechanism of injury
- A timeline of events
- Any information regarding the hazardous material involved
- Treatment thus far and the patient's response to the care
- Your impression of the severity and progression of the injury

As a result of this information two events occur. The first is that the pilot notes the limited exposure (flash fire) to the hexane and the telltale gasolinelike odor associated with this chemical is not present in the closed ambulance. The pilot is also informed of the decontamination process that has occurred and decides that it is safe and legal to fly this patient. The second event is based on the medical report to the flight crew. Your therapy thus far has had little effect on the patient and you suspect that the patient has a pending airway occlusion due to laryngeal edema from thermal or chemical insult. This information guides the flight crew to opt for an RSI procedure and secure the airway prior to moving the patient.

Had this information not been presented to the flight crew in a complete and direct manner, it may have led to a repetition of care that had not produced optimal results and valuable time needed to secure the swelling airway would have been lost. This situation could result in a hypoxic patient becoming combative in flight and causing a safety issue for the crew and aircraft. At the very least the flight crew will be faced with a difficult intubation, surgical cricothyrotomy, or needle cricothyrotomy while in flight. The motion, vibration, and noise of the aircraft will contribute to the difficulty involved in these therapies.

Due to quality assessments initially and serially, you have been able to supply the flight team with a clear picture of this patient's injury and response to care. The judgment to perform an RSI in this case proves appropriate as the airway is viewed to be edematous upon direct laryngoscopy during the intubation procedure.

The patient is transferred without further incident to a burn-trauma center 20 minutes by air (estimated 60 minutes by ground) from the scene. While en route to the burn center, the flight crew gives a detailed report to the receiving team, complete with chemical name and number. The flight crew continues to ventilate the patient easily with 100% oxygen and a pulse oximetery reading of 100%. The patient's heart rate decreases to 88 bpm, indicating a reduction in oxygen demand and pain. Additional doses of morphine are given at 5-minute intervals per the program's standing orders.

The receiving center, as per its protocols, opts for another decontamination prior to entering the facility. The patient is admitted, extubated 4 days later, and is discharged within 2 weeks after treatment for his burns. No other injuries or issues related to his chemical exposure are noted.

In this case the clear and concise style of communication between the ground and aviation crews has led to rapid intervention for a potentially fatal complication of an airway burn. Although no specific complaint was made regarding mouth or airway pain, the paramedic's total assessment told a different story. The combination of mechanism of injury, anxiety, tachypnea, wheezing, and low pulse oximetery pointed to a patient in distress. Quick assessment and treatment coupled with a clear, concise report to the flight crew complete with the medic's notation that the patient was *not improving* with therapy, led to the early intubation and a patent airway. The second issue regarding the chemical exposure was also handled well. Identification, decontamination, and assessment led to an informed decision by the pilot to fly the patient.

The combination of the above actions led to early intervention, rapid and safe movement to an appropriate tertiary care center with a continuum of quality patient care, and accurate information throughout the episode.

REFERENCES

Bledsoe, Bryan E., Robert S. Porter, and Richard A. Cherry. *Special Considerations/ Operations.* Vol. 5 of *Paramedic Care: Principles & Practice.* Chapter 8, "Ambulance Operations, Chapter 11, "Hazardous Materials Incidents." Upper Saddle River, NJ: Brady/Prentice Hall Health, Pearson Education, 2001.

McSwain, Frame, Paturas, ed. *PHTLS: Basic and Advanced Trauma Life Support.* 4th ed. Akron: Mosby, 1999.

Preparing a Safe Landing Zone. Alexandria, VA: NEMSPA, 2002.

Varela, Joe, ed. *Hazardous Materials: Handbook for Emergency Responders.* Indianapolis: Wiley, 1997.

42

C. Crawford Mechem, MD

Exposure to Hazardous Materials

CASE PRESENTATION

Paramedics are called to a small farm for a patient in respiratory distress. Two farm workers were involved in an altercation inside a tool shed. One worker grabbed a bottle from a shelf and threw the liquid contents on the other and fled the scene. When the police arrived, they found the patient on his hands and knees retching and gasping for air. The bottle was lying on the floor next to the patient. One of the officers examined the label and saw that it was a stock solution of diazinon, an insecticide that is used as a dilute solution for spraying agricultural plants. He radioed this information to his dispatcher so that it could be forwarded to the paramedic unit. He also requested that a hazardous material (hazmat) unit be dispatched.

When the paramedics arrive, they find the patient lying on his side outside of the shed. He has a brownish liquid on his clothing and skin. His respirations are labored. They also find one of the police officers leaning against a tree and breathing heavily. The hazmat unit has not arrived and is expected to be delayed at least 30 minutes. The paramedics are hesitant to approach the patient and the officer because of the known exposure to an insecticide. However, they recognize that the patient is in serious condition.

QUESTIONS

1. Should the paramedics wait for the hazmat unit to arrive or initiate immediate care?
2. What safety measures, if any, should the paramedics take in approaching the patients?
3. How do insecticides exert their toxic effects?

225

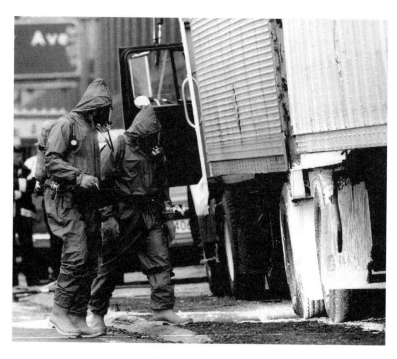

Rescuers wearing encapsulating suits and SCBA on a hazmat scene.

DISCUSSION

The case presents two separate issues that need to be addressed. First is how to care for the farm worker and the police officer who both appear to be suffering from insecticidal poisoning. The second and broader issue is how emergency medical personnel should respond to hazmat incidents and care for victims without jeopardizing their own safety in the process.

According to the Department of Transportation (DOT), a hazardous material is "any substance or material in a form which poses an unreasonable risk to health, safety, and property when transported in commerce." DOT places hazardous materials in eight different categories: (1) explosives and blasting agents; (2) gases; (3) flammable and combustible liquids; (4) oxidizers and organic peroxides; (5) poisonous and infectious substances; (6) radioactive substances; (7) corrosives; and (8) other regulated materials. Although prehospital care providers may encounter any of these potentially toxic substances in the course of their work, most hazmat incidents involve four broad categories of substances: corrosives, pesticides and herbicides, gases, and fuels. The majority of exposures occur at fixed sites, whereas a minority involve transportation accidents. These materials may result in serious toxicity and even death; however, strict adherence to a few simple procedures and precautions will in most cases protect the providers and allow them to care for victims.

The key to a safe and appropriate response to a hazmat incident is preplanning. According to Occupational Safety and Health Administration (OSHA) regulations, any employee who is expected to respond to a hazmat incident is required to attend training appropriate to his or her anticipated level of response. For most EMS personnel, hazmat awareness or hazmat operations training is adequate. EMS personnel should also have a basic familiarity with the types of hazardous materials that may be encountered in their jurisdiction. In addition, ambulances should be equipped with appropriate personal protective equipment and other items to protect their crew. These items include plastic bags for storing contaminated items; plastic sheets and duct tape to cover surfaces within the ambulance to minimize further contamination; rubber boots and suits made of water-impermeable material such at Tyvek®; gloves made of rubber, nitrile, or another chemical-impermeable material (latex does not afford adequate protection); face and eye protection; some form of respiratory protection; and reference materials.

The first step in responding to a hazmat incident is for the emergency responder to recognize that an incident exists and call for appropriate back-up according to local protocols. Emergency vehicles should be parked upwind from the spill. In addition, if the hazardous material is a flowing liquid, vehicles should be parked uphill. However, they should be parked on the same level if gases or fumes that may rise are present. Emergency responders should also be cognizant of the three zones of a hazmat incident: the hot, warm, and cold zones. The hot zone is the area of actual contamination and is the most dangerous to the responder. In most cases, EMS personnel should not enter this zone, leaving this task to specially trained and equipped hazmat personnel. The warm zone is adjacent to the hot zone and is less dangerous to responders. However, protective clothing is still necessary to operate in this zone. Decontamination and limited life-saving therapy are conducted in the warm zone. Finally, the cold zone is contaminant-free and is where normal EMS activities, such as patient triage and treatment, will be conducted.

The second step in the response to a hazmat incident is isolating the contaminant and preventing further spread. This involves cordoning off the area and limiting access. In addition, those who have been potentially exposed should not be allowed to leave the area until they have been adequately decontaminated. Law enforcement officers may need to assist with this.

Once steps have been taken to limit contamination, the emergency responder should attempt to identify the agent involved and determine its toxicity, the best way to perform decontamination, and how to treat any victims. Identification of the agent should be made at a safe distance from the source. Binoculars may be useful for this purpose. Placarding, bottle labels, bills of lading on trucks, shipping manifests on trains, and material safety data sheets (MSDSs) are potential sources of information. Additional resources for information on toxicity, decontamination, and therapy include DOT's *2000 Emergency Response Guidebook: A Guidebook for First Responders During the Initial Phase of a Dangerous Goods/Hazardous Materials Incident,* local poison control centers, and the Chemical Transportation Emergency Center (CHEMTREC). CHEMTREC operates a 24-hour toll-free telephone number that can provide valuable information on managing specific hazmat incidents. The number is 800-424-9300.

Only after the substance has been identified and its toxicity determined can a decision be made about patient rescue, decontamination, and treatment. The material may be deemed too dangerous for medical personnel to approach. In that case, the scene should be secured until hazmat personnel arrive. On the other hand, depending on the material involved, it may be safe for medical personnel to perform patient rescue, decontamination, and subsequent care, provided they wear appropriate personal protective equipment

(PPE). In all circumstances, the safety of emergency responders must take precedence over patient care. The urge to rush in to save a critical patient should be avoided if, in so doing, emergency personnel may become contaminated and sickened as well.

Decontamination is begun by removing the patient's clothing and jewelry. In most cases, this will eliminate approximately 80% of the contaminant. These items should be sealed in labeled plastic bags. Particulate matter should be removed with a brush. The skin may then be decontaminated by flushing with large quantities of water for at least 20 minutes. Whereas containing the resultant run-off water is ideal, in many situations this is neither practical nor necessary. The use of water is contraindicated in a small number of exposures. The optimal way to decontaminate a patient exposed to such a material is best determined by consulting one of the resources listed above.

Although in some cases it may be necessary to initiate life-saving interventions and administer antidotes before or during decontamination, in most cases decontamination can be completed prior to patient care. After the patient has been decontaminated, medical personnel will also need to remove PPE and undergo decontamination. Patient care may then be administered.

Most insecticides fall into one of two categories, organophosphates and carbamates. Diazinon is an organophosphate insecticide used to control pest insects on food crops, in gardens, and in the home. It is commonly sold as a 90% solution that is pale to dark brown. Its mechanism of action is the inactivation of the enzyme cholinesterase, which breaks down the neurotransmitter acetylcholine into choline and acetic acid. Inhibition of cholinesterase therefore leads to an accumulation of acetylcholine at nerve junctions. After 24 to 48 hours, this inhibition becomes irreversible. Although potentially fatal for insects, this may also have serious consequences for humans. Signs and symptoms of organophosphate poisoning include hypertension, bradycardia or tachycardia, bronchospasm, altered mental status, seizures, and muscle fasciculations and weakness. Other manifestations can be remembered by the mnemonic, SLUDGE, which stands for salivation, lacrimation, urinary incontinence, diarrhea, gastrointestinal distress, and emesis. Blurred vision and pinpoint pupils are also commonly seen. Death usually results from respiratory failure.

The toxic effects of carbamates are similar to those of organophosphates. However, there are fewer central nervous system manifestations, and seizures do not occur. Unlike organophosphates, carbamates cause only temporary inhibition of cholinesterase, lasting about 6 hours. This distinction has an important impact on therapy.

Emergency management of patients manifesting toxicity from organophosphates or carbamates involves decontamination, supportive care, and administration of antidotes. Rescuers should avoid direct contact with contaminated clothing and vomitus by wearing chemically impermeable clothing, rubber or nitrile gloves, and face and eye protection. Patients with any respiratory compromise should be put on high-flow oxygen. In the setting of copious airway secretions or impending respiratory failure, endotracheal intubation may be indicated. Hypotension is treated with fluid resuscitation and pressor agents. Seizures are managed with IV diazepam or lorazepam.

Atropine is administered to reverse pulmonary and gastrointestinal symptoms. An appropriate starting dose for adults and children older than 12 years is 2–4 mg intravenously and may be repeated every 15 minutes until bronchospasm and pulmonary secretions resolve. The dose for children under 12 years is 0.05–0.1 mg/kg. Doses of up to several hundred milligrams per day may be necessary. Atropine may also be administered via the intramuscular or endotracheal route if IV access is not immediately available.

Atropine has no effect on respiratory depression or muscle fasciculations and weakness. Therefore, in the case of organophosphate toxicity, pralidoxime (2-PAM) is also administered. This prevents the irreversible inactivation of cholinesterase and is best given within 24–36 hours of exposure. The recommended dose for adults and children older than 12 years is 1 gm IV over 30 minutes. The dose for children under 12 years is 20–50 mg/kg in 100 cc of normal saline infused over 30 minutes. The dose may be repeated in 1 hour, and then every 6–8 hours for the next 24–48 hours or until signs and symptoms resolve. Because the binding of carbamates to cholinesterase is complete within 30 minutes and is reversible, 2-PAM is not indicated in cases of carbamate toxicity.

RETURN TO THE CASE

The medics contact the regional poison control center for advice. Based on the information they receive, they don Tyvek suits, shoe covers, nitrile gloves, and face masks with shields. They remove the clothing from the patient on the ground and instruct the police officer to undress. They then decontaminate both with large quantities of water from a nearby garden hose. The patient is complaining of trouble breathing and tightness in his chest. He denies any other medical problems, but his breathing is too labored for him to provide other information. His vital signs are blood pressure 160/96, pulse 64, and respiration 28. The paramedics note copious secretions from the nose and mouth. Auscultation of the lungs reveals diffuse wheezing, and his oxygen saturation is 91%. Assessment of the officer reveals blood pressure 136/80, pulse 96, and respiration 18. His examination is significant for rhinorrhea and soft bilateral wheezes, and his oxygen saturation is 94%. He is able to speak in complete sentences and says that he has a history of asthma. They place both patients on 100% oxygen and establish IV access. They administer 4 mg IV atropine to the farm worker, 2 mg to the police officer, and dress both patients in Tyvek suits. They then remove their own Tyvek suits and transport the patients to the nearest hospital. En route, they give an additional 2 mg of atropine to the farm worker and administer 2.5 mg of nebulized Albuterol to the officer.

The police officer's symptoms are improved on hospital arrival, but the farm worker continues to be in respiratory distress. Emergency department staff repeat the decontamination of both patients prior to bringing them into the department. The farm worker subsequently undergoes endotracheal intubation and is given additional doses of atropine. One gram of IV 2-PAM is also administered. He is transferred to the intensive care unit (ICU), where he receives a total of 48 mg of atropine over the next 24 hours. The police officer is also given IV 2-PAM and is admitted to a step-down ICU bed. There he is given additional doses of atropine and Albuterol. Both patients recover uneventfully.

REFERENCES

Bledsoe, Bryan E., Robert S. Porter, and Richard A. Cherry. *Special Considerations/Operations.* Vol. 5 of *Paramedic Care: Principles & Practice.* Chapter 11, "Hazardous Materials Incidents." Upper Saddle River, NJ: Brady/Prentice Hall Health, Pearson Education, 2001.

Cox, R. "Hazmat." *eMedicine Journal* 2 (2001). Available at http://www.emedicine. com/emerg/topic228.htm.

Dickinson, E. T. "EMS Special Operations." In E. T. Dickinson, *Fire Service Emergency Care*. Upper Saddle River, NJ: Prentice Hall, 1999, 732–742.

Reigart, J. R., and J. R. Roberts. *Recognition and Management of Pesticide Poisonings*. Office of Prevention, Pesticides, and Toxic Substances of the United States Environmental Protection Agency, publication EPA 735-R-98-003, March 1999. Available at http://www.epa.gov.

Slaper, D. "Toxicity, Organophosphate and Carbamate." *eMedicine Journal* 2 (2001). Available at http://www.emedicine.com/emerg/topic346.htm.

43

Jonathan Politis, BA, NREMT-P

EXTRICATION

CASE PRESENTATION

Your shift started at 0600 (6 A.M.) today and it's now 0845 and you are finally ordering some breakfast. Just as your food is delivered your pager starts beeping: "Medic 1, Medic 2, Rescue 7, Engine 3 and Battalion 1 respond to an MVA with entrapment at Central Avenue and Fuller Road."

Oh well, that food will have to wait! It's a 3-minute response to the scene and you are the first arriving unit. You radio back, "Firecom, this is Medic 1 arriving and establishing command. We have a two-vehicle collision, heavy damage, with entrapment in the intersection. Send two additional medic units and have them park in sequence behind my vehicle." Immediately, you and your partner don command and triage bibs and start the triage process at the scene. The initial triage sweep has found three Priority 3 walking injured whom you place in the Medic 1 patient compartment. The car with the most serious damage has massive front-end deformation with intrusion of the firewall and driver's door into the patient compartment. There is a center console and the passenger side door opens easily.

Within minutes, Battalion 1 arrives and you transfer command to her after a brief face-to-face transition of command. Command assigns Medic 3 and 4 to the Priority 3 patients and Medic 2 to assist you with the entrapped patient. You have gained access to the backseat and manually stabilized the head while your partner starts the assessment. You find a 35-year-old female who is verbally responsive but has altered mental status, a barely palpable radial pulse, and a respiratory rate of 36. She is restless, and has an obvious fracture of the left femur. Vitals are respirations 36, pulse 140, and blood pressure 110/90. The oxygen saturation registers error and she has equal breath sounds bilaterally.

Command assigns Rescue 7 to your vehicle and the extrication officer completes the vehicle stabilization and asks, "OK, what do you guys want us to do?"

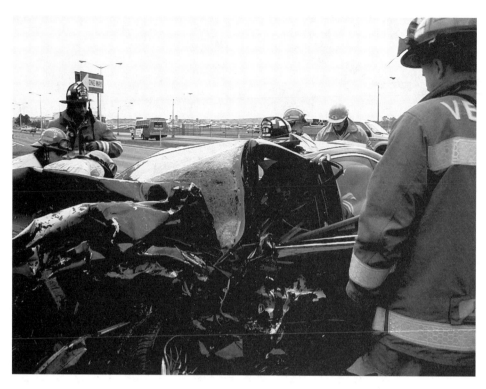

A heavily entrapped patient.
Courtesy of Jon Politis.

QUESTIONS

1. What triage levels should be assigned to the entrapped and ambulatory patients?
2. What is the significance of the patient's restlessness?
3. What is the most appropriate way to extricate the entrapped patient?

DISCUSSION

Regardless of the EMS system, the first arriving EMS unit must ensure scene safety and personal safety and size up the situation. In this case, their standard operating procedure (SOP) required them to establish command, provide a brief arrival report, and begin the initial triage of the patients. Using START (Simple Triage And Rapid Treatment) triage they asked those who could walk to report to one of their medic units. In START, these patients are initially triaged as Priority 3 "green" patients. This leaves all other patients who can move under their own power as Priority 1, 2, or 0. Moving them to the back of an ambulance is a safety tactic to get them out of traffic as soon as possible and keep them in one place. A better alternative might be to have them go to a nearby building or other area of safety. In START, the first step is to assess breathing and, if there is none, make an attempt to open the airway. If there is no breathing after opening the airway then the patient is Priority 0 (P-0). If respirations are over 30, patients are tagged as P-1; if less than 30, they are tagged as P-2. The next step is to assess circulation. If the radial pulse is present, they are tagged as P-2; if absent, they are tagged as P-1. The final criteria is the level of consciousnes (LOC): If alert, they are tagged as P-2; if LOC is altered, they are tagged as P-1.

START TRIAGE RECAP

Priority 1—Red

- Altered mental status
- Radial pulse absent
- Respirations over 30

Priority 2—Yellow

- Alert
- Radial pulse present
- Respirations under 30

Priority 3—Green

- Able to follow commands and walk

Priority 0—Black

- Unresponsive
- No breathing
- No pulse

An important point to remember is that P-3 green patients on secondary triage may be categorized as P-1 or P-2. Just because patients can follow commands and walk does *not* mean they lack serious injuries. It is essential that secondary triage of P-3s take place as soon as possible after resources can be assigned to them. What priority is the entrapped patient? She has altered mental status and a respiratory rate of over 30. Both of these physiologic parameters call for immediate tagging as P-1.

Looking at the photograph at the beginning of the case, did you notice the heavy intrusion into the occupant compartment? What about the fractured femur? She has significant mechanism of injury to the left side of her body. Blunt trauma is very deceptive. A broken femur alone can cause significant blood loss and a fracture of the pelvis alone can be life threatening. Impact to the left torso can cause pulmonary contusion and injury to solid organs such as the spleen. Any of these can cause significant blood loss and cellular hypoxia.

The first response to blood loss is compensation by increasing the heart rate and peripheral vasoconstriction. Until a person reaches Grade 3 hemorrhage, which is about at 25%–30% blood loss, the systolic blood pressure remains close to normal. Once in Grade 3 hemorrhage, the blood pressure starts to fall. The important message here is this: Always look for early signs of compensated shock—sustained tachycardia, vasoconstriction, restlessness, and thirst! In this patient the sustained tachycardia, restlessness, and thready pulse are all signs of significant occult bleeding and compensated shock. She is so vasoconstricted that the pulse oximeter will not sense blood flow in the fingertip. If this patient has these obvious signs of bleeding within 8 minutes of the crash, she has lost a significant amount of blood quickly. There is no time to waste! If you wait until the patient's blood pressure falls to start taking aggressive action, the patient may not survive. This patient needs "bright lights and cold steel"—in other words, the hospital operating room.

In this case the extrication officer asked the paramedics what they wanted done. The whole purpose behind all of the tools and extrication technology is to free patients so they can get to definitive care early. There is a tendency to use tools and equipment even when they are not really necessary. If the patient is stable, then a slower, more careful approach in using tools to clear the easiest extrication pathway is called for. However, if the patient's condition is serious or critical, the patient must be extricated in the fastest way possible! The old saying that "we tear the car apart from around the patient" no longer holds true. The reality of modern trauma care is that we need to move only what metal is necessary to extricate quickly. The extrication officer and paramedics in this case are working as a team to benefit the patient by extricating quickly. Because of her condition and minimal entrapment they make a decision to rapidly extricate her out the passenger side door. There is minimal tool work done except to stabilize the car and have a charged line ready in case of a fire. What is the best way to extricate? The method that is best for the patient! If the patient can withstand waiting a few minutes, clear an easy pathway and minimize the pain. If the patient is bleeding to death, don't waste time! Effective rescue is a balance of medical and mechanical skills focused on the patients' needs.

RETURN TO THE CASE

You and your partner recognize this woman as a P-1 trauma patient who has obvious signs of bleeding because she is in compensated shock. A rigid collar is applied, her airway is managed, and oxygen by nonrebreather face mask is applied. With the help of the rescue company crew, she is rapidly extricated out the passenger door and immobilized on a long spine board. During the extrication, the P-3 patients are moved to the other arriving medic units. The woman is moved to the back of Medic 1 and a crew member from Medic 2 drives to the trauma center as both paramedics continue assessment and treatment in the back of the unit. Her clothing is removed and IV access is gained enroute to the trauma center. She is in intense pain from the femur fracture so a traction splint is applied en route that provides considerable pain relief. Vital signs are reassessed as she is continually monitored. She arrives at the trauma center where the trauma team continues the resuscitation. She is found to have a ruptured spleen, a pulmonary contusion, and a midshaft fracture of the left femur. The total scene time was 11 minutes and transport time to the trauma center was 16 minutes. In total, she crashed, was assessed, extricated, treated, and delivered to the trauma center in just over 30 minutes.

REFERENCES

Bledsoe, Bryan E., Robert S. Porter, and Richard A. Cherry. *Special Considerations/ Operations.* Vol. 5 of *Paramedic Care: Principles & Practice.* Chapter 10, "Rescue Awareness and Operations." Upper Saddle River, NJ: Brady/Prentice Hall Health, Pearson Education, 2001.

Campbell, John Emory. *Basic Trauma Life Support.* 5th ed. Upper Saddle River, NJ: Brady/Prentice Hall Health/Pearson Education, 2004.

Vivian Hwang, MD

44

NEAR-DROWNING

CASE PRESENTATION

You and your partner are riding along through the park when you get a call from the dispatch center that a middle-aged man just fell into the local river and is in distress.

You arrive at the scene within 2 minutes and find the patient on the ground next to the river with bystander CPR in progress. As you approach the patient, a witness quickly tells you that they were all at a picnic when they heard a splash in the water. Their friend had a few too many drinks and must have stumbled into the water which was approximately 3 feet deep. They were able to drag him out within 5 minutes, but it looked like he wasn't breathing so they started CPR.

Primary survey reveals an unresponsive patient with poor inspiratory effort. Breathing is shallow and irregular at a rate of 6 breaths per minute. Breath sounds are present and equal on both sides. Skin is cool, clammy, and cyanotic appearing. There is a slow, palpable radial pulse present. You smell alcohol on his breath and do not see any external signs of trauma.

Your partner begins BVM ventilation with 100% oxygen. A second paramedic crew arrives. They help you place a C-collar and logroll the patient onto a backboard. A large-bore IV is established. You recheck and cannot feel a pulse. ETA to the nearest hospital is 6 minutes. You proceed with ACLS protocol.

QUESTIONS

1. What is the pathophysiology of drowning?
2. What are the key components to initial resuscitation of drowning and near-drowning patients?

Drowning is a major cause of accidental death in the United States and is the second most common cause of death in those under 44 years of age. *Drowning* is defined as death by suffocation after submersion in a liquid medium within 24 hours. *Near-drowning* describes a patient who survives for 24 hours or more after submersion whether the victim ultimately survives or not. The incidence peaks during the summer months. Sites of drowning include pools (most common), any natural body of water, bathtubs, buckets, and septic tanks. Conditions that predispose to drowning include use of intoxicants, diving and boating accidents, hypothermia, medical conditions such as seizure disorder, electrical shocks, and overestimation of swimming ability.

Submersion in a liquid medium will ultimately lead to hypoxemia and cerebral hypoxia. When a conscious victim becomes submerged, breathholding will reflexively occur for up to 3 minutes. Panic ensues, and the victim will then make inspiratory and swallowing efforts, causing water to stimulate severe laryngospasm and bronchospasm. Approximately 15% of drowning victims will develop laryngospasm that prevents aspiration of liquid, termed "dry drowning." The majority of patients will aspirate a significant quantity of liquid leading to "wet drowning." This results in hypoxia, and the patient will ultimately become unconscious. The victim will continue to swallow water, resulting in gastric distention increasing the risk of vomiting and aspiration. If untreated, hypotension, bradycardia, and death will result in a short period.

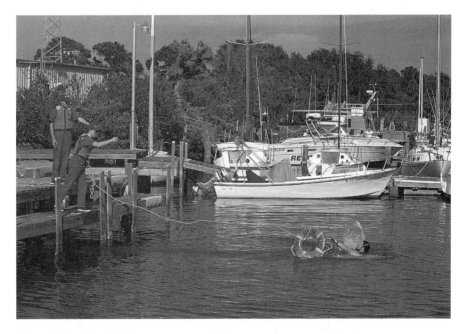

Flotation device being thrown to a victim in distress.

In the past, distinctions were made between freshwater and saltwater drowning because of animal studies showing physiologic and biochemical differences between the two. In freshwater drowning, aspiration of a large amount of hypotonic water can diffuse into the vascular space causing hemodilution. This can then result in hypervolemia and dilutional hyponatremia; however, it has been shown that aspiration of large volumes would be needed to cause clinically significant electrolyte changes. In saltwater drowning, aspiration of hypertonic fluid creates an osmotic gradient drawing water from the blood stream into the pulmonary interstitial space, resulting in pulmonary edema. It is clear that both freshwater and saltwater drowning have the effect of washing out surfactant and creating the potential for developing noncardiogenic pulmonary edema. The clinical management of these patients is thus fairly similar. It has also been observed that the temperature of the water and possible contaminants within the water have become more important factors in determining the morbidity and mortality of these patients. Chlorine in pools is especially deleterious on pulmonary tissues.

There are three prehospital factors that can alter outcome of victims of near-drowning: water temperature, duration of submersion, and duration of resuscitation. Submersion in icy water (less than 41°F/5°C) does result in a higher chance of survival, especially in children. Duration of submersion is often difficult to determine, but in a small study, submersion longer than 10 minutes led to death or severe neurologic deficits in 6 out of 6 children. The duration of resuscitation also plays a role in outcome; Quan and Kinder showed that field resuscitation longer than 25 minutes resulted in a poor outcome in 17 out of 17 patients. Kyriacou and colleagues showed in a retrospective study that 126 (85.1%) out of 148 patients had good clinical outcomes if they received some type of resuscitation compared to 10 (55.6%) out of 18 patients who received no resuscitative intervention. Unfortunately, there is no standard medical index or score that can be applied to patients who experience drowning or near-drowning that can predict with 100% accuracy those who will or will not survive with good neurologic outcomes. Thus, all drowning victims should be treated aggressively unless rigor mortis, putrefaction, or excessively prolonged submersion is present.

When approaching a drowning or near-drowning victim, it is important to be aware of the environment that the victim is found in to ensure safety for yourself and other rescuers. The goal of treatment is to establish ventilation and perfusion to the patient as rapidly as possible. If the victim is found in the water, a water rescue should be attempted only if the appropriate resources are available including proper training, equipment, and sufficient personnel. Patients should be removed from the water as soon as possible by a trained rescue swimmer. If a patient is found unconscious and without respirations, ventilation should be initiated while the patient is still in the water. It is important to maintain spinal cord precautions especially if there is a mechanism for traumatic injury (i.e., diving or mechanism of drowning is unknown). It may be necessary to place the patient on a long backboard while in the water.

Once the patient is out of the water, quickly assess ABCs. Assume that all patients are hypoxic, acidotic, and hypothermic. CPR should begin as soon as possible for those who have arrested. Remember to maintain C-spine precautions if indicated. Administer oxygen at 100% FIO$_2$ using BVM ventilation with proper positioning of jaw and tongue. Jaw thrust is the ideal maneuver for positioning of the airway, especially when C-spine precautions are indicated. Maneuvers to empty the lungs of water, such as the Heimlich maneuver, are of unproven benefit and are not recommended unless there is airway obstruction. These maneuvers may delay early intubation and lead to an increased risk of aspiration as well as arrhythmias in the hypothermic patient.

Patients with evidence of respiratory failure require immediate tracheal intubation to secure the airway and prevent risk of aspiration during resuscitation. Near-drowning patients with hypothermia may have sinus bradycardia or atrial fibrillation and have very weak and difficult to palpate pulses. Before initiating compressions, it is important to search carefully for pulses for at least 1 minute. Patients who are extremely hypothermic (with core temperatures less than 77°F/25°C) are also at risk for asystole and ventricular fibrillation. Importantly, ventricular fibrillation can be precipitated by rough handling of the patient. If a patient is in arrest, initiate the ACLS protocol. Patients in arrest should get one or two attempts at defibrillation and administration of drugs through a large-bore IV. If attempts at defibrillation for patients with core temperatures less than 82.4°F/28°C are not immediately successful, discontinue until temperature is over 84.2°F/29°C. Core temperatures are difficult to determine in the field, but patients who have had prolonged immersion are probably severely hypothermic. Passive external warming measures include removing wet clothing and wrapping patients in blankets. Lactated Ringer's or normal saline should be run at 75 ml/hr. These patients should be rapidly and gently transported to the nearest emergency department maintaining insulation against further heat loss. Some authorities advocate transfer of all severely hypothermic and clinically lifeless patients to the nearest facility with cardiopulmonary bypass. Overall, 92% of near-drowning survivors recover neurologically intact. A small study by Habib et al. showed that patients who were not comatose on admission to the intensive care unit or who had a pulse and detectable blood pressure on admission to the emergency department survived neurologically intact. Those who arrived pulseless and comatose died or had severe neurologic impairment.

RETURN TO THE CASE

The cardiac monitor and pulse oximeter are placed on the patient. The monitor shows sinus bradycardia in the 40s. A palpable pulse is confirmed within 1 minute. The patient remains unconscious with minimal respirations and the decision to intubate the patient is made. No medications are needed. One paramedic applies anterior cricoid pressure (the Sellick maneuver) while another maintains cervical stabilization. The patient is intubated using direct laryngoscopy and a 7.5 mm endotracheal tube. Tube placement is confirmed by direct visualization, a colorimetric end-tidal CO_2 monitor, and by the presence of bilateral breath sounds. The tube is secured with tape. Normal saline at 75 ml/hr is run through a large-bore IV. The wet clothes are gently and quickly removed, and the patient is wrapped in warm blankets. The patient is transported to the nearest emergency department.

The patient is received at the local emergency department. Initial vital signs include a temperature of 92.5°F/69.2°C, pulse of 40, blood pressure 90/50, O_2 saturation 94% on 100% FIO_2. His GCS improves to 8. The patient is warmed using passive external warming techniques. The CXR reveals bilateral fluffy infiltrates and a normal-sized heart. Head CT and C-spine series are negative for any acute findings. The patient is transferred to the ICU where the patient continues to get aggressive pulmonary toilet.

The patient is extubated on the sixth hospital day and is discharged to a rehabilitation facility with mild neurologic impairment. One year later, he has fully recovered.

REFERENCES

Bledsoe, B. E., R. S. Porter, and Shade, B. R. *Near-drowning and Drowning in Paramedic Emergency Care*. 3rd ed. Upper Saddle River, NJ: Brady/Prentice Hall, 1997, 877–880.

Bledsoe, Bryan E., Robert S. Porter, and Richard A. Cherry. *Special Considerations/ Operations*. Vol. 5 of *Paramedic Care: Principles & Practice*. Chapter 10, "Rescue Awareness and Operations." Upper Saddle River, NJ: Brady/Prentice Hall Health, Pearson Education, 2001.

DeNicola, L. K., J. L. Falk, M. E. Swanson, and N. Kisson. "Submersion Injuries in Children and Adults." *Critical Care Clinics* 13, no. 3 (1997): 477–502.

Dickinson, E. T. *Water-Related Emergencies in Fire Service Emergency Care*. Upper Saddle River, NJ: Brady/Prentice Hall, 1999, 398–403.

Golden, F., M. J. Tipton, and R. C. Scott. "Immersion, Near-drowning and Drowning. *British Journal of Anesthesia* 79, (1997): 214–225.

Habib, D. M., F. W. Tecklenburg, S. A. Webb, N. G. Anas, and R. M. Perkin. "Prediction of Childhood Drowning and Near-drowning Morbidity and Mortality." *Pediatric Emergency Care* 12, no. 4 (1996): 255–258.

Kyriacou, D. N., E. L. Arcinue, C. Peek, and J. F. Kraus. "Effect of Immediate Resuscitation on Children with Submersion Injury. *Pediatrics* 94 (1994): 137–142.

Quan, L., and D. Kinder. "Pediatric Submersions: Prehospital Predictors of Outcome." *Pediatrics* 90 (1992): 909–913.

Weinstein, M. D., and B. P. Krieger. "Near-drowning: Epidemiology, Pathophysiology and Initial Treatment." *Journal of Emergency Medicine* 14, no. 4 (1996): 461–467.

Ken Campbell, RN

45

NEEDLE-STICK INJURIES

CASE PRESENTATION

It's almost 0345 (3:45 A.M.), the shift has been busy with typical calls of chest pain, diabetic emergencies, a motor vehicle crash, a COPD patient, and a new-onset CHF patient. Thoughts are about tomorrow, your first day off in 6 days, when the alert sounds. There's a multivehicle crash with entrapment at an approach street near the interstate. Rescue, fire, police, and additional EMS units are simultaneously dispatched.

As your partner and you respond, police have arrived on the scene confirming multiple patients and entrapment. Your initial scene evaluation indicates two upright patients entrapped in a sport utility vehicle (SUV) broadsided at the intersection to the interstate entrance ramp. Another compact car is several yards away, with heavy damage to the front crumple zone and windshield. A single occupant is identified lying across the front seat, unresponsive.

The second EMS unit arrives with multiple personnel and focuses on the SUV while you gain access through an opened passenger door on the compact car. Your patient is pale, with lacerations and abrasions to the forehead, and his respiratory effort appears adequate. While in-line traction is maintained, your assessment identifies a patient who was a sole occupant, unrestrained driver, speaking to you, but slurring speech and confused. His trachea is deviated and breath sounds are significantly diminished on the right with obvious respiratory distress. The decision is made to immediately needle decompress your patient's chest because of a presumed tension pneumothorax. The needle decompression has good results with return of breath sounds on the right and decreased respiratory distress. Secondary survey reveals bilateral upper arm swelling and potential humerus and clavicular fractures, abdominal tenderness, and abrasions over the forearms, chest, and abdomen. His Glasgow Coma Scale remains at 12. No medical history can be obtained.

With the assistance of fire rescue personnel, further immobilization and extrication are completed and you are en route to the hospital with an ETA of 4 minutes. IV access is gained using the external jugular vein and a normal saline bolus is initiated, stabilizing the patient's blood pressure.

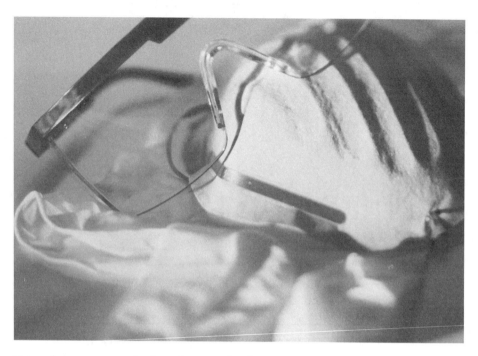

Universal precautions must be observed in caring for all patients.

Then, as you arrive at the hospital, it happens: As you lift and center the backboard on the stretcher, you suddenly feel what we all fear—a needle stick in the palm of your hand. You look down to see the bloody stylet of an angiocath pointing up from the stretcher.

QUESTIONS

1. How did this happen? What was I exposed to?
2. What do I do now and whom should I tell? Is there a policy? What are my rights?

DISCUSSION

Needle-stick injuries are preventable. Our daily prehospital routine includes multiple potential exposures to blood and body fluids either through excretions or needle sticks. The latter is highly preventable and can be significantly minimized through awareness, technique, and equipment choices. Once a needle-stick occurs, it is essential that the provider seek immediate medical attention. Initial medical evaluation and treatment is the first step in a process that will include extensive documentation of the incident, initiation of workers' compensation, and potential ongoing medical monitoring.

Under OSHA's Bloodborne Pathogen Standard published in 1991, as an occupational injury, your employer must keep a log of sharps injury as well as exposure to body fluids and infectious materials. Since that initial legislation, at least 21 states have passed legislation regarding the health care worker and bloodborne pathogen exposures. Common provisions, although varying from state to state, include

- Listing of safety devices as engineering controls
- Listing of available safety devices by the state for employer use
- Development of a written exposure plan requiring periodic review and update
- Development of protocols for safety device identification and selection by employers and frontline employees
- Development of a sharps injury log and reporting requirements of log information
- Development of methods to increase use of vaccines and personal protective equipment
- Waivers or exemptions from safety device usage under certain circumstances
- Placement of sharp containers in accessible positions
- Training for workers regarding safety device usage

The Ryan White Comprehensive AIDS Resource Emergency (CARE) Act of 1990, through federal legislation, establishes funding for primary health care and support services for people with HIV. Within this act are several areas of interest for EMS providers. The act mandated that a list be developed containing potentially life-threatening infectious diseases to which emergency personnel may be exposed. It further identified methods of exposure and guidelines that medical facilities must follow when occupational exposures occur. The final listing of these diseases, published in 1994 by the CDC, included the following:

- Infectious pulmonary tuberculosis
- Hepatitis B
- AIDS
- Diphtheria
- Meningococcal disease
- Plague
- Hemmorrhagic fevers
- Rabies

If it is determined that a patient has any of the listed infections and an exposure risk has occurred, notification of designated EMS officers or exposed EMS personnel must be made within 48 hours. Furthermore, the designated EMS officer or personnel themselves who have potentially been exposed, through transport, may request from the medical facility determination of actual exposure. Response to the inquiry must be made within 48 hours. Further appeal processes have also been identified.

Management guidelines for exposure and postexposure prophylaxis to hepatitis B and C viruses and HIV have been identified to minimize conversion. These guidelines, updated by the U.S. Public Health Service in 2001, were modified from their 1998 release and include establishment of bloodborne pathogen and management policies, bloodborne pathogen testing, and postexposure prophylaxis (PEP).

PEP management may differ based upon consideration of known HBV, HCV, or HIV status or risk factors in the source person. The algorithm for exposure should include immediate washing of wounds and skin with soap and water and copious flushing with water of any mucous membranes exposed. There is no support in the medical literature for the use of antiseptic washes as no study has documented their benefit over simple soap and water. Identification of the risk associated with exposure can be made by knowing whether blood, body fluid, or tissue was contacted. PEP decision-making also takes into account the type of exposure: human bites, sharp penetrating injuries via hollow or solid needle, mucosal membrane, or broken skin need to be considered for risk evaluation. For example, hollow needle exposures are generally considered higher risk than solid needle exposures due to the risk of increased blood inoculum in hollow needles.

Obviously, certain patient populations are more likely to be carriers of certain infectious diseases. Patients who have received extensive blood transfusions, are users of intravenous illicit drugs, or who practice unsafe sexual behavior, are commonly identified as patients with an increased risk of being carriers of HBV, HCV and HIV. However, many other patients are also potential carriers of these diseases. Treat all patients as likely carriers and maintain universal precautions. A treatment algorithm should include appropriate blood tests that should be done for a provider with an occupational exposure. Testing can include antihepatitis B surface antigen with follow-up testing 1 to 2 months later. If exposure to hepatitis C virus is suspected, hepatitis C antibody and alanine aminotransferase (ALT) should be drawn. Follow-up labs should be done 4 to 6 months later. Pregnancy testing of women of childbearing years should be done if applicable. HIV antibody testing should be done at exposure, 6 weeks, 3 months, and 6 months after exposure. In addition to these tests, baseline labs may also be drawn at the time of initial evaluation, because certain PEP medications may have adverse effects on subsequent blood chemistries.

Many EMS personnel have already received hepatitis B immunization through a series of injected vaccines, lessening the risk of conversion as a result of an occupational exposure. In cases where the provider has not been vaccinated, the U.S. Public Health Service recommends hepatitis B immune globulin (HBIG) and hepatitis B vaccine series after evaluation of the surface antigen testing. Studies have shown that HBIG treatment, when given within the first week postexposure, is 75% effective in reducing hepatitis B conversion in the occupational exposure.

Treatment for exposure to hepatitis C virus is not currently recommended, partially due to inconclusive studies as to the effectiveness of treatment. Contracting the hepatitis C virus after a percutaneous exposure carries a lower risk than exposures to hepatitis B virus, about 1.8%. According to the *New England Journal of Medicine* (1997), the risk of acquiring HIV is even less, about 0.3%. Prophylactic treatment for potential HIV exposure is recommended. The CDC recommends a basic 4-week regimen of the drugs zidovudine and lamivudine, commonly distributed as Combivir. Be aware that there are alternative and expanded treatment regimens that may include didanosine, indinavir, nelfinavir, stavudine, efavirenz, abacavir, as well as several others and combinations. When it is determined that postexposure prophylaxis is appropriate, it should be started as soon as possible (within hours of the exposure).

One of the key determinants used by physicians to decide whether PEP is indicated is an assessment of the source patient's identifiable risk factors for being infected with either HIV or viral hepatitis. Intravenous drug users, for example, would be considered high-risk source patients that would likely require initiation of PEP. In addition, when available, the serology (specifically, whether the patient has antibodies or antigens in his or her blood that indicate exposure to HIV or viral hepatitis) of the source patient is of great importance in determining the need for PEP. Unfortunately, the serology of the source patient is often difficult to obtain: The physician treating the exposed health care worker may be unable to obtain blood samples from the source patient for testing. In the obvious case, if a paramedic is stuck by a needle from an unknown patient (such as being stuck by a dirty needle while cleaning the rig at the start of a shift), it will be impossible to determine the source patient's risk factors or serology. In cases where the identity of the source patient is known, depending on state laws, the physician may or may not be able to obtain a blood sample for testing depending on the patient's willingness to consent to the blood draw. Finally, it is always helpful when the exposed paramedic can be treated in the same emergency department as the source patient to help facilitate the treating physician's ability to obtain an accurate history and potential serology from the source patient. In cases where the source patient's serology is drawn, the treating physician may start PEP drugs and potentially discontinue their use if the source patient's serology is found to be negative for HIV or viral hepatitis infections.

Prevention of needle sticks has been made easier in the prehospital environment. Recent advances in sharps safety include needleless IV sets, self-covering and self-retracting IV catheter needles, prefilled medication syringes, and better disposal containers. Having multiple disposal containers available for use will increase compliance for proper disposal of sharps. No matter which devices are used, awareness remains the foremost tool to protect against accidental exposure. Proper handling and disposal of sharps will prevent almost all adverse events. Disciplining yourself against any needle recapping will also eliminate needless exposure in either a moving or a stationary environment.

RETURN TO THE CASE

After providing a bedside report to the trauma team, you immediately remove your glove and wash your hand thoroughly, noting a puncture wound in the center of your left palm. You then notify the emergency department attending physician that you have sustained a needle stick. She places you in a separate examination room and a clerk registers you as a patient. As per your departmental policy, you notify your on-duty supervisor who responds to the ED to take a report.

After being examined by the physician (who has also examined and obtained a history from the trauma patient and his family) it is recommended that you begin PEP with Combivir. This is deemed appropriate because the trauma patient's family has informed the ED physician that he may have "done some drugs" in the past. The patient is too confused to be able to provide any history as his GCS fell to 10 after arrival in the trauma room and he is now intubated. The trauma surgeon advises the trauma patient's family that an occupational needle stick has occurred and he would like permission to draw serology for HIV and hepatitis testing, and the family agrees. You have your own blood drawn for baseline serology, complete blood count and liver functions (the latter being drawn as part of starting the Combivir), and receive your first dose of PEP. You are then discharged from the ED.

The only good news was that your hepatitis B and tetanus immunizations are up to date so you do not need additional shots.

Three days later you are called back to the hospital's occupational medicine department. The doctor informs you that all HIV and hepatitis serology on the source patient was negative and you may now stop taking the Combivir.

In your agency's follow-up of the incident it cannot be determined whether you or your partner was the one who left the bloody stylet on the stretcher. You and your partner both receive counseling memos in your personnel files for failing to comply with the department's needle-stick prevention policy.

REFERENCES

Bledsoe, Bryan E., Robert S. Porter, and Richard A. Cherry. *Introduction to Advanced Prehospital Care*. Vol. 1 of *Paramedic Care: Principles & Practice*. Chapter 2, "The Well-Being of the Paramedic." Upper Saddle River, NJ: Brady/Prentice Hall Health, Pearson Education, 2000.

National Institute for Occupational Safety and Health. *Overview of State Needle Safety Legislation*. Available at http://www.cdc.gov.niosh.topics/bbp/ndl-law.html.

Ridzon, R., K. Gallagher, C. Ciesielski, E. E. Mast, M. B. Ginsberg, B. J. Robertson, C. C. Lou, and A. Demaria Jr. "Simultaneous Transmission of Human Immunodeficiency Virus and Hepatitis C Virus from a Needle-Stick Injury." *New England Journal of Medicine* 336 (1997): 919–922.

The Ryan White CARE Act: A compilation of the Ryan White CARE Act of 1990 (PL.101-381), as amended by the Ryan White CARE Act amendments of 1996 (PL.104-146) and the Ryan White CARE Act amendments of 2000 (PL.106-345). Available at ftp://ftp.hrsa.gov/hab/compile.pdf.

"Updated U.S. Public Health Service Guidelines for the Management of Occupational Exposures to HBV, HCV, and HIV and Recommendations for Postexposure Prophylaxis." *MMWR Recommendation and Reports* 50, no. RR11 (June 29, 2001): 1–42. Available at http://www.cdc.gov/mmwr/preview/mmwrhtml/rr501al.htm.

U.S. Department of Labor Occupational Health and Labor. *Bloodborne Pathogens Standard 1910.1030*, Retrieved April 18, 2001, from http://www.osha.gov/pls/oshaweb/owadisp.show_document?p_table∇STANDARDS&p_id=10051.

Derek J. Tenhoopen, MD

46

PREECLAMPSIA/ ECLAMPSIA

CASE PRESENTATION

You are dispatched to the local health club where you are told that a "very pregnant-looking woman" in the yoga class almost fainted, and now she just "doesn't feel right."

You approach the patient, who is obviously pregnant. She tells you her due date is in 3 weeks. She complains of a severe headache and "spots in front of her eyes" that will not go away. She had not eaten breakfast this morning because she had experienced significant indigestion. On physical examination you note edema of her hands and face in addition to dependent edema. Her vital signs reveal a blood pressure of 140/88, a pulse of 102, and a respiratory rate of 28. On lung exam, you note fine bibasilar crackles. However, other than upper and lower extremity edema and mild hyperreflexia, the remainder of her examination is unremarkable. Your partner obtains a finger stick blood glucose of 90.

Your initial impression was near syncope from hypoglycemia. Now that she has been off her feet for almost 15 minutes, she states she feels much better and insists she will follow up with her obstetrician tomorrow, as scheduled. As she stands up, she suddenly collapses to the ground again complaining of a severe headache. A repeat blood pressure is now 184/108. As you consider placement of an IV, she develops a grand mal seizure.

QUESTIONS

1. What is the drug of choice for the treatment of severe preeclampsia/eclampsia
2. How do you reverse the effects of this drug when symptomatic overdose (the presence of apnea, obtundation) is suspected?

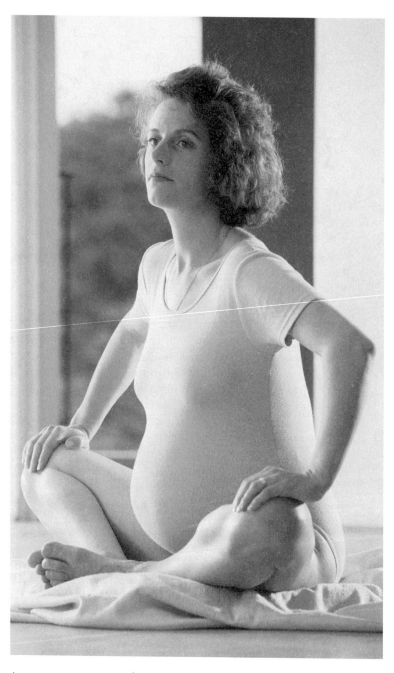

A pregnant woman in yoga class.
Courtesy of Romiily Lockyer and Getty Images, Inc.—Image Bank

DISCUSSION

Hypertensive disease complicates approximately 12%–22% of pregnancies in the United States and is the second leading cause of maternal mortality. In fact, it is directly responsible for 17.6% of maternal deaths in this country. Maternal hypertension is also an important cause of perinatal morbidity and mortality of the newborn, secondary to both direct fetal effects and iatrogenic preterm delivery performed for maternal indications such as eclampsia. Despite the importance of this condition, its origin remains somewhat obscure, and the disease process is ultimately reversed only by delivery.

Hypertension in pregnancy can be classified into four disorders: preeclampsia/eclampsia, chronic hypertension, superimposed preeclampsia on chronic hypertension, and transient or late hypertension. However, in clinical practice two distinct entities are commonly encountered in pregnant women: chronic hypertension and gestational hypertension (this term has replaced "pregnancy-induced hypertension"). Hypertension is defined as a sustained blood pressure increase to levels of 140 mmHg systolic or 90 mmHg diastolic. Although results of earlier reports suggested that an increase in blood pressure of 30 mmHg systolic or 15 mmHg diastolic from second trimester values to third trimester values was also of diagnostic value, this concept is no longer considered valid.

Preeclampsia/eclampsia is a disorder unique to human pregnancy. This disease predominately affects first pregnancies and develops after 20 weeks of gestation. Preeclampsia is a syndrome defined by hypertension and the appearance of protein in the urine (proteinuria). Preeclampsia may also be associated with myriad other signs and symptoms, such as edema, visual disturbances, headache, and epigastric pain.

Eclampsia is defined as the presence of new-onset grand mal seizures in a woman with preeclampsia. It continues to be an important cause of maternal mortality. The optimal choice of anticonvulsant therapy for the patient with eclampsia has been the subject of ongoing debate for several decades. The most commonly used drugs for the treatment and prevention of eclampsia are magnesium sulfate, diazepam, and phenytoin. In June 1995 the results of the Collaborative Eclampsia Trial were reported. This prospective randomized study provided compelling evidence that magnesium sulfate was superior to either diazepam or phenytoin in the prevention of recurrent convulsions in eclamptic patients. There was also a significant reduction in the perinatal morbidity of patients receiving magnesium sulfate.

Within the obstetric community, parental magnesium sulfate is now considered the drug of choice for both the prevention and treatment of pregnancy-induced seizures. This is most commonly given as an intravenous loading bolus (4 gm over 20 minutes) followed by a continuous infusion (2–3 gm/hr) administered via a controlled infusion device. Infusion of magnesium sulfate should be discontinued and a serum magnesium level obtained in any patient with loss of deep tendon reflexes, respiratory rate of less than 12 per minute, and a decrease in urinary output to below 25 cc/hr. Magnesium sulfate can also be administered via the intramuscular route.

When symptomatic magnesium overdose is suspected (e.g., the presence of apnea, obtundation), it can be reversed by the intravenous administration of 1 gm (10 ml of 10%) calcium gluconate intravenously over 2 minutes.

Although magnesium is the preferred agent for the control of seizures in the setting of eclampsia, many EMS systems opt to use a benzodiazepine such as diazipam or lorazepam to control the acute seizure, especially if the patient is in status seizures. Most EMS systems will require consultation with the base station physician in this setting for the administration of either magnesium or a benzodiazapam.

Any patient with active generalized seizures must receive meticulous monitoring of the airway status and administration of supplemental oxygen. In addition, because of the advanced pregnancy and the potential that compression of the inferior vena cava will occur in the supine position leading to hypoperfusion, make all reasonable efforts to shift the gravid uterus to the left side of the abdomen, away from the vena cava. This can be accomplished by placing a rolled-up blanket under the right hip.

Magnesium sulfate, although an effective anticonvulsant agent, does not substantially affect blood pressure; therefore, if blood pressure control is necessary, additional agents are mandatory. Loss of autoregulation may predispose the preeclamptic/eclamptic patient to a cerebral accident. Although no large randomized clinical trials have compared treatment with placebo, antihypertensive therapy is generally recommended for a diastolic blood pressures that exceed 105–110 mmHg. Hydralazine and labetalol are the two agents most commonly used for this purpose. The usual treatment dose for labetalol is 20 mg intravenous bolus followed by 40 mg if not effective within 10 minutes; then, 80 mg every 10 minutes to a maximum total dose of 220 mg.

RETURN TO THE CASE

In our case of the primigravida woman in yoga class, preeclampsia should be immediately suspected. This pregnancy was her first and she was close to term. In addition, this woman presents with significant neurologic (headache and visual problems) and gastrointestinal (severe epigastric pain) complaints and her blood pressure is markedly elevated. Furthermore, she has nondependent edema. (Her initial blood pressure reading was falsely decreased because she had been off her feet for a prolonged period before the arrival of paramedics.)

In this case, the paramedics administer 5 mg of IV diazepam on their standing orders for seizure control, which stops the patient's seizure within 2 minutes. In consultation with the online physician at the hospital, a loading dose of 4 gm of magnesium sulfate is prepared by placing 4 gm in a 100 cc mini-bag and infusing over 15 minutes. This infusion is completed just as the ambulance arrives at the hospital. While the EMS unit is en route to the ER, the emergency medicine physician mobilizes the on-call attending obstetrician and neonatal team who respond to the ER and take over the care of the patient from the paramedic crew.

After a brief assessment in the ER, the patient is transferred to the labor and delivery floor and undergoes an emergency cesarean section. Her baby is admitted to the neonatal ICU for observation and discharged home on the fifth postoperative day. The mother continues to have problems with hypertension even after delivery, which require her to take oral antihypertensive medications for several weeks after discharge.

REFERENCES

American College of Obstetricians and Gynecologists. "Diagnosis and Management of Preeclampsia and Eclampsia." ACOG Practice Bulletin 33. Washington, DC: American College of Obstetricians and Gynecologists, 2002.

American College of Obstetricians and Gynecologists. "Hypertension in Pregnancy." ACOG Technical Bulletin 219. Washington, DC: American College of Obstetricians and Gynecologists, 1996.

Bledsoe, Bryan E., Robert S. Porter, and Richard A. Cherry. *Medical Emergencies:* Vol. 3 of *Paramedic Care: Principles & Practice.* Chapter 14, "Obstetrics." Upper Saddle River, NJ: Brady/Prentice Hall Health, Pearson Education, 2001.

Walker, J. J. "Preeclampsia." *Lancet* 356 (2000): 1260–1265.

47

Douglas M. Wolfberg, JD

REFUSAL OF CARE

CASE PRESENTATION

You and your partner, a paramedic and an EMT, respectively, are dispatched to the scene of a two-vehicle collision at an intersection adjacent to a shopping center. Upon arrival, you observe two vehicles pulled to the side of the road, with what appears to be minimal damage to each. Some of the occupants appear to be out of their cars and walking around the scene, exchanging insurance information. The scene appears to be secure and there are no obvious hazards, so you and your partner approach the various individuals who appear to have been involved in the accident.

You approach the person identified as the driver of vehicle 1, a 17-year-old female. She appears to be alert and oriented, though exhibiting some signs of emotional distress and states that she is worried about telling her mother, with whom she lives, that she has been in an accident with her mother's car. She mentions that she does not live with her father but sees him every other Saturday afternoon. Your partner approaches the patient identified as the driver of vehicle 2, a 29-year-old woman who has a 2-year-old child in the backseat of her minivan. You and your partner observe that the child appears to be properly secured in a child safety seat. The 29-year-old female appears alert, oriented, and calm.

Your assessment of the 17-year-old reveals a small contusion on the right side of her cheek and she reports slight pain in her chest. She states that she was not wearing a seat belt and that she was traveling at about 20 miles per hour at the time of the crash. She cannot recall whether her chest impacted the steering wheel because "things happened so quickly." Her pulse is 120, her respirations are 30, and her blood pressure is 140/90. Her pupils are equal and reactive. There is no evidence of external bleeding. The 17-year-old clearly tells you that she does not wish to go to the hospital. You ask for her mother's phone numbers at work and at home, and you are unable to reach her. You are, however, able to reach her father at work and explain the situation to him. He strongly indicates that he wants you to take his daughter to the hospital. She continues to refuse treatment and trans-

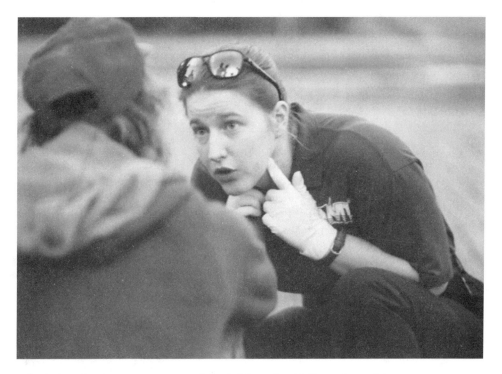

Refusal of care by patients can pose a significant liability risk to EMS providers and their agencies.

portation to the hospital, and tells you that her father is not the one who makes her decisions, and that her mother would agree with her not going to the hospital.

Your EMT partner's assessment of the 29-year-old reveals no complaints and no signs of trauma. She indicates that she was wearing a seat belt and that her minivan was struck on the front passenger side. She reports that she was not moving at the time of the crash, but estimates that vehicle 1 was traveling at about 10–15 miles per hour when it struck her minivan. Her pulse is 72, her respirations are 16, and her blood pressure is 120/70. Upon assessment her 2-year-old child, who has now been taken out of the car seat, is playing happily and giggling in his mother's arms and appears to have no signs of trauma. The 29-year-old indicates that neither she nor her 2-year-old son requires any medical attention and tells you that she will sign any form she has to so she can be on her way and get her groceries home and put her son down for a nap.

QUESTIONS

1. Can you legally accept the 17-year-old's refusal of care?
2. Can you legally treat and transport the 17-year-old on the permission of her father, who is divorced from her mother and not the primary custodial parent?

3. Can your partner, an EMT, accept the refusal of care for the 29-year-old patient, both for her and her 2-year-old child, or must you, as the paramedic, perform an assessment and obtain the woman's signature on your refusal form?

DISCUSSION

Refusal of EMS care and transportation by patients is an important medical–legal issue routinely confronted by EMS providers. Because refusals of care have the potential to give rise to litigation down the road, it is important that EMS providers understand the concepts of patient refusals and proper documentation of refusal cases to maximize their liability protection while ensuring that their patients receive appropriate care when necessary.

To begin, the general rule regarding refusals is that a competent person has the right to refuse medical treatment, even potentially life-saving emergency medical care. The treatment of a patient without consent may constitute an actionable tort under state law, such as battery or negligence.

Determining whether a patient is competent requires assessments of the person's legal capacity and mental capacities.

"Legal capacity" refers to whether the person has the legal right to make health care decisions. The most common issue in terms of legal capacity is whether or not a person is a minor. In most states, a minor is someone under the age of 18. Some states permit minors to make health care decisions under certain circumstances, but the general rule is that a person must be 18 to make their own health care and other legal decisions. Another example of someone who lacks the legal capacity to make a health care decision is someone who has been declared "incompetent" or "incapacitated" by a court of law.

"Mental capacity" refers to the person's ability to effectively receive and process information about their condition and proposed treatment and weigh the risks and benefits both of treatment and refusal in making a decision. Persons should be assumed to possess mental capacity unless your assessment, and documentation, clearly indicate otherwise. To determine mental capacity in the field, evaluate the person's ability to recall basic information, such as their name, the date or day of the week, their location, their address, the name of the current president of the United States, and so on. Determine if the person has any known conditions that might affect mentation, such as senile dementia, Alzheimer's, or other organic brain syndrome. Finally, when assessing a person's mental capacity, be sure to consider whether there are any other situational factors affecting their mental abilities. For instance, a hypovolemic or hypoxic person's mental capacity may temporarily be affected by his or her condition, and metabolic conditions like hypo- or hyperglycemia may also affect mentation.

A person should possess both legal and mental capacity to make a decision to accept or refuse medical care. If a person has both legal and mental capacity, the EMS personnel should take the time to explain the benefits of EMS treatment and transportation, the potential injuries or conditions that the patient might have, and the inherent limitations of EMS personnel to make definitive diagnoses in the field. If a patient has legal and mental capacity, and has been properly been informed of things like his or her possible condition and proposed treatment, the person may refuse EMS care and transportation.

Once a properly informed person who is both legally and mentally competent decides to refuse care, the EMS personnel should thoroughly document the person's refusal. Documentation of these encounters should include a description of the scene, the findings upon assessment, the specific words used by the person to refuse care, the steps you took to inform the person of the risks of and alternatives to refusal, and follow-up instructions you provided to the person in case of further problems. The legally and mentally competent person who is refusing care should be asked to sign a refusal of care form, which contains specific instructions and clear, detailed language protecting the EMS providers from liability arising out of the person's informed refusal.

EMS providers should also understand when persons other than the patient may legally refuse emergency care and transportation. If a person lacks legal capacity, for example, because of minority (under the age of 18 in most states), generally the person's parent or legal guardian may consent to or refuse care on the minor's behalf. Whether a parent has the legal right to consent or refuse care for their child varies under state law, but as a general rule, either parent may consent for care for their child, even if the parent is himself or herself a minor. Unless a parent's custodial rights have been completely severed, that parent may still provide consent or refusal for their child's care, even if he or she is not the primary custodial parent.

In most states, a person who has temporary legal custody of a minor child may also consent for or refuse care under certain circumstances. For instance, school administrators in most states may consent for care of a minor student under their charge at school or at an extracurricular school event, which is the legal concept of *in loco parentis*.

In some states, minors do have certain rights to consent to or refuse health care. For example, some states permit pregnant or married minors to consent to health care. In other states, minors may consent to care if they are a certain age (say, 14, for example) and no one else who may give legal consent is available to do so. Again, this varies from state to state and you should consult with your ambulance service's management or legal counsel for more specific information.

Other individuals may consent to or refuse care on behalf of an incapacitated person in certain situations. For instance, a person may execute a "durable power of attorney" or "health care power of attorney" (POA) document. The person who executes the POA is called the "principal," and the person to whom decision-making authority is given is called the "agent" or the "attorney-in-fact." The precise powers granted to the agent or attorney-in-fact will vary both by the language of the actual POA document and by state law, but as a general rule the agent or attorney-in-fact is empowered to make the principal's health care decisions. You should obtain a copy of the POA document whenever possible and include it with your patient care report and signed refusal form.

Other individuals may consent to or refuse care on behalf of a person in other situations depending upon state law. For instance, in some states an adult child may make medical decisions for a parent, or adult siblings or spouses may be able to legally make health care decisions on behalf of a patient.

Another principle to keep in mind is the concept of "implied consent." Under implied consent, as it exists in nearly every jurisdiction, a person who is (1) seriously ill or injured, and (2) unconscious or otherwise unable to speak for himself, may be treated and transported in an emergency situation without the express consent of the patient or of another legally authorized decision maker.

Assessments in a refusal case and the documentation of these incidents falls within the scope of practice of both EMTs and paramedics. However, some EMS systems have specific policies or protocols in place that require interaction with online medical command by a paramedic before an ALS provider can accept a patient's refusal or release a patient to BLS. Where paramedics and EMTs run together on a crew, the paramedic should conduct the assessment and complete the appropriate refusal documentation whenever possible.

RETURN TO THE CASE

The paramedic wisely refuses to accept the refusal of the 17-year-old patient, who is exhibiting some signs of possible trauma and who lacks the legal capacity to refuse care. Although the father is not the minor's custodial parent, the paramedic clearly explains the circumstances to the father by telephone, documents the father's identity and telephone number, as well as the specific consent for treatment and transportation given by the father. It would be reasonable for the paramedic to accept the consent of the father under these circumstances.

The EMT accepts the refusal of the 29-year-old mother both for her and for her 2-year-old son. The EMT completes a patient care report detailing the history of the incident, the physical presentation at the scene, and the assessment of the mother and son and obtains a signed refusal of care form from the mother specifically including her 2-year-old son. Upon retrospective review of the call with the ALS service medical director, the paramedic is counseled to review all assessments and refusals by his EMT partner and to sign off on the patient care report as having done so.

REFERENCES

Bledsoe, Bryan E., Robert S. Porter, and Richard A. Cherry. *Introduction to Advanced Prehospital Care*. Vol. 1 of *Paramedic Care: Principles & Practice*. Chapter 6, "Medical/Legal Aspects of Advanced Prehospital Care." Upper Saddle River, NJ: Brady/Prentice Hall Health, Pearson Education, 2000.

Lazar, R. A. *EMS Law: A Guide for EMS Professionals*. Rockville, MD: Aspen, 1989.

Page, Wolfberg & Wirth, LLC. "Practical Pointers for Patient Refusals." Retrieved October 25, 2000, from http://www.pwwemslaw.com.

Wolfberg, D. M. "Refusing Emergency Medical Care: How Far Do a Patient's Rights Go?" *Journal of Emergency Medical Services* (January 1995): 133–136.

Wolfberg, D. M. "Sign Here and We're Gone—Practical Tips for Handling Patient Refusals." *Journal of Emergency Medical Services* (March, 2000): 140–141.

Elizabeth M. Datner, MD
Iris Reyes, MD

48

SEXUAL ASSAULT

CASE PRESENTATION

You are called to the scene of a college dorm room at 4 A.M. for the complaint of a distraught college student. You arrive to find a tearful, withdrawn 18-year-old female sitting on the floor. She appears disheveled and tired. Obvious bruises are evident on her inner thighs, which you can see below her shorts. She is not wearing a shirt and a bite mark is apparent low on her chest above her bra. She does not make eye contact with you when you arrive or offer any explanation. Her roommate and resident supervisor are present. They state that she returned home about an hour previously and hasn't moved since or said what happened to her. She was seen earlier that night at a fraternity party where she was drinking and dancing.

After asking her friends to leave, you approach the student. You sit down on the floor and ask her what happened. She doesn't answer. You ask her if someone hurt her, and assure her that she is safe now and that you are there to help her. She begins to cry. You again ask if someone hurt her and she nods yes. You ask her to tell you what happened so that you can help her stay safe, also noting that she can take her time and tell you only what she wants to tell.

The student begins to talk slowly telling of how she was at a frat party, drinking, and the next thing she knew she was in a utility closet with a boy that she knew and he was ripping off her clothes. She states that she then blacked out and awoke as he was leaving the closet; her clothes were off and she was in pain. She vaguely remembers trying to resist his taking off her clothes, but notes that she was unable to fight. She frequently repeats "It was my fault, I shouldn't have been drinking." When asked, she denies anything other than superficial injuries and soreness in her genital area.

You offer to take her to the hospital. She says she will go to student health in the morning and that she doesn't want anyone to know what happened. She refuses to talk to the police.

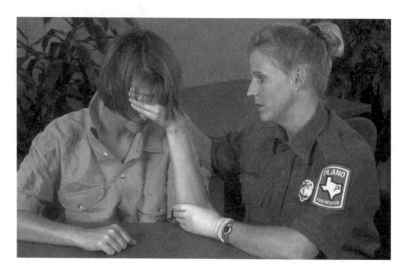

Prehospital providers must be sensitive to the wide range of demeanors exhibited by victims of sexual assault.

QUESTIONS

1. Because the student has no acute medical complaints, should you leave and advise her to go to student health the next day?
2. What is the role of the EMS provider with respect to the rape victim?
3. Because the patient doesn't really know what happened, what should you document?

DISCUSSION

The prevalence of sexual assault is tremendous. According to Linden, in the United States 1 in 6 women and 1 in 33 men will be the victim of a sexual assault during their lifetime. Despite this high prevalence, Feldhaus states that fewer than half of these assault victims report the crime to the police or seek medical care. Unless associated with significant physical trauma, victims of sexual assault rarely seek help within 72 hours. This makes identification, treatment, and conviction of the assailant more difficult. Reporting of rape cases is often hindered by inappropriate myths, misplaced shame, and social stigmas that unfortunately incriminate the victim rather than the perpetrator. Prehospital personnel must be particularly aware of their approach to the patient so that they do not imply blame on the part of the victim. A sexual assault is *never* the fault of the victim regardless of the victim's background, race, or lifestyle. Responsibility for the rape lies completely with the assailant.

The role of the prehospital care provider in the case of sexual assault is to provide safety, security, and support to the victim in addition to providing medical services. A secondary but extremely important role is to identify and preserve forensic evidence. The provider must approach the patient in a nonjudgmental way with sensitivity to the victim's feelings of lack of control. Asking permission before touching the patient and allowing the victim to determine the pace of the interview and the surroundings in which it takes place allows the victim to regain a sense of control over his or her environment. The provider must gather information required to appropriately care for the victim and collect evidence, but should refrain from asking more detail than is necessary to care for the medical injuries so that later confusion or contradictory statements do not result. Only injuries that need immediate intervention should be treated. Pressure should be applied to bleeding wounds with a clean, dry gauze pad. Wounds should not be cleaned because they will be sampled for forensic evidence during the rape exam. All clothing or personal belongings that were involved in the assault should be taken with the victim. They should be placed in clean, dry paper bags to protect evidence. Victims should be encouraged to remain in the clothing in which the attack occurred and refrain from washing, urinating, defecating, douching, brushing their teeth, or otherwise cleaning or grooming. Evidence rapidly deteriorates (within 24–72 hours) and should be collected as soon as possible. Victims should be encouraged to be evaluated as soon after the incident as possible so those samples can be collected. Evidence collection does *not* obligate victims to pursue the case either legally or criminally, but allows them to keep their options open in the future if they decide to pursue the case. If possible and if acceptable to the victim, he or she should remain at the current location until police arrive to initiate an investigation.

Documentation is extremely important in caring for rape victims. The record of the EMS provider is evidence. It should reflect the facts that were observed rather than conclusions drawn or judgment or belief of the occurrence of the event. Statements that are not supported by facts should be avoided. For instance, documenting that the victim was sitting on the floor, crying, wearing no shirt and with bruises on her legs is appropriate. Describing the victim as "hysterical" or "out of control" or wearing "skimpy" or "seductive" clothing is not appropriate.

Rape victims can display a variety of demeanors. Reactions differ from person to person and emotional, behavioral, and analytical responses may vary dramatically between victims. The circumstances of the event and the psychological situation of the victim add to the diverse range of reactions. Reactions will vary depending on whether perpetrators were strangers, acquaintances, spouses, family members, same gender, opposite gender, or if multiple perpetrators are involved. The extent of physical injury and level of violence will also affect the reaction of the victim.

Victims may appear calm and controlled or may display intense expressions of emotion. According to Burgess and Holstrum, the Rape Trauma Syndrome (RTS) describes victims' general reactions to sexual assault. Initially, the victim experiences the acute phase of RTS, a period marked by disorganization and a broad range of emotions. The initial reactions can vary from strongly expressive reactions such as tenseness, crying, restlessness, and even smiling to a more controlled reaction with subdued affect, calmness, and composure. These reactions are often related to the fear, anxiety, humiliation, self-blame, shame, and anger experienced by victims. Immediate behavioral responses may display disturbances in concentration, ability to form cohesive sentences, and focus on questions and statements.

Weeks to months after the event the long-term reorganization process begins. Kirkpatrick and colleagues state that victims may experience feelings of depression, restlessness, and exhaustion, similar to those who have experienced posttraumatic stress disorder (PTSD). Symptoms can include nightmares, flashbacks, disturbed eating and sleeping patterns, sexual dysfunction, and difficulty in social adjustments. Over time, the process of reorganizing victims' understanding of the world pre- and posttrauma and potentially finding some degree of resolution and integration of the event into their life may occur.

RETURN TO THE CASE

You convince the student to go with you to the hospital. You inform her that you will be taking her to the local hospital that has the rape crisis center rather than the closest emergency department because they have specialized care. You also inform her that you will stay with her until she is comfortably situated, that she will be safe with you, and that everything she tells you or the rape crisis team is confidential. She does not have to decide anything about pursuing the case from a legal standpoint immediately. She will have a full examination and treatment for her injuries.

The student requests to take a shower before you go. You inform her that she should not shower, go to the bathroom, or brush her teeth to preserve possible evidence. You ask her to bring her shirt if she has it and place it in a clean paper bag. You ask her to keep her clothes on as they are (with a clean shirt), and tell her to bring a change of clothes with her because her clothes will be kept for evidence. You offer to bring someone with her for support and she requests that her roommate accompany her.

You transport the student to the hospital that is the rape crisis center in your area. You have the patient give her shirt in the bag to the health care team that will evaluate her. Prior to leaving the patient you give her a resource card you carry that has rape crisis center information on it as well as hotline numbers in case she decides against evaluation. You wish the patient good luck, carefully complete your prehospital care report, and return to your base station.

Three days later you read in the paper that an arrest was made on campus for the rape. Six months later you receive a letter from the district attorney requesting your presence at the trial of the student to testify to your findings that morning. She notes that she has obtained your report and you should review it prior to testifying.

REFERENCES

Bledsoe, Bryan E., Robert S. Porter, and Richard A. Cherry. *Special Considerations/Operations*. Vol. 5 of *Paramedic Care: Principles & Practice*. Chapter 4, "Abuse and Assault." Upper Saddle River, NJ: Brady/Prentice Hall Health, Pearson Education, 2001.

Burgess, A., and L. Holstrum. "Rape Trauma Syndrome." *American Journal of Psychiatry* 131 (1974): 981–986.

Feldhaus, K. M., D. Houry, and R. Kaminsky. "Lifetime Sexual Assault Prevalence Rates and Reporting Practices in an Emergency Department Population." *Annals of Emergency Medicine* 36, no. 1 (July 2000): 23–27.

Kilpatrick, D. G., C. N. Edmunds, and A. K. Seymour. *Rape in America: A Report to the Nation*. Charleston: National Victim Center and Crime Victims Research and Treatment Center, Medical University of South Carolina, April 1992.

Linden, J. A. "Sexual Assault." *Emergency Medicine Clinics of North America* 17, no. 3 (August 1999): 685–697.

Iris Reyes, MD

49

VAGINAL BLEEDING

CASE PRESENTATION

You are called to the home of an 18-year-old female whose boyfriend answers the door. You are taken to her bedroom where you find a young woman who appears apprehensive, weak, pale, and slightly diaphoretic. She is alert and appropriately responsive. She states that she has had a heavy period with vaginal bleeding for 2 days. You ask her how many sanitary pads or tampons she has used per hour. Her boyfriend laughs and says that he has gone to the store twice today to buy more pads.

She reports a mild crampy pain in her lower belly for the past 2 days and has passed large clots today. You ask her if she is pregnant. She replies that she does not think so and that she has recently started taking birth control pills. The boyfriend states that she always has heavy periods, but has never bled like this.

Before leaving for the hospital, she insists on checking on her child who is asleep in the next room. Upon standing, she complains of feeling very dizzy and then faints onto her bed. She awakens almost immediately but now reports worsened belly pain.

Your partner checks her vital signs while you go out to get the litter. He obtains the following results: blood pressure 80/45, heart rate 126, and respiratory rate 16. Her skin is pale and clammy. There are no visible bruises and no bleeding gums. Her abdomen is soft and nondistended, but she has lower abdominal tenderness.

You immediately place her in a supine position and remove her blouse to place a large-bore intravenous catheter in her right arm. She sees the IV and pulls away saying that she is afraid of needles and refuses to allow you to stick her. She states that she will go to the hospital, but not with an IV.

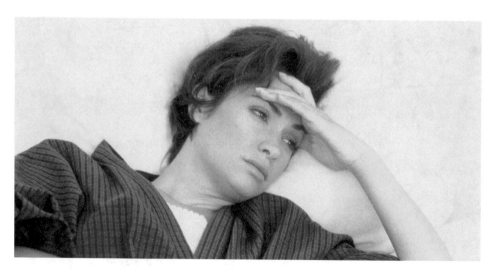

Ectopic pregnancy must be considered in all women of child-bearing age who present with vaginal bleeding and/or abdominal pain.
Courtesy of James Darell and Getty Images, Inc.–Stone Allstock.

QUESTIONS

1. Should you allow the patient to be transported to the hospital without IV access?
2. What other questions should you ask the patient that might help you determine the cause of bleeding?

DISCUSSION

Two key points to remember when assessing a patient complaining of vaginal bleeding is that all women of childbearing age are presumed to be pregnant until proven otherwise. Also, pregnancy cannot be ruled out even if the patient reports normal menses, regular contraceptive use, history of tubal ligation, or no recent sexual intercourse.

Initial management at the scene of an unstable patient requires following the ABCs of resuscitation. The establishment of two large-bore IVs and fluid resuscitation with 1–2 L of normal saline is essential in the hypotensive patient. Supplemental oxygen and cardiac monitoring should be instituted in the management of the unstable patient.

The initial evaluation should also include a focused assessment of the patient's reproductive history. This should specifically address menstrual regularity, last normal menstrual period, history of ectopic pregnancies or miscarriages, history of past treatment for venereal diseases, recent termination of pregnancy, and contraceptive use. Questions about the patient's medical history include the presence of diabetes, hypertension, and thyroid illness, bleeding disorders, and liver disease. Medication usage, particularly anticoagulant, aspirin, antibiotic, and anticonvulsant use, can also be medically relevant.

The amount of bleeding can be misleading when assessing patients with this complaint. Without a pelvic exam, it is impossible to know if the bleeding is from the vagina, cervix, uterus, or placenta. Life-threatening conditions, such as ruptured ectopic pregnancies, may produce only scant vaginal bleeding, if any. Determining the number of pads used per day can assess the volume of blood lost. A soaked pad is suggestive of approximately 20 to 30 ml of blood loss.

Although the most common cause of vaginal bleeding is menstruation, atypical bleeding should be investigated. The abnormal causes can be divided into the following categories: hormonal, infectious, organic, traumatic, and pregnancy related. In postmenopausal women, neoplastic or medical causes are more likely. Women of childbearing age should have pregnancy and its related complications considered as a possible cause of bleeding or pelvic pain. Trauma to the pelvic region is more likely to be the cause of bleeding in the younger patient, but can occur at any age.

Ectopic pregnancy, or pregnancy implanted outside the uterus, is increasingly common. It is the second leading cause of maternal death. The incidence of ectopic pregnancy has quadrupled over the past 20 years. Risk factors associated with this condition include prior ectopic pregnancy, history of pelvic inflammatory disease, history of infertility (no prior pregnancies despite 3 years of unprotected sex), prior tubal ligation, intrauterine device use for contraception, in vitro fertilization, and elective abortion within the past 1–2 weeks. It has also been reported that patients who have undergone a recent elective abortion may in fact be carrying an ectopic pregnancy that has progressed to rupture. The clinical presentation of patients with ectopic pregnancy can be variable. Patients most commonly develop pelvic pain following a missed period. Vaginal bleeding may not even be a presenting complaint. They may have normal vital signs and physical exam findings until they actually rupture. A pelvic ultrasound can be diagnostic when considering an ectopic pregnancy. Delay in diagnosis can lead to rupture of the fallopian tube, hemorrhage, and death.

Retained products of conception after an incomplete elective abortion can serve as a nidus for infection. These patients present with continued bleeding, fevers, pelvic pain, malaise, and nausea. If left untreated, severe complications and even death can result.

Spontaneous or threatened abortions also present with pelvic pain and vaginal bleeding in early pregnancy. It is estimated that 15%–20% of all known pregnancies end in miscarriage. Most spontaneous abortions or miscarriages occur at approximately 8 or 9 weeks of gestation. Some patients may be unaware that they are pregnant at the time of presentation. These patients typically develop mild spotting that progresses to heavy bleeding and the passage of clots and fetal tissue.

Vaginal bleeding in the late second or third trimester pregnancy can be due to placenta previa or placental abruption. Placenta previa occurs in approximately 1 in 250 births. It involves the implantation of the placenta over the cervical os (mouth). Bleeding is usually painless but can be associated with uterine irritability.

Placental abruption occurs when a normally implanted placenta separates from the uterus lining. Blood accumulates in the space created and the portion of the placenta involved may be unable to transport necessary nutrients and oxygen to the fetus. This condition has an incidence of between 1 in 86 to 1 in 200 live births. Trauma accounts for approximately 2% of all abruptions. Patients with abruption will typically present with vaginal bleeding associated with abdominal pain. The pain can mimic the contractions of early labor but can also be severe, sharp and acute. The amount of blood lost vaginally is not indicative of the amount concealed in the uterus. Abruptions can be mild to severe and require prompt evaluation in labor and delivery units.

Vaginal bleeding is a common presenting complaint for emergency medical services. In some patients, however, life-threatening conditions exist and appropriate early intervention can significantly reduce morbidity and mortality.

RETURN TO THE CASE

With the help of her boyfriend, you convince the patient of the gravity of the situation. She allows you to put in only one IV. After drawing a full set of blood tubes (to later be used for a CBC and a type and cross), you begin to infuse 1 L of normal saline wide open and transfer her to the ambulance. You advise the boyfriend to proceed to the hospital in his car.

Once alone with you, the patient volunteers that she had an abortion 2 days ago and that she did not want her boyfriend to know. She states that he would have made her keep the baby. She asks that you not tell him about the abortion. You inform her that you will maintain her confidentiality but ask if you can relay the information to the physicians at the hospital. She agrees to this, but only if they also promise to maintain her confidentiality. You reassure the patient and proceed to the hospital. En route to the ED you advise the base station physician of the inbound hypotensive and tachycardic patient with vaginal bleeding.

Upon arrival at the emergency room, you provide a report to the accepting physician and specifically address the patient's request of confidentiality regarding her recent abortion.

Evaluation in the emergency department includes the prompt placement of a second large-bore IV and the request of uncrossmatched blood from the blood bank. A pelvic examination reveals large clots in the vaginal vault and a closed cervical os. The patient has significant tenderness to palpation of the left adnexa. She undergoes an emergent pelvic ultrasound that reveals a ruptured left ectopic pregnancy. The gynecology consultant is en route from the labor floor and directs immediate transfer of the patient to the OR. She is successfully treated and survives, despite significant blood loss.

REFERENCES

Bledsoe, Bryan E., Robert S. Porter, and Richard A. Cherry. *Medical Emergencies*. Vol. 3 of *Paramedic Care: Principles & Practice*. Chapter 13, "Gynecology." Upper Saddle River, NJ: Brady/Prentice Hall Health, Pearson Education, 2001.

Eisinger, H. E. "Early Pregnancy Bleeding: A Rational Approach." *Clinical Family Practice* 3, no. 2 (June 2001): 225–249.

Ettner, F. M. "The Obstetrical Care of Young Women." *Clinical Family Practice* 2, no. 4 (December 2000): 1017–1035.

Owen Traynor, MD

50

VIOLENT PSYCHIATRIC PATIENT

CASE PRESENTATION

You are dispatched to a reported behavioral emergency. The scene is secured by the local police department prior to your arrival. You arrive on scene and are met in front of the residence by the patient's mother. She states that her 25-year-old son has been acting strangely for the past 2 or 3 weeks. "He can't stay here with me anymore—I can't live like this," she says.

Before you enter the residence you ask the patient's mother to describe her son's behavior. She tells you that he has become anxious and agitated. He has not been sleeping very much in the past week. He angers easily and is "out of control," at times.

Tonight the patient's behavior frightens her. She reports that he threatened to kill her if she nagged him again.

The mother states that he is in his room at the rear of the house. You ask about past medical and psychiatric history, medications, allergies, and substance abuse history. She tells you that he does have a history of asthma and uses an albuterol metered dose inhaler. He has no history of mental illness and she knows of no drug allergies. She believes that he drinks too much alcohol, although she is not aware of any other substance use. She tells you that she has been asking him to get some help for the past 2 weeks, but he has refused.

QUESTIONS

1. How does the paramedic assess a patient's risk of violence?
2. What steps can be taken to facilitate a safe patient encounter?
3. How can a paramedic identify medical causes of behavioral emergencies?

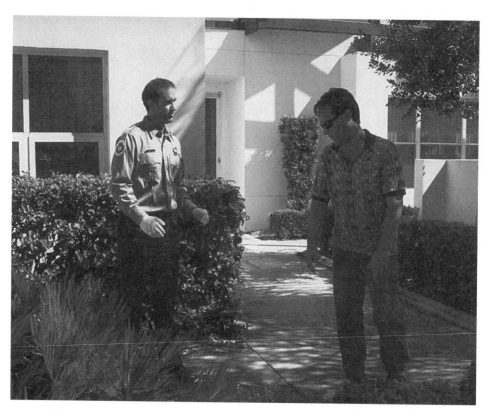

Assuring the personal safety of the EMS provider is the first step in approaching a behavioral emergency.

DISCUSSION

EMS providers frequently respond to behavioral emergencies. Like other EMS calls, there is a risk that the patient may be suffering from a serious illness that may be life threatening. An important feature of behavioral emergencies is that the EMS crew and other bystanders may be at risk of injury or death, as well. A key consideration, then, is not only an ongoing assessment of the patient's safety and risk of violent behavior but also an ongoing assessment of crew safety.

Safety assessment begins with the review of dispatch data. The caller may identify potential violent behavior as the reason to call 911. EMD dispatch protocols typically send police assistance when violent behavior has been reported. It is generally prudent for EMS units to await arrival of police units before approaching the scene. In many jurisdictions, EMS units are instructed to stage a safe distance from the scene and await notification from law enforcement prior to proceeding into the scene.

The scene survey provides additional safety information. The 911 caller and other bystanders may be available to answer questions about the patient. The nature of the patient's behavior, presence of weapons, possible hostages, and the location of the patient should be obtained. If possible, find out about entrances and exits to the patient's location. If there are no indications that the scene is unsafe, or if the scene has been secured by law enforcement personnel, then paramedics may proceed to meet the patient.

TABLE 50-1

CHARACTERISTICS AND PREDICTORS OF VIOLENT BEHAVIOR

History	Childhood abuse or neglect
	History of prior suicide attempts or self-mutilation
	Prior violence or family violence
Age/gender	13–25-year-old males
Psychiatric factors	Active symptoms of psychiatric disorders (command hallucinations, paranoid delusions, psychotic disorganized thought, excitability)
	Combination of serious mental illness and substance abuse
	Personality disorders
	Substance abuse-related disorders—intoxication or withdrawal
	Note: Chronic alcoholism is more predictive of violence than acute intoxication. The higher the number of comorbid psychiatric disorders, the greater potential for violence.
Emotional factors	"Acting out" behavior
	Angry or rageful effect
	Emotional lability
	Irritability or impulsivity
	Poor frustration tolerance
Social factors	Limited or poor social supports
	Low socioeconomic status
	Medication noncompliance
Neurobiological factors	Delirium
	HIV/AIDS
	Mental retardation
	Neurologic diseases
	Seizures
	Structural brain abnormalities
	Traumatic brain injury

It can be difficult to predict violent behavior. Although there have been many characteristics identified (Table 50-1), the best predictors of violent behavior are the patient's current state and a prior history of violent behavior.

The first goal of this patient encounter is to reduce the risk of injury to all involved. This will require a well-thought-out approach. Risk reduction will be most effective if we are able to promptly recognize the potential for violent behavior and act in a preemptive fashion to defuse the situation.

It may be helpful to think of violent behavior as a continuum of behavior ranging from mild agitation or anger to outright physical violence. Thus, interventions may be employed that correspond to the patient's current behavior along the continuum.

Consider first a patient whose behavior leads you to think there may be potential for escalation to violence. You may choose to manipulate the environment to help the patient remain calm. Move to quiet surroundings with ready access to an exit. Never allow the potentially violent patient to position himself between you and your exit. Ensure that you have adequate assistance available including police personnel. Make sure there are no weapons available. Your interview techniques should be direct and empathetic. Assure the patient of his safety. At times you may have to set limits on what behavior is acceptable. Respect the patient's personal space. Avoid assuming a confrontational posture. At this point you may be able to complete your patient assessment.

Should the patient's behavior reveal increased agitation or loss of control you may wish to offer the option of medications to help the patient remain calm and in control. Medications such as haloperidol, or benzodiazepines such as diazepam or lorazepam, may be helpful.

Once the behavior deteriorates sufficiently to indicate that the patient lacks capacity for rational decisions, chemical and physical restraints may be necessary. The medications above may be given via intramuscular or intravenous routes. Once the decision for physical restraints has been made, negotiations with the patient cease. Adequate assistance must be available to safely restrain the patient. Restraints should be applied only by those who are trained and skilled in their safe use. At all times, the least restrictive and most effective means of control should be employed.

Carefully monitor all patients who are physically or chemically restrained. There have been cases in which restrained patients have died. Never hog-tie or restrain a patient in a prone position. The lateral recumbent position, or the supine position with the head elevated, are generally the safest positions. In general, once physical restraints are applied, they should rarely be removed in the prehospital setting.

Many of the patients with behavioral emergencies seen by EMS providers will have a medical diagnosis (Table 50-2) as the cause of their abnormal behavior.

It may be difficult for EMS providers to distinguish between medical and psychiatric causes of the abnormal behavior. The history of the present illness is usually the best assessment tool. However, the patient may not be the best source of this information; ask family members and bystanders. Medical illness usually develops quickly, over hours to days, whereas psychiatric illness may develop over days to weeks. The psychiatric patient is likely to have had abnormal behavior in the past. Noncompliance with psychiatric medications can be associated with a behavior change.

Perform a thorough physical examination, looking for physical findings that suggest a medical or traumatic etiology. Some prehospital diagnoses associated with abnormal behavior include

- Head trauma
- Stroke
- Hypoxia
- Myocardial infarction
- Diabetic emergencies
- Sepsis
- Shock
- Dehydration

TABLE 50-2

SOME MEDICAL DISORDERS THAT MAY BE ASSOCIATED WITH BEHAVIORAL EMERGENCIES

Endocrine disorders	Hypo- or hyperthyroidism
	Hypo- or hyperglycemia
	Hypo- or hypercalcemia
	Steroid-induced psychosis
Infectious diseases	AIDS
	Subacute bacterial endocarditis
	Encephalitis
	Urinary tract infections
	Pneumonia
Substance abuse-related problems	Intoxication
	Withdrawal
Other organ systems disorders	Chronic obstructive pulmonary disease (COPD)
	Acute liver disease
	Chronic renal disease
	Myocardial infarction
	Pulmonary embolism
	Intracranial hemorrhage
	Malignant hypertension
	Electrolyte abnormalities
	Metastatic cancer or intracranial tumor

Although psychiatric patients may have abnormal vital signs, a medical cause should be sought when they are present. Diagnostic testing, such as pulse oximetry, blood glucose determination, and cardiac monitoring, should be performed as needed to exclude hypoxia, hypo- or hyperglycemia, and cardiac ischemia.

Specific therapy can be implemented when a medical diagnosis is discovered.

RETURN TO THE CASE

Two police officers arrive while you are completing your discussion with the patient's mother. You decide to enter the home with the police officers and meet a 25-year-old male who appears mildly anxious. He is willing to be evaluated by you and your partner. He indicates no intention to harm you or the others present to help him.

The patient visibly relaxes as you demonstrate calm, compassionate care. He admits that he has been drinking a lot lately and that he has been having trouble controlling his anger. The physical examination discovers no acute abnormality. The patient is not hypoxic and his blood glucose is within normal limits.

The police ensure that the patient has no weapons. The patient agrees that getting some help now is a good idea. You transport him to the local emergency department without further incident. One year later, the patient is continuing outpatient counseling for anger management. He has been alcohol free for 8 months.

REFERENCES

Bledsoe, Bryan E., Robert S. Porter, and Richard A. Cherry. *Medical Emergencies*. Vol. 3 of *Paramedic Care: Principles & Practice*. Chapter 12, "Psychiatric and Behavioral Disorders." Upper Saddle River, NJ: Brady/Prentice Hall Health, Pearson Education, 2001.

Citrome, L., and J. Volavka. "Violent Patients in the Emergency Setting." *Psychiatric Clinics of North America* 22, no. 4 (1999): 789–801.

Hill, S., and J. Petit. "The Violent Patient." *Emergency Medicine Clinics of North America* 18, no. 2 (2000): 301–315.

51

Jonathan L. Burstein, MD

WEAPONS OF MASS DESTRUCTION

CASE PRESENTATION: CHEMICAL

It is a warm and breezy fall evening. You are finishing your dinner break when you and your partner get a radio call to respond to the local high school playing field for a person with seizures. As you get moving, the dispatcher calls you again to say that multiple calls are coming in, and "it sounds like something bad is going on."

On arrival at the gate to the field, you see a mob of several hundred people running toward you. In the grandstand are at least 10 or 15 people lying still or twitching occasionally. Your partner jumps out of the unit and runs up to the stands. Suddenly you see him jerk back, fall to the ground, and seize. A police officer pulling up with you runs forward to grab him, and she collapses as well.

You radio to dispatch that you have a possible hazmat event with multiple casualties and need help.

QUESTIONS

1. How could you safely enter the scene to rescue your partner and the other victims?
2. Based on what you have seen so far, what are likely the most useful treatments for this exposure?

DISCUSSION

This is the classic presentation of a nerve agent exposure, such as the sarin event in Tokyo in 1996. Nerve agents are organophosphates, and typically cause salivation, lacrimation, urination, defecation, and gastric emptying (SLUDGE syndrome), papillary constriction, bronchoconstriction and wheezing, seizures, muscle weakness, apnea, and death.

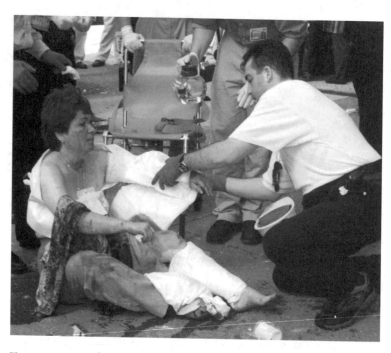

Treating injuries at the scene of a terrorist bombing.

When entering a scene that is likely dangerous (multiple victims down, possible hazmat), your first priority is always self-protection. If you become a casualty, you are helping no one. Most EMS care, including IVs and intubation, has been shown to be feasible in level B hazmat gear (chemically resistant suit, self-contained breathing apparatus) and that is the minimum level needed for entering a potentially contaminated area. For entering the "hot zone" of greatest contamination, level A is required (fully encapsulating suit, self-contained breathing apparatus).

Nerve agent symptoms are caused by blockade of the enzyme acetylcholinesterase. This causes acetylcholine, a neurotransmitter, to build up to dangerous levels in both "nicotinic" receptors in voluntary muscle tissue (causing muscle weakness), and "muscarinic" receptors in the autonomic nervous system (causing the other symptoms). Atropine, in doses of 2–6 mg IM or IV in adults, will reverse the autonomic effects; pralidoxime, in doses of 1 to 3 gm IM or IV, will reverse the voluntary muscle weakness. Seizures, if prolonged, can be treated with benzodiazepines such as lorazepam or diazepam. These drugs are available in standard dosage forms (bottles, syringes) and are also available in autoinjectors for use by non-ALS-trained personnel.

RETURN TO THE CASE

The hazmat team and numerous other units quickly arrive. Meanwhile, you had suited up in level B gear and, with an armful of autoinjectors, had started treating all the victims you could reach. You knew better than to walk into the plume of vapor you saw issuing from what looked like an ordinary Styrofoam cooler in the stands.

With the rapid atropine and pralidoxime treatment you and the other rescuers provide, 8 of the 17 people down survive. Your partner is one of them.

At the two nearest hospitals, numerous slightly contaminated patients get into the ED without decontamination. At one of these hospitals, one nurse and one aide become ill due to off-gassing of sarin vapor from the patients. No one dies, however, and both hospitals make plans to be better prepared next time.

REFERENCES

Brennan, R. J., J. F. Waeckerle, T. W. Sharp, and S. R. Lillibridge. "Chemical Warfare Agents: Emergency Medical and Emergency Public Health Issues." *Annals of Emergency Medicine* 34 (August 1999): 191–204.

Macintyre, A. G., G. W. Christopher, E. Eitzen Jr., R. Gum, S. Weir, C. DeAtley, K. Tonat, and J. A. Barbera. "Weapons of Mass Destruction Events with Contaminated Casualties: Effective Planning for Health Care Facilities." *Journal of the American Medical Association* 283 (January 2000): 242–249.

Office of the Surgeon General, Department of the Army. *Medical Aspects of Chemical and Biological Warfare.* Part I, Vol. 5 of *Textbook of Military Medicine.* Washington, DC: TMM Publications, 1997.

CASE PRESENTATION: BIOLOGICAL

It's been a busy few days. Your last two shifts seem to have been an endless litany of "I feel like crap." "I'm coughing like crazy." "Can't shake this fever." "I hate the flu!" Now you have just been called for another one—a young man coughing up blood at his office.

When you arrive, the patient is in the downstairs lobby and looks terrible. He's maintaining his airway, but has a respiratory rate of 36, and you soon discover his blood pressure is 70/palp. He's holding a handkerchief coated in bloody mucus.

QUESTIONS

1. You are beginning to suspect that something unusual is going on. With whom might you discuss your concerns?
2. What information might help to sort out what is happening in town?
3. What risks might this patient pose to your health? How can you protect yourself?

DISCUSSION

This is one way in which a bioterrorism attack, or a natural epidemic, may present. In general, the most concerning situation would be airborne spread of either a particularly lethal agent (such as anthrax) or a contagious agent (such as smallpox or plague). The most likely major natural event would be an outbreak of pandemic influenza.

Response to such an event would generally be coordinated by the local public health agency with state and federal support. Most patients would in fact *not* likely use EMS, and would probably present directly to EDs or physician offices and clinics. Every locality therefore needs to have some sort of surveillance system to detect such outbreaks early; EMS runs will often be included in the data such a system collects. In the event an area does not have an active public health agency, hospital resources such as infection control officers may play a similar role.

Most bioterrorism agents are not truly contagious; rather, they are infectious, requiring blood or body fluid contact. Thus, standard precautions would be sufficient to protect yourself. For smallpox or pneumonic plague, a high-efficiency particulate air (HEPA) filter mask, appropriately fitted, is needed. In addition, for smallpox, all mucous membranes need to be covered. In essence, TB precautions are enough for plague, whereas smallpox requires more extensive protective gear.

In general, bacterial bioterrorism agents will be treatable with antibiotics. Viral agents will usually be prevented by vaccination. It is possible that EMS personnel will be pressed into service to distribute antibiotics or give vaccinations in the event of a large-scale outbreak. Local protocols may have to be altered to allow these types of specialized medical interventions.

RETURN TO THE CASE

You quickly put a nonrebreather on the patient with 100% oxygen, and cover the filter port with a HEPA mask. Unfortunately you are worried that you have been exposed anyway, and you're not surprised when your supervisor calls you back to the station and hands you a packet of antibiotic pills to start taking. You find out later that the patient had to be intubated in a few hours and expired shortly thereafter of what appears to be pneumonic plague.

By a week later, several thousand people have gotten sick, and several hundred have died. Local hospitals are overwhelmed, and the federal government has brought in several disaster medical assistance teams and supplies from the national pharmaceutical stockpile to provide medical care. You've been working 12 hours on, 12 hours off for 9 days, and are glad to finally get a full 24 hours off to sleep. Because you got antibiotics early, both you and your partner do fine.

REFERENCES

DeLorenzo, Robert A., and Robert S. Porter. *Weapons of Mass Destruction Emergency Care.* Upper Saddle River, NJ: Brady/Prentice Hall Health, Pearson Education, 2000.

Franz, D. R., P. B. Jahrling, A. M. Friedlander, D. J. McClain, D. L. Hoover, W. R. Byrne, J. A. Pavlin, G. W. Christopher, and E. M. Eitzen Jr. "Clinical Recognition and Management of Patients Exposed to Biological Warfare Agents." *Journal of the American Medical Association* 278 (August 1997): 399–411.

Office of the Surgeon General, Department of the Army. *Medical Aspects of Chemical and Biological Warfare.* Part I, Vol. 5 of *Textbook of Military Medicine.* Washington, DC: TMM Publications, 1997.

Richards, C. F., J. L. Burstein, J. F. Waeckerle, and H. R. Hutson. "Emergency Physicians and Biological Terrorism." *Annals of Emergency Medicine* 34 (August 1999): 183–190.

LIST OF ABBREVIATIONS

ABBREVIATION	MEANING
2-PAM	pralidoxime
AAA	abdominal aortic aneurysm
AAMS	Association of Air Medical Services
ABCDE	airway—breathing—circulation—disability—exposure or environment
ABCs	airway—breathing—circulation
AC	antecubital
ACE Inhibitors	angiotensive converting enzyme inhibitors
ACLS	Advanced Cardiac Life Support
ACS	acute coronary syndrome
AD	advanced directive
AED	automatic external defibrillator
AF	atrial fibrillation
AIDS	Acquired Immunodeficiency Syndrome
ALS	advanced life support
ALT	alanine aminotransferase
AMI	acute myocardial infarction
AV	arteriovenous; *also* atrioventricular
AVB	atrioventricular block
AVM	atriovenous malformation
AVPU	Alert—Verbal—Painful—Unresponsive
Bi-PAP	bi-level positive airway pressure
BLS	basic life support
BP	blood pressure
BPM	beats per minute; *also* breaths per minute
BSA	body surface area
BSI	body substance isolation
BVM	bag valve mask
CA	cyclic antidepressant
CABG	coronary artery bypass graft
CBC	complete blood count
cc	cubic centimeters
cc/hr	cubic centimeters per hour
cc/kg	cubic centimeters/kilogram
cc/kg/hr	cubic centimeters per kilogram per hour
CCU	Coronary Care Unit
CDC	Centers for Disease Control and Prevention

ABBREVIATION	MEANING
CHEMTREC	Chemical Transportation Emergency Care
CHF	congestive heart failure
cm	centimeter
CO_2	carbon dioxide
COPD	chronic obstructive pulmonary disease
CPAP	continuous positive airway pressure
CPR	cardiopulmonary resuscitation
CT Scan	computerized tomography
CUPS	Critical—Unstable—Potential Unstable—Stable
CVA	cerebral vascular accident
CXR	chest x-ray
°C	degrees Celsius
°F	degrees Fahrenheit
D_5W	5% Dextrose in water
DKA	diabetic ketoacidosis
DNR	Do Not Resuscitate
DV	domestic violence
ECG	electrocardiogram
ED	emergency department
ELM	external laryngeal manipulation
EMD	Emergency Medical Dispatch
ER	emergency room
ESRD	end-stage renal disease
ET or ETT	endotracheal tube
ETA	estimated time of arrival
FIO_2	fractional concentration of inspired oxygen
GCS	Glasgow Coma Scale
gm	grams
gm/hr	gram per hour
GSW	gunshot wound
HAZMAT	hazardous material
HBIG	Hepatitis B immunoglobulin
HCTZ	hydrochlorothiazide
HD	hemodialysis
HEPA	high efficiency particulate air
HIV	Human Immunodeficiency Virus
HR	heart rate
IC	incident commander
ICP	intracranial pressure
ICU	Intensive Care Unit
IM	intramuscular
IV	intravenous
J	joules
JVD	jugular vein distention

ABBREVIATION	MEANING
kg	kilogram
km	kilometer
KVO	keep vein open
L	liter
L/hr	liters per hour
L/min	liters per minute
LPM	liters per minute
LZ	landing zone
MAST	medical antishock trousers
mcg	micrograms
MCP	Medical Command Physician
mcg/kg/min	micrograms per kilogram per minute
MDI	metered dose inhaler
MDMS	Material Safety Data Sheets
mEq/L	milliequivalent per liter
mg	milligram
mg/dl	milligrams per deciliter
mg/kg	milligrams/kilograms
mg/min	milligrams per minute
min	minute
ml	milliliter
mL	milliliter
ml/hr	milliliters per hour
mm	millimeter
mmHg	millimeters of mercury
MMWR	Morbidity and Mortality Weekly Report (published by CDC)
MONA	morphine—oxygen—nitroglycerin—aspirin
MRI	magnetic resonance imaging
ms	millisecond
msec	millisecond
MVA	motor vehicle accident
MVC	motor vehicle crash
NAEMSP	National Association of EMS Physicians
NHTSA	National Highway Traffic Safety Administration (federal agency)
NIOSH	National Institute for Occupational Safety and Health
NRB	non-rebreather mask (for oxygen administration)
NS	normal saline
NSAID	nonsteroidal anti-inflammatory drug
NTG	nitroglycerin
OPA	oropharyngeal airway
OR	operating room

OSHA	Occupational Safety and Health Administration (federal agency)
PALP	palpation
PASG	pneumatic antishock trousers
PAT	Pediatric Assessment Triangle
PD	peritoneal dialysis
PEA	pulseless electrical activity
PEP	post exposure prophylaxis
PICC	peripherally inserted central catheter
POA	power of attorney
PPV	positive pressure ventilation
prn	as necessary
PTCA	percutaneous coronary angioplasty
PTSD	post traumatic stress disorder
PTX	pneumothorax
q	every
RCA	right coronary artery
RR	respiratory rate
RSI	rapid sequence induction; *also* rapid sequence intubation
RTS	rape trauma syndrome
SABCDE	securing—airway—breathing—circulation—disability—exposure or environment
SAMPLE	signs/symptoms—allergies—medications—previous medical history—last meal
SBP	systolic blood pressure
SC	subcutaneous
SCI	spinal cord injury
SE	status epilepticus
SL	sublingual
SLUDGE	Salivation—Lacrimation (tears)—Urination—Diarrhea—Gastrointestinal—Emesis
SOB	shortness of breath
sol	solution
SpO$_2$	oxygen saturation using pulse oximetry
SQ	sublingual
SSRI	serotonin selective reuptake inhibitors
START	Simple Triage and Rapid Treatment
STAT	immediate
SUV	sport utility vehicle
SVT	supraventricular tachycardia
TPA	tissue plasma activator
VF	ventricular fibrillation
WPW	Wolff-Parkinson-White Syndrome

INDEX

Hematoma, epidural, 160
Hemodialysis, 67, 70
Hemodilution, 238
Hemodynamically unstable
    patient, 113–114
Hemopneumothorax, 145
Hemoptysis, 178
Hemorrhage
    acute subarachnoid, 132
    exsanguinating, 184
    grade 3, 234
    intracranial, 84
Hemorrhagic fevers, 243
Hemorrhagic strokes, 25
Hemothorax, 143, 145
Hepatitis B immune globulin
    (HBIG), 244
Hepatitis B vaccine, 244
Hepatitis B virus, 243
Hepatitis C virus, treatment of
    exposure for, 244
Herniation, 158
    cerebral, 158
Hexane, 223
Hickman catheter, 43, 44
High-Altitude Pulmonary Edema
    (HAPE), 52
High efficiency particulate air
    (HEPA) filter mask, 274
HIV antibody testing, 244
Host carrier sources, 244
Hostile environment, rendering
    aid in, 200–205
Hot zone, 202, 227
Household chemicals poisoning
    from, 108
Huber point needles, 43
Human bites, 244
Humidification, 9
Hydrochlorothiazide (HCTZ), 58
Hyperglycemia, 63
Hyperkalemia, 68
Hypernatremia, 58
Hypersensitivity, 9, 97
Hypertension, 52, 84
    chronic, 249
    essential, 84
    gestational, 249
    malignant, 84
    in pregnancy, 249

Hypertensive crisis, 83–86
Hypertensive emergency, 84
Hypertensive encephalopathy, 84
Hypertensive urgencies, 84
Hyperthyroidism, 52
Hyperventilation, 159, 160
Hypocalcemia, 113
Hypoglycemia, 63
Hypohydration, 58
Hypokalemia, 113
Hypomagnesemia, 113
Hyponatremia, 58
Hypotension, 6, 114
    after dialysis, 68
    orthostatic, 132
    postintubation, 183–184
    systemic, 5
Hypothermia, 172
    with altered mental status,
    87–90
Hypoxemia, 9, 237
Hypoxia, 157–158
    cellular, 233

I
Icy water, submersion in, 238
Immunoglobulin E (IgE)
    receptors, 30
Implied consent, 255
Incomplete spinal cord lesions, 154
Indinavir, 244
Induction agents, 80
Infection at fistula site, 68
Infectious endocarditis, 52
Infectious pulmonary
    tuberculosis, 243
Informed consent, patient
    participation, 104
Inhalation injury, signs of
    potential, 148–149
Inhaled beta-agonists, 20, 32
Insecticidal poisoning
    categories of, 226
    defined, 226
Insecticides, categories of, 228
Insulin, 64
Insulin-dependent diabetics, 61, 63
Insulin shock, 63
Intoxication, violent behavior
    and, 269

Intracranial hemorrhage, 84
Intracranial pressure (ICP), 159
Intrauterine device (IUD), 263
Intravenous drug users, 244
Intubation
    difficult, 71–76
    facilitated, 78–82
Intussusception, 209
Ipratropium bromide (Atrovent),
    20–21
Ischemia, 46
    muscular chest wall, 46
    myocardial, 47, 114, 443
Ischemic cardiac disease, 4
Ischemic strokes, 25
Isoproterenol, 15

J
Jaw-thrust method, 78, 162, 238
Jugular venous distention (JVD),
    6, 114, 144, 163

K
Kernig's sign, 93
Ketamine, 21
Ketorolac (Toradol) in pain
    management, 102
Kussmaul's respirations, 64
Kussmaul's sign, 6

L
Labetalol, 85
Laryngotracheal disruption, 74
Lasix (furosemide), 53
Left-tube thoracostomy, 179
Legal capacity, 254, 256
Lidocaine, 37
Line sepsis, 43
Living wills, 189, 191
Lorazepam, 47–48, 272
    for seizures, 120

M
Macintosh blade, 74
Macroglossia, 73
Magnesium
    for control of seizures, 249–250
    overdose of, 249
Magnesium sulfate, 21, 37, 250
    for eclampsia, 249